Working More Creatively with Groups

In this classic text Jarlath Benson presents the basic and essential knowledge required to set up and work with a group. He looks at how to plan and lead a group successfully and how to intervene skilfully. As well as covering the different stages in the life of a group, the book emphasizes the various levels of group experience and gives suggestions for working more creatively with them.

For this new edition the author has added two new chapters reflecting how his own thinking and practice have developed since the book was first published. In the first he presents his new model for planning, setting up and working with reflective practice groups which are increasingly used in professional settings and agencies across the public sector and health care. In the second he considers why some groups fail and offers practical and helpful ideas and insights to guide agencies and groupworkers to think and plan more systemically, and provides a series of clinical vignettes that facilitate each of these contexts and perspectives.

There is also an expanded section on how to plan and conduct the sophisticated art of co-working and again a series of clinical vignettes that illustrate best practice.

Working More Creatively with Groups is well known to countless social workers, psychologists, teachers and community workers and many other professionals who utilize and employ groupwork in their practice. This new edition not only provides the basic guide to groupwork but also shows how to move on to more in-depth and intensive work.

Jarlath Benson is a psychotherapist working in private practice in Belfast and London for the past 35 years.

Working More Creatively with Groups

Jarlath Benson

Fourth Edition

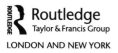

Routledge
Taylor & Francis Group

LONDON AND NEW YORK

Fourth Edition published 2019
2 Park Square, Milton Park, Abingdon, Oxon, OX14 4RN

and by Routledge
52 Vanderbilt Avenue, New York, NY 10017

Routledge is an imprint of the Taylor & Francis Group, an informa business

First Edition published by Tavistock Publications Ltd 1987

Third Edition published by Routledge 2010

British Library Cataloguing-in-Publication Data
A catalogue record for this book is available from the British Library

Library of Congress Cataloging-in-Publication Data
Names: Benson, Jarlath F., author.
Title: Working more creatively with groups / Jarlath Benson.
Description: 4th Edition. | New York : Routledge, 2019. | Revised edition
   of the author's Working more creatively with groups, 2010. | Includes
   bibliographical references and indexes.
Identifiers: LCCN 2018032885 | ISBN 9781138321922 (hardback) | ISBN
   9781138321946 (pbk.) | ISBN 9780429452369 (ebook)
Subjects: LCSH: Group counseling.
Classification: LCC BF636.7.C76 B45 2019 | DDC 158.3/5—dc23

ISBN: 978-1-138-32192-2 (hbk)
ISBN: 978-1-138-32194-6 (pbk)
ISBN: 978-0-4294-5236-9 (ebk)

Typeset in Bembo
by Apex CoVantage, LLC

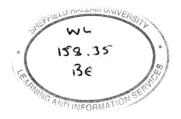

For Judy who after all these years still really does make it all worthwhile – the best groupworker I have ever known!

Contents

Acknowledgements

Many people have contributed to the making of this book and I have acknowledged them in previous editions. Of those important people Bill Schwarz and Fr Miceal O'Regan OP and Tom Hamrogue have sadly passed away and I still miss them very much.

My wife Judy Kennedy continues to be an enduring source of inspiration as do my daughters Emer, Orla and Lia. They constitute my primary group and have provided profound love, insight, practice and learning over the years. I have had another group to study and work with since the last edition who have given me enormous joy and insight – my grandchildren Cal, Jamie and Lola.

The Institute of Psychosynthesis in London where I have taught since 1990 continues to provide me with many fine colleagues who have helped me distil my ideas and develop my practice. To them I offer thanks and deep respect. Sincere thanks and gratitude again go to Joan and Roger Evans for their endless and continued stretching of my mind. A particular word of thanks again must also go to Dr Michael Kelly who has helped me think about my groupwork. His calm and wise mentorship has helped me greatly through the years.

Dr Deyra Courtney has continued to support me in the group analytic psychotherapy programme in the Centre for Psychotherapy in Belfast and her steady professionalism and encouragement is a great comfort to me and the group members. For nearly ten years now Chris Fry, a psychoanalytic psychotherapist and group psychotherapist trained in the American school of Modern Group Analysis, and I have co-led a group in the Centre for Psychotherapy. This has been a wonderful experience and I have learned so much about co-working in groups alongside Chris who is a very fine group psychotherapist. I thank him for sharing his skill and insights with me and teaching me so much about co-working and for his friendship.

Dr Mary Ryan is a group analyst and co-director of a counselling skills course in Maynooth University in Ireland which has been an inspiration to many people over years. For the past ten years she has tasked me with providing group supervision to her team of teachers. I have enjoyed working with this highly professional group of people and have learned as much if not more from them than they have from me. My thanks to Mary for her support and friendship.

A word of thanks must also go to Kate and Gordon Oswald my dear in-laws who put up with me working on the new chapters and offered insights when my wife and I were staying with them in May 2018 in their beautiful home in Castine, Maine, USA.

Finally I wish to thank all my readers who have let me know in so many ways over the years how helpful and encouraging they have found this book. It has been immensely gratifying to hear how people have valued the previous three editions and how the book has accompanied them on their first tentative steps into groupwork. I am deeply honoured that this text has been so valued by its readers for the past 30 years.

Jarlath F. Benson
July 2018

Introduction

Many of the problems and questions of group life can be dealt with in one of two ways – either by giving prescription and information or by creating opportunities in which personal and direct experience itself reveals meaning and suggests resolution. For example, a leader can respond to a new and anxious group where members are asking endless questions:

- Let's not ask any more questions for now and find something to do together

  or

- I think the answer to your question is this . . .

And here is another way:

- I notice that many of you are asking a lot of questions today. What is it like for you that you don't know all the answers about this group?

The first two answers can deal with the situation but may miss or avoid what is really happening. By contrast the third answer endeavours to lead the enquirer into her own experience, open up, and involve her in the real nature of her need to know. From such experience and awareness of events may emerge meaning and more suitable ways of handling situations in groups.

In essence this is the central thesis and belief advanced in this book: that it is desirable, more respectful, and more creative to involve the whole person in interaction and inquiry and makes most sense to involve the group in its own development, learning, and resolution.

The need for context

The first thing that one needs is a context, a frame of reference which informs and disciplines, and so I want to put forward some of the principles which underpin and guide my own approach to working with groups.

Such a context was not immediately evident when I first started working with groups. As a newcomer to the groupwork scene I might have been excused for feeling that I would be more at home in a Martian supermarket. Knowing what type of groups there were, which theory to choose, how to discriminate between technologies, selecting appropriate methods for use in a particular situation appeared to me to require the wisdom of Solomon. I felt very confused and uncertain as to what approach or line was best to take, so what I did was to try a little bit of everything. I operated on the principle – if it works use it, if it doesn't junk it!

As it turned out, this proved not to be such a bad idea as it might first appear. I experimented, both as member and practitioner with various brands and schools of groupwork and adapted their insights and techniques to fit my particular circumstances. I read widely and was not afraid to raid other fields and disciplines for ideas or tools which I could use. I plagiarized, improvised, and synthesized and always allowed practice to determine what was true. Gradually out of this intensely pragmatic approach there began to emerge a rationale and recurrent working principles which I found could 'travel' and could provide me with a framework for intervening in a wide variety of group environments. Here are some of the more important of these principles:

- Group experience is fundamental
- The group provides consistency and predictability
- The group is organic and natural
- The group is an energetic experience
- The 'here and now' is important
- The 'hidden' must be made visible
- Experience in the group is multidimensional
- There is an organizing principle in the group

I want to make some brief statements about these principles in turn.

Group experience is fundamental

At birth we are introduced into our first, small, and intensely personal group, called the family. This group offers the new human being protection and identity. It also offers an opportunity to develop and individuate from the mass experience of humanity as well as providing a qualitative aspect to life.

In its turn the family is dependent for its survival, identity, beliefs, and behaviour on membership of a wide range of formal and informal groups in the larger society – school, church, political, friendship, interest, leisure, and work groups. So from birth we are enlisted in, and gradually committed to, group living in a variety of forms.

Some areas of group influence

• Learning	• Habits
• Attitudes	• Achievement and Performance
• Values	• Mental and emotional well-being

Here are some of the practice applications of this first principle that we will look at in later chapters.

- Developing a sense of identity, support, belonging
- Negotiating the beginning stage of work
- Establishing cohesion, trust, interdependence
- Developing norms, values, rules
- Identifying and meeting individual and group needs

The group provides consistency and predictability

Because of the sheer scope and mass of human experience, group relationships are vital in the birth, nurturing, and maturing of the individual's sense of self. Modern writers in the field believe, like Hargreaves,[1] that the 'self arises from the social experience of interacting with others'. Bernard Davies[2] is even more explicit. Interaction with other selves is not merely a process which releases the 'core' features and attributes of a person. The individual 'is actually *constructed* in relations with others'. Interaction among humans is what 'defines' and 'creates' a person's experience of self.

But interaction does not occur in a vacuum. Individuals need to engage in interaction frequently and over a period of time if these social interactions are to become patterned and if expectations concerning each other's behaviour are to develop. Without the *consistency* and *predictability* which comes with patterned and regular interaction, the self which emerges from such transactions is weak, diffuse, and prone to chaos, as anyone who has worked with highly disturbed children, or psychiatric patients, can attest.

The function of the group

And this is where the experience of group is so important. The group is a unique way of transforming or stepping down the mass potential and chaos of undifferentiated human contact into manageable units of predictable and consistent interaction, shared experience, and normative behaviour within which the self can arise. The group provides the context within which socialization and the formation and development of self occurs. Without the group the individual cannot emerge from mass humanity and without the individual the group is just another amorphous mass of living matter.

Practice applications

- Developing a sense of identity and belonging (page 83–86)
- Establishing cohesion and trust (page 99)
- Making contracts, using power and authority (page 46–48, 94–98)
- Creating context, boundary, structure (page 197–206)
- Identifying and working with roles (page 68–72)
- Developing norms and values (page 65–72)

The group is organic and natural

There are a bewildering number of definitions of what a group is, and as a result, there seem to be many apparently conflicting definitions. The reason for this is that an author often selects the relations or properties that are of special importance in his work and then posits these as the criteria for group existence. We can, however, identify a list of attributes that various theorists agree are especially important features of groups.[3]

Key concepts

- A set of people engage in frequent interaction
- They identify with one another
- They are defined by others as a group
- They share beliefs, values, and norms about areas of common interest
- They define themselves as a group
- They come together to work on common tasks and for agreed purposes

What emerge from this list are three very important characteristics of a group:

- There are parts
- There is relationship between the parts
- There is an organizing principle

In other words a group is organic and intentional and not just some random experience.

People come together in a group to satisfy some common need or interest that can be expressed as the group purpose. A network of social relationships is generated within which members accept or reject each other and engage in selected activities. As they do so, *roles* become established and *values* and norms of behaviour emerge, through which individuals can modify and influence each other over time.

This is the understanding I have in mind whenever future reference is made in this book to a group. I am talking about a group as a natural and purposeful experience, involving people in mutual interaction and acceptance, over a period of time, and not just any arbitrary massing of people, a bus queue or shoppers in a supermarket.

Practice applications

- Negotiating beginnings, middles, and ends (page 77–79, 165–166)
- Learning how to pace, maintain individual and collective action (page 74–79)
- Clarifying purpose and goals (page 12–17, 93)
- Developing interaction and 'right relationship' (page 149–151)
- Understanding individual and collective behaviour (page 65–66)

The group is an energetic experience

Individual and group experience and interaction change in condition and quality over time. Because the group is organic and natural there is an ebb and flow that we can call process. This group process can be emotionally and physically felt and the worker should aim to develop skills of working with process in order to facilitate group interaction and goal achievement. In particular you will need to learn to work with the two core experiences of group life – the urge to be separate and the need to belong. Let me explain.

The momentum to differentiate from mass consciousness is experienced by the individual as a need to detach and separate (initially from 'mother'). This drive towards independence is clearly beneficial as it widens horizons, provides new learning situations, and opens up contact with an ever-decreasing range of novel objects and situations.

The urge to detach gives rise to one dimension of the experience of self which is a uniquely personal one of distinction, aloneness, and separation. And yet, at the very least human beings are dependent on each other for survival and identity. So there is a contrary pull back towards mass, attachment, dependence, and being a part of something bigger than self. This attachment process refers to one of the simplest and yet most fundamental elements in social behaviour – the tendency to seek the proximity of other members of the species. Again this is a relatively clear-cut principle, occurring almost universally in animals as well as in man. It gives rise to the other dimension of the self – the need to be dependent and in relationship with others. As we will see in Chapter 3, it is the tension generated between these two poles of human experience – the urge to be separate and the need to be attached – which is the drive mechanism for movement and growth in groups.

Each participant in a group experience, and every group if it is to survive and evolve, has to reconcile the urge to separate with the need to be attached. Failure to resolve or even recognize these fundamental human drives results in warped and anti-human experience in groups and gives rise to the fears and anxieties many people express about involvement in collective situations. Chapters 4 to 8 provide ideas and suggestions to help you work with these ideas in practice.

Practice applications

- Understanding and managing behaviour at beginning, middle, and end of group (page 77–79)
- Working with conflict, tiredness, boredom, being stuck (page 49–53, 94–98)
- Teaching process analysis (page 168–170)
- Teaching group maintenance skills (page 163–167)
- Balancing individual and group needs (page 65–74)
- Co-operating with and facilitating love and will energies (page 74)

The 'here and now' is important

Individual and group experience and interaction is continuously unfolding in the present tense of group life. Because of the 'nowness' of process, every experience is open to change and development. While this means that I tend to focus primarily on what is happening 'here and now' in the group for each member, it does not mean that I exclude reflexive or historical perspectives. There are many times and situations where exploration of past experience or 'out-of-group' experience is necessary as a way of helping members understand and deal with present time concerns in the group.

But there are other times when it is necessary to attend to the quality of group experience, the levels of trust, hostility, silence, superficiality, and so on if the group is to progress towards its goals. By looking at what is happening in the 'here and now' situation you can help group members become aware of their responsibility for their own behaviours and experiences and determine more appropriate options and strategies. Asking questions like:

- How are you feeling now?
- What is happening in the group now?
- What do you want now?
- What does this behaviour experience mean for us/you?

has the powerful effect of focusing members' attention in the session. In this way it is possible to utilize and build on the present behaviours and experience of members in the group.

Practice applications

- Problem solving and decision making (page 112)
- Helping members make choices (page 216)
- Improving communication and interaction (page 205–208)
- Helping members be more authentic (page 214)
- Developing a sense of personal power and self-responsibility in members (page 214–217)
- Emphasizing the importance of themes and patterns in collective behaviour (page 220, 222–226)

The 'hidden' must be made visible

In groups people play 'games' with each other in order to produce certain responses which will reinforce and confirm their beliefs about themselves. These 'games' are also a way of dealing with situations and interactions which might prove fearful, anxious, or involve anger, dependency, helplessness, and aloneness. The result is to distort reality and perception and inhibit creativity and authenticity.

Part of your job as leader is to engage people in the business of making explicit the hidden messages in communications within the group so as to reveal and open up for resolution the problems and difficulties faced by members. Sometimes these messages and feelings are unconscious – members are unaware of what they are feeling or doing in certain situations and at these times a lot of work has to go into uncovering individual and group dynamics in order to create insight and understanding and work more effectively.

Making hidden thoughts, feelings, and desires visible so as to facilitate interaction and activity is one of the most important and frequent tasks you will be called on to perform in the group and Chapters 4 to 8 contain much that will help you with this task.

Experience in the group is multidimensional

To be more accurate I should say that each group member operates or experiences the world on a number of different levels and the coming together of people can give an aggregate level or dimension of experience in a group. It is possible to talk about these levels as if they were separate, since each has different functions and requirements. They each need to be addressed if the individual and group experience is to be complete and meaningful. At the physical level members are sensitive to light, heat, cold, noise, hunger, the type of seating, the need for movement, activity, and the like. All these factors have a major influence on the ability of members to participate and on the quality of interaction. It is important that you recognize people's needs at the physical level and respond accordingly.

At the emotional level members find that they have various feelings about the work, the leader, and each other which can enhance, but more often interrupt proceedings. Again, it is essential that you are able to recognize this, and provide ways and means of channelling and transforming emotional energy if your group is not to get stuck or torn apart by violent and conflictual feelings.

There is an intellectual level of experience at which members need to know the objectives and purpose of the group, understand, and comprehend different aspects of the work and generally hold opinions, beliefs, and attitudes. Much of your work in the group at this level will be geared to helping members generate ideas, formulate plans, anticipate consequences, and understand the meaning of their actions.

It is important to be able to work at these different levels and Chapters 4 to 8 give clear suggestions and hints for practice at various stages of the group's development. In Chapters 9 and 10 I offer ideas and guidelines which will help you move from one mode of experience to another. This is particularly useful when working with people who are not very verbally proficient or who find it hard to conceptualize. I have talked a little about Maslow's ideas regarding human needs in Chapter 3 and this will give you a context within which you can understand the importance of the physical, emotional, and intellectual levels of individual and group experience. If you want to read more about the influence of these three aspects at the level of individual personality some of the psychosynthesis books are very interesting and have ideas that transfer naturally to group settings.[4]

There is an organizing principle in the group

What brings a number of individuals together to form a group is their belief and hope that the group can offer means of satisfying their particular needs. This belief and hope is institutionalized in the 'group purpose' and it is this purpose which I see as the principle of organization in any group. Without a purpose the group has no meaning or relevance and is a sterile, usually chaotic experience. Purpose engages members at the level of will to plan objectives and strategies, to organize, make choices, and execute in action. Purpose creates boundary, structure, parameter and really provides the conditions and circumstances within which the other principles referred to can operate.

A slightly different perspective on purpose is yielded by my use of the word 'vision'. The concept of vision recurs continually throughout this work and refers to the range of possibilities that a group can open up for its members. I use the notion of vision to convey a deeper sense of the group purpose. Vision points to the potential inherent in collective action and indicates what we may be if we choose accordingly. Vision sustains the group through the dark and stormy periods of its life when it is all too easy for members to slip into despair and hopelessness. Vision provides the values and beliefs by which group members decide to live and work together. Of course the vision of possibility indicated in a particular group must be incarnated in everyday group experience if it is not to remain at an abstract and intangible level.

Together vision and its more solid manifestation, purpose, provide a 'centre' or organizing principle in the group which becomes more real and strong as it is used. Initially this vision or purpose is carried by the worker for members only until such time as they can begin to develop and formulate their own personal vision of what the group means. This theme is more fully developed in Chapter 8 so that it is only relevant here to emphasize the importance of ensuring that you can clearly articulate why it is that you believe a group can help these particular people at this time.

A definition

Putting all these principles together, it is possible to see now what the context for practice is and even make a clear statement about what is meant by groupwork practice:

> Groupwork practice refers to the conscious, disciplined, and systematic use of knowledge about the processes of collective human interaction, in order to intervene in an informed way, or promote some desired objective in a group setting. In the sense that it is used in this book, groupwork practice is a *helping process designed to correspond to specific instances of individual and group need, based on a view of human beings as in constant interaction and relationship with others.* Groupwork is a productive, healthy, and creative experience, carried out on the basis of *explicit agreements,* openly pursued and clearly arrived at, about the purpose and task of the group, rights, and responsibilities of members.

References

1 Hargreaves, D.H. (1972) *Interpersonal Relations and Education (PH)*, London: Routledge & Kegan Paul.

2 Davies, B. (1975) *The Use of Groups in Social Work Practice*, 58, London: Routledge & Kegan Paul.

3 For a review of definitions of groups see Cartwright, D. and Zander, A. (eds) (1968) *Group Dynamics, Research, and Theory*, London: Tavistock.

4 Ferrucci, P. (1982) *What We May Be*, Wellingborough: Turnstone Press. Whitmore, D. (1986) *Psychosynthesis in Education*, Wellingborough: Turnstone Press. Assagioli, R. (1975) *Psychosynthesis*, Wellingborough: Turnstone Press.

Chapter 1

How to plan the group

The importance of planning cannot be emphasized enough – as our traditional folk wisdom shows. Foresight and organization are the basis of many of our favourite proverbs: 'Look before you leap', 'A stitch in time saves nine', 'Prevention is better than cure', and so on.

Yet despite the abundance and richness of these traditional insights many groups still fail to get off the ground or splutter into anonymity after a few sessions, due simply to the fact that not enough attention was given, before the group even started, to its planning and organization. There are many reasons for this. From time to time, I still come across the 'It'll be all right on the day' types or the leaders who believe that planning the group is manipulative or will detract from the involvement of members. Even some who do conscientiously try to organize their thinking about their reasons and purposes for using groupwork, often generate goals and objectives for a group that are unrealistic or grandiose. Much of the conflict and hostility which can then ensue in those groups is simply a product of the leaders' resentment and frustration with members who won't seem to 'work', and members' anger and confusion about the discrepancy between what they are capable of, or willing to do, and what is expected of them.

Before we go on to look at some procedures for planning the group let me say a bit more about why it is important to plan.

Why plan a group?

Whatever their ages, interests, or concerns, individual members come to the group with their own perception of what they want, or do not want from the experience. As the group develops, a common perception of need or interest emerges, which may or may not be compatible with the wants and desires of members (see page 65–66). At some point both individual and group perceptions of needs and goals will be tested against the worker's perception of the group purpose.

As Whitaker says, if a worker is not clear in his mind about the sort of group he wishes to conduct, 'he will almost inevitably present mixed cues and signals to the group'.[1] Douglas goes even further. A group leader has got to have a 'reasonable certainty about what he intends to do'.[2] Particularly where a group leader is working with suspicious, disbelieving, or hostile clients, 'if his own ideas and values are hazy then he will not be convincing'.[3]

But there are other reasons for planning a group:

- To assess the degree of need and plan a response
- To determine if groupwork is appropriate in the circumstances
- To clarify the purpose of the group
- To focus on members' needs
- To identify specific outcomes
- To determine how these will be achieved. (A plan is the means employed to achieve particular ends or outcomes.)
- To help potential members see the group as a means of meeting their needs
- To pinpoint difficulties or obstacles and develop coping strategies
- To identify resources
- To clarify roles, expectations, tasks of workers and members

Clearly we could extend this list. The point is that leaders who start groups without being clear about their reasons for using groupwork, without adequate planning, or whose desired outcomes are vague are bound for trouble. In my introduction I said that my own style of groupwork was concerned with the 'here and now' of individual and group experience. This does not mean that I walk into a group without having considered why I am there, what I can or cannot offer, or without having done some preparation to help group members use a particular experience or activity to achieve an agreed objective.

My own experience is that the ability to work creatively and spontaneously in a group, and use the unexpected incidents that frequently occur, is based on a solid foundation of advance planning and consideration. In architecture there is a dictum, 'Form follows function', and this is good advice for group workers. We need to spend time identifying the function of the group in order to arrive at the most appropriate form for realizing our purposes.

A guide to planning

If Douglas is right that a group leader ought to have a 'reasonable certainty about what he intends to do' then we need to look at what activities the leader engages in to acquire this conviction. In the following sections I want to explore in some detail what I consider are the major planning activities of the group leader. My intention is not to suggest that planning a group is an operation which is absolute and definitive or precludes negotiation and agreement with members. The focus throughout is on the worker and what he can do before the first session to help the group become more effective. But first let us ask a question:

Is planning for an existent group different from planning for a group convened by the leader?

There are two ways in which a worker can engage with a group. Either she can convene the group herself or she can be invited or required to work with an already existing group.

If a leader works with an existent group she has not convened, the only difference this makes to the planning process is that:

- The group leader does not select group members. They are already selected
- She does not determine the goals or purposes of the group though she may help to clarify them
- She may have her role prescribed though she may be free within limits to perform it as she sees fit
- The programme may be prescribed although the group leader may have some control over content

---

With these constraints in mind I want to suggest a method which can apply to the planning of any group whether it already exists or has yet to be formed. There are six stages in this formulation:

- Researching and justifying the need for groupwork
- Attending to membership
- Programming the group
- Leading the group
- Presenting the group
- Planning the first session

The first three stages will be discussed now and the final three explored in the next chapter.

Researching and justifying the need for groupwork

There are a number of steps in this phase of planning.

Becoming aware of the need or problem

The first point to consider is *how the demand* for group service or membership *comes to your attention*. Is it a *request* from an already existing group for help with, let's say, programme design; from a colleague who wants you to work with some of the children on his caseload because 'you are good with kids', or from a woman you know who is socially isolated and wants to join a group to make friends? Perhaps the provision of a group service is a *requirement* of your job. You may be expected to reach out to young people through groupwork or required to encourage and facilitate the work of community action groups or work with a diabetes group or post cancer group. Is the idea of groupwork a *response* on your part to emerging client needs or recognized themes in team, office, agency work-load? Considering how the demand for groupwork comes to your attention is important because it raises some important points:

- Who makes the application?
- For whom?
- Why?
- What do they want?
- What do the beneficiaries of the group service actually need?

If you think for a moment you will realize that there are many people who did not origi-nally request help but who are now receiving it and occasionally the demand for a group service represents more the needs of workers or an organization to maintain its grant aid or be seen to provide certain services than it does the real needs of potential group mem-bers. This is a recurring factor in why some groups just don't work and will be explored more fully in Chapter 16.

In other circumstances people can ask for help with no real understanding of an agen-cy's services or obligations and then find themselves caught up in a programme they are unwilling to be involved in. The point is this, by carefully and thoughtfully assessing how and why you became aware of a particular demand for a group service you can:

- Begin to establish the motivations of yourself and colleagues to offer a service
- Decide that there really is a need that can be met by groupwork and which justifies time, resource, and expenditure
- Gather preliminary information about possible goals for a group
- Make it easier for people to participate in relevant programmes
- Highlight the range and functions of agency provisions and the consequences of involvement

Considering the proposal and testing alternatives

Having established that a social situation exists which might prove amenable to group-work intervention, the next step is to consider if groupwork is in fact the desired or most appropriate response. Ask questions like:

- Is there a clearly demonstrable group need or problem?
- Does a shared need or problem exist among enough people to warrant groupwork?
- Can I identify a common aim which is likely to get agreement?
- Can groupwork really achieve gains for these potential members?

- What sort of gains?
- What special properties of the group do I wish to make use of?
- Are potential members likely to see the group as relevant and helpful?
- Will the group damage or label or stigmatize any member?
- Is there another medium or form of intervention that can achieve the desired outcome as well as the group?
- Why is the group setting more effective than the one-to-one setting?
- Can I make reasonable estimates of time involved, programme, cost?
- Can I get agency approval for the group in terms of use of time, finance, resource?

From the answers to these questions I try to establish that there is a need which is shared by people, is best met by working in a group, and that I can contribute in some way to this need. I find it useful to identify a *general aim* for the group such as:

- Providing social activity for isolated people
- Helping a community group clarify its goals
- Providing emotional support for depressed men and women

Having a general aim for the group focuses thinking and makes it easier to locate relevant literature or talk to other group leaders who have worked in this area, in order to obtain a better understanding of the needs of the group and learn about more effective and appropriate ways of working. However, aims are often stated in such general terms that it is not possible to evaluate whether they have been achieved or not. Subsequently I try to break aims down into narrower, more specific goals or objectives. This goal setting is important because:

- Goals motivate behaviour. An *individual goal* is the reason why a member joins a group. A *group goal* is a future state of affairs desired by enough members of the group to motivate them working towards its achievement.
- Goals are guides for action. Goals indicate to worker and members the tasks that must be performed, the behaviours and processes of interaction that must be engaged in if the goal is to be achieved.
- Goals are a way of attaining agreement and resolving conflict.
- Goals are a way of evaluating the effectiveness of group procedures. Without goals there is nothing to evaluate (see page 333–337).

Examples of goals in a group might be:

> - To help John improve his conversational skills
> - To prevent children going into care
> - To clarify role requirements in the team

Some goals which might refer to the worker's desired outcomes can be specified at this stage; other goals require the approval and adoption by members and must be negotiated in the group itself. Louis Lowy suggests a number of principles that should be adhered to by the group leader when identifying goals for the group.[4]

> - Worker goals should be based on assessment of group members and stage of group development
> - Goals should be stated in behavioural terms
> - Goals should refer to the state of improved functioning of members and group
> - Goals should be realistic and achievable
> - Goals should be prioritized
> - Goal formation should be a shared process involving members and worker

By pinpointing some goals at this stage you can begin to see if, how, and why groupwork is an appropriate method to use in a particular setting.

Justifying the group

The final area of importance in this research phase of group planning concerns the relationship of the group to the agency, institution, or community of which it is a part. Whitaker suggests that, 'There are many settings in which it is not prudent to undertake groupwork until after one has thoroughly explored one's plans with one's colleagues.'[5] There are good reasons for this.

Professionals are often deeply suspicious of groups, sometimes even hostile. I have worked with many who have been exposed to groupwork 'teaching' on their training courses, which has left them embittered and cynical because of what they regard as the manipulativeness of group workers, the potential for damaging group experience, or the impenetrable mystique which surrounds groupwork. Parsloe talks about the 'shared fantasy amongst social workers about what goes on in groups', and suggests that some elements of this fantasy are believed to be that the group leader never breaks a silence, seldom speaks, is apparently always free from anxiety, and able to expose the raw feelings of an individual or the group, at a stroke.[6]

No doubt some professionals have experienced this sort of groupwork and it creates in them a wish to protect their clients from similar experiences. It is important to reassure these workers, if you can; and discuss with them how you see the group and what it can offer members in terms of gains. Unless you deal with colleagues' reservations or mixed feeling about groups you can find that they pass their fears on to clients; they are dilatory in making referrals to you or they just simply refuse to co-operate.

One way of securing the support of colleagues is to demonstrate to them that the involvement of clients in a group can actually contribute to and enhance their work. To do this you should determine what the objectives of the agency or institution are in respect of the potential group members. Ensure that the general aim and the goals for your group are compatible with agency objectives and you are not proposing to work in an area that is the concern of another organization (social worker intending to teach children literacy and numeracy skills, youth worker offering a therapy group for depressed youngsters). This is important because crossing professional boundaries or working in grey areas can undermine your credibility and expose you to charges that the proposal is irrelevant to the remit of the agency and cannot justify resource and expenditure.

You should identify the agency's actual operational concerns in relation to potential group members and establish what the priorities are. Try to work out the contribution your group can make to the service being offered by the agency and pinpoint where the group will enhance, back up, or confirm the work of colleagues.

It is worth putting this information on paper even though at this stage it may represent only brief outline thinking about the proposed group, its aims, and its contribution to agency delivery of service. Here is part of an actual outline proposal from my own work which illustrates thinking at this stage.

EXAMPLE

Outline plan for working with depressed women on a group therapy basis. A definition of problem and focus of work: A number of women have been identified on existing casework loads by individual caseworkers as in need of involvement in a therapeutic peer group, which would help them deal with their depressive feelings.

The background of these women could be summarized as follows:

- Single parent and usually with child management difficulties
- A number of women have children on the NAI register (non–accidental injury register: a list of children abused by parents and held by the social services)
- Marked degree of social isolation due to poor family relationships, lack of social support, etc.
- Poor housing conditions, low income

Against this background the following responses have been observed in the women:

- A perception of self as of low value and worth
- An ineffective or inadequate presentation and use of self
- An inability or reluctance to assume an appropriate degree of responsibility for their selves and their behaviour

These three responses would appear to produce problematic behaviour such as depression, communication and relationship problems, poor motivation, poor child management.

Possible goals for group

> - To begin to relieve the distress that these women are obviously experiencing by offering a group support
> - To bring together women who live in the same neighbourhood in order to jointly tackle problems encountered in their mutual experience
> - To help the women work on what they identify as the painful and distressing areas of their life
> - To help the women develop strategies for dealing more effectively with distress and depression

Why a group?

> - The women all come from the same neighbourhood although only one or two know each other
> - They have similar problems: single parents, child management difficulties, depression, social isolation
> - The group can offer companionship, support, encouragement to work on depression, feedback, opportunities to make relationships
> - The women would be willing to attend the group
> - The group offers the caseworker another therapeutic option, assessment facilities, as well as providing additional monitoring of high-risk cases

An outline like this is not a final plan with estimates of cost, resource, programme details, methodology, and worker's role clearly delineated. It is merely a proposal which helps your colleagues and managers understand more about your project, enables them to express their views and feel involved. Whitaker believes that a group is more likely to be successful if colleagues 'accept and support its aims and general procedures and value its potential contribution to the shared goals of the organization or institution'.[7] With an outline like this you can ask for permission to gather referrals, secure a promise of resources and funding, and move to the next phase of planning. Even in situations where you do not have to persuade colleagues or superiors of the need for groupwork you should still commit early thoughts to paper.

Attending to membership

The constituency of group membership can exercise a powerful effect on the interaction that ensues and can facilitate or inhibit the progress of the group towards the goals for which it was formed. Whether you form a group for the first time or are working with an existent group it is important to pay attention to the implications of membership for group effectiveness. As Behr and Hearst assert "A group starts with a vision of its membership."[8]

Knowing something about who is in the group, and why, can help you:

- Identify individual motivations and needs
- Plan individual goals, where appropriate
- Formulate group goals
- Select members, where appropriate
- Assess the likely effect of members on each other
- Anticipate unhelpful behaviour and interaction
- Encourage facilitative behaviour and interaction
- Plan a relevant programme
- Pitch the programme at a suitable level
- Suggest a particular leadership style

Recruitment

Some workers take an active part in recruiting and selecting members for the group. There is general agreement that decisions about size and potential membership in such groups are based on:

- The agency's goals and expectations of the group
- The worker's goals for the group
- The needs and goals of potential members
- Group goals that are likely to emerge over time

Another widely accepted principle is that groups should be *similar* enough to ensure commonality of need and compatibility but *disparate* enough to ensure that members will be stimulating and useful to each other.[9] Some leaders will select particular individuals for a group because of their similarity or disparity on certain *descriptive* and *behavioural* attributes. Descriptive attributes 'classify an individual as to age, sex, marital status, occupation, or other "positions" he may be said to occupy', while behavioural attributes 'describe the way an individual acts or can be expected to act based on his past performance'.

Paradise and Daniels list 18 descriptive and behavioural attributes they take into consideration when selecting children for group membership.[9] These attributes include: need to belong to the group, ability to communicate, ability to tolerate behavioural differences, level of dependency, level of aggression, ability to delay gratification, age, sex, and socioeconomic status.

Bertcher and Maple suggest that a group is more effective if members have *similar descriptive attitudes* as this encourages cohesion, interactiveness, and compatibility, and *disparate behavioural attributes* because this increases 'the behavioural repertory that will be useful to the group' and fosters interest and responsiveness.[10]

Groups will not be effective if there is:

- Too much compatibility – can become 'samey' and stagnant
- Too much or too little stress
- Not enough creativity or novelty
- Negative or dissenting subgroups

Important descriptive attributes group leaders often consider are:

- *Age and developmental level*: When working with children and young people I tend to keep to a narrow age band – usually two years between oldest and youngest – in order to capitalize on similar interests and abilities when programming and making decisions. Often an older but emotionally less developed child can be placed in a younger age group where he can feel more comfortable. In adult groups a wider age-spread is more usual and can be valuable to teach younger adults from the experience of older adults. These older members can also learn from younger members how to resolve problems or difficulties left over from an earlier stage. Rutan and Stone suggest that groups for 20- to 30-year-old adults operate best in an age band of ten years and groups of older members can easily manage the wider age range.[11]
- *Sex*: While my own preference is to work with mixed-sex groups where possible, as being more normal in relation to social life, there are situations where it can be more advantageous to work in single-sex groups. For example, my experience with groups of eight- to ten-year-old and 11- to 13-year-old children is that they tend to split into subgroups along sex lines and it can be very hard to develop cohesion particularly where the purpose of the group is to focus on a task. It is often just better to work in a single-sex group with these age-sets. I find that five- to seven year olds and 14 to 17 year olds can better manage the inter-sex relationships in a group and this can be used to good effect. With some adult groups, women's consciousness-raising groups, groups who explore sexual issues, or whose purpose is to express the trauma of rape, incest, or sexual assault, there may be good reasons to work in a single-sex setting where the presence of members of the opposite sex would be embarrassing, provocative, or counterproductive.
- *Geographical proximity*: In some circumstances leaders like to work with people from the same neighbourhood as a way of consolidating and transferring the learning that goes on in the group setting to the domestic environment. Many youth and community workers seek to work with adolescent peer groups as a way of countering deviant norms, believing the groups if modified will be more resistant to the delinquent subculture than lone individuals. Where people join groups

to deal with the problems created by social isolation it makes sense to work with them if they all live in a neighbourhood where they can continue contact between meetings.

In other instances geographical proximity can be a disadvantage. When confidentiality is important, as in a therapeutic group, members' relationships, previous knowledge of each other, or even just knowing that another member lives in the same estate can be an impediment to self-expression and the development of trust. My experience is that confidentiality is more likely to break down in groups where members are drawn from the same vicinity, for obvious reasons.

Behavioural attributes that are considered important by many leaders are:

- *Ability to communicate*: If a potential member finds it hard to verbalize his feelings and thoughts it could be damaging to him and inhibitive of the group to place him in a setting where the major activity is intended to be discussion. He may require a group more suited to his ability and level of communication.
- *Degree of disturbance*: This has to be carefully assessed in treatment contexts if individuals are not to be scapegoated or provoked and the group is not to be severely impeded or held up.
- *Motivation to work or join in group activity*: If the group is to be successful it is important to be able to gauge how willing each individual is to be in the group and involve himself in its work. In many groups members attend reluctantly, to appease parents, social workers, probation officers, or authority figures; such groups rarely work.
- *Ability to relate to others*: It is important to know that an individual is able to relate to others even minimally, because of the interpersonal nature of the group. Paradise and Daniels point out four aspects of this variable.[12]

    1　How *sensitive* is the individual to the feelings and behaviour of other people?
    2　Does the individual have adequate defence mechanisms to fall back on in adversity?
    3　How able is the individual to *delay gratification* particularly in a setting where shared experience is emphasized?
    4　*How dependent* is an individual in relationships?

There is an alternative view to the active recruitment and selection of members by the group leader. Some other leaders simply form the group by taking whoever is available at the time and responsive to the stated group goal. Tropp states that 'There is no point in trying to determine what combination of particular individual characteristics would make the most effective group composition.'[13] He believes that it is 'undesirable to collect all this data' because it is not possible to predict future group behaviour of an individual and because, ' . . . it creates a contaminating process whereby the members become aware of the leader's prior knowledge and judgements about them,' and tend to behave in ways that fulfil these expectations.[14] All that needs to be known is that there is commonality of need and that no member 'is going to be clearly harmful to or harmed by the group experience'.[15]

This is a viewpoint on recruitment that I have a lot of sympathy with. When I first started working with groups I used to ask for referrals that gave me information on such variables as age, sex, intelligence, language ability, degree of disturbance, sociability, and so on. I then rigorously combed these referrals trying to create the optimum combination of members for the group. I have been repeatedly surprised when individuals did not behave as was predicted from the referral. Now I am more cautious about information on a potential group member that may have been gleaned from a formal one-to-one setting. Even when I know information comes from seeing the individual in the collectivity of school, family, or institution I am aware that the spontaneity, informality, and egalitarian nature of the group setting can release different and previously unseen qualities in the person which can make reliance solely on *historical* factors for selection unwise.

Sometimes there are situations in which there is a commonality of need but there are such marked differences that it is important to think carefully about their possible consequences. These may be differences of race, religion, or political affiliation, known rivalries and tensions which normally would make it very difficult for the group to work. On these occasions I check with the potential members beforehand if they feel that these differences will affect them adversely but usually I find that people's need for the group service is sufficient to overcome these apparent barriers. Infrequently a potential member will refuse to join because of such factors but only rarely in my experience have these differences disrupted a group. As far as possible I now prefer to let group purpose and the setting I am operating in determine how members are recruited.

To give an example: there are often occasions in which I will make an offer of a group-work service to people I have no first-hand knowledge of, to deal with a certain need or problem in a particular neighbourhood. In response to a community request I will let it be known that I am forming a group to help addicted youngsters stop glue-sniffing, or provide single parents with social support and contact. In these circumstances I would follow Tropp's suggestions and work with whoever responded to the group objective if it was at all clear that they could benefit by, and contribute to the group experience. The only criterion I would apply after this would be numerical. If too many turn up I suggest either a second group to run concurrently or if this isn't possible I ask members present to decide among themselves the urgency of their need to be in the group, and offer a placement to those who can wait until the first group has ended. This is usually a satisfactory arrangement for all concerned.

While I do not ignore completely what descriptive and behavioural attributes are available I am much more concerned with the needs of individuals to be in the group, and their motivation to be there and to use the experience. To this end it is important to have contact where possible with potential members before the group starts in order to clarify expectations, responsibilities, requirements, and objectives (see 'Presenting the group', page 45).

Structural issues

SIZE

The purposes and needs of the group should determine its size. In a therapy group where the emphasis is on self-disclosure, intimacy, and support, membership would be smaller (eight and under) than in an activity group where a larger membership (up to 12 and often more) would ensure more variety, skills, and resources. An educational group can have more members (up to 25) because there may be more passivity and reliance on a leader or teacher than a work group (under seven) where energy and attention tends to be focused on the doing of certain tasks. Here are some variables to think about when considering size.

- Intimacy
- Support   } Decreases as numbers get larger
- Satisfaction
- Opportunity to participate   } Increases as numbers get smaller
- Consensus

- Personal recognition decreases   As numbers increase
- Number of personal relationships increase
- Subgroups emerge
- More reliance on leader
- More need for formal procedures and rules
- Ability to tackle more complex problems develops
- Problem solving takes longer
- More creativity

There is general agreement that an optimum size for a group is seven members.[16] This is large enough to allow recognition, intimacy, and involvement. In the learning group seven to 13 seems to work out best while five is a good size for a work group although larger numbers do provide more resource and skills.[17]

FREQUENCY AND NUMBER OF MEETINGS

Again this is something which is determined by group purposes and needs. Generally I find that the deeper I need to go in exploring interpersonal or ego issues the more time is required to build up trust, cohesion, and safety. For individuals to take risks with increasingly private material, the group needs the consistency and predictability that comes with regular and patterned interaction (see page 23–24). In the more overtly therapeutic group setting I go for weekly meetings held over a six-month period (25 sessions) for adults, or nine months (36 sessions) for children.

For more task-oriented groupwork such as team development, social skills training, or educational groups, I again choose a weekly meeting, but over a shorter time span – anything from six to 12 weeks depending on the availability of time, group needs, and purpose. The reason for this is that there is quite a different emphasis on relationships in the work group than in the therapy group.

Sessions in the therapy context last for one and a half hours and I find that this permits a maximum number of group members to participate. Work groups I usually fix at two and a half hours and very occasionally two hours. I almost never work a shorter session. Many other leaders prefer to have a session lasting between one and two hours because they are afraid that members will get bored or tired with a longer session. In my experience group members do respond to the longer sessions, and boredom or tiredness, when they occur, become an opportunity to help the group acquire maintenance skills (see page 163).

Flexibility and creativity in the use of managing time is important in most groupwork settings. Weekly and fortnightly meetings sustain the momentum and build up a sense of belonging and commitment as well as the consistency and predictability which is so important if a group is to be healthy and productive. But there are many situations in which it is difficult or inappropriate to use normal time determinants and you may have to be more inventive. In times of crisis – such as sexual assault, death of a relative, sudden mental stress, or terminal illness – an otherwise emotionally destabilizing or hazardous situation can be facilitated by sensitive and flexible groupwork offered within 24 to 72 hours of 'the cry for help'.[18] One or a number of group sessions lasting from a few hours to a day, a weekend, or spread over some weeks can be offered to crisis victims and their families depending on their need.

In other settings, such as a hospital where patients attending a specialized support group may live in a wide geographical area, occasional one-day or weekend sessions can top up the monthly or (more often) infrequent meetings. Residential and education settings can also respond to more intensive group meeting. In teaching groupwork skills to social work students I will often use a 'ten-hour session'. With work teams where the emphasis is on developing and strengthening work relationships, I always start with a one- or two-day 'nutcracker' intensive as a way of loosening up rigid procedures and ways of thinking before going into the more usual weekly sessions. I have observed an increasing use of reflective practice groups where professional staff gather to consider the impact and interactions of agency, clients and other factors on their practice. Because of the pressures of resources and demands such groups often meet bimonthly for an hour and a half. With motivated groups in my experience these longer intervals can still produce satisfying results. See Chapter 14 for a fuller discussion of such groups.

Don't be afraid to experiment with the length of session, number and frequency of meetings to suit your group needs. You will find that most people are fairly adaptable and open to new approaches designed to facilitate them.

CLOSED OR OPEN GROUPS

A closed group is one that starts and finishes with the same people and is run for a fixed number of sessions. In an open group members may come and go at different times for various reasons. The time span for the group may be set beforehand or may be left indeterminate. The classic long-term psychotherapy group is generally referred to as a slow-open group.[19] The lifetime of the group is open-ended and members arrive and leave when their therapeutic work is achieved. The ongoing pattern of joining and leaving provides rich opportunities for working through a series of psychological events such as rivalry, competition, anxiety and loss.

Advantages	
Open group	*Closed group*
• Constant modification of group culture • Greater variety of resource and skill • Can be more creative, imaginative • Good for work on initiating and terminating relationships • Issues of separation, termination, inclusion • Issues around change, adaptability	• Consistent and predictable • Can be more cohesive and intimate • Easier to balance

Disadvantages	
Open group	*Closed group*
• Can be more unstable, less predictable • Lacks depth, intimacy of closed group • Subgrouping, cliques, alliances • Hard to balance	• Tendency to get into conformity and 'group think' • Lacks the range and variety of the open group • Less able to deal with change and adaptability • Limited opportunity to deal with termination issues

Programming the group

Programming is a highly skilled part of working in a group. It demands imagination, flexibility, assessment, selection-design, and interventional skills as well as an ability to co-ordinate human and material resources in a manner which meets the needs of the individual and the group. According to Vinter, the word programme denotes 'a class of group activities', which 'follow a pattern, unfolding in a rough chronological sequence and sometimes reaching a definite climax or conclusion'.[20] Examples of programme activities would be a game, role-play exercise, group discussion, or making a meal together. Programme in some groups is a structured procedure. In other types of groups the programme is unstructured for it is in fact the work of the group to study its own dynamics and process as in a psychotherapy group (page 249) or reflective practice group (page 265).

Why use programme?

A programme of activities is not an end in itself. Group leaders use programme consciously and carefully in order to influence groups and individuals and achieve specific outcomes. Perhaps the most important reason for using programme is to provide a point of focus – a context for group members to come together and provide a rationale for work. Context creates boundaries and boundaries create rules and structure, consistency and predictability. The work of the group can proceed:

> - To acquire new skills
> - To learn new behaviours
> - To engage in therapy
> - To study group dynamics
> - To reflect on professional practice

As we saw earlier (page 3), without the consistency and predictability that comes from patterned interaction and context, human interaction tends to be weak, diffuse, and anarchic. Children and adults get a sense of who they are and learn by doing and working with others in settings where there is a degree of structure.

When children and adults suffer from relationship difficulties or have a poor image of themselves as a result of missed or absent life-opportunities they can benefit enormously from a carefully structured group experience which aims at rebuilding self-confidence or improving social skills. In other situations where resolution of a problem or task is the reason for the group's existence thoughtful selection of activity by the leader can provide the necessary structure and procedure for helping the group to achieve its objectives. We can list some of the reasons for using programme in the group:

> - To provide a medium or context in which members can engage and interact
> - To provide the group with structured experience
> - To influence directly or indirectly the group or individuals
> - To achieve particular results or desired objectives
> - To modify or control undesirable behaviour
> - To facilitate the growth and development of a group

The important point to remember is that programme should always be related to individual and group needs and goals. The programme is not an end in itself. As a leader you should always be able to say why you are using a certain activity or engaging the group in a particular project.

Creative programme design in structured groups

Creative programme design is about responding to people in a way that enables them to meet their needs while at the same time helping you achieve group tasks and purposes. To do this the group worker requires certain skills and knowledge. Ross and Bernstein suggest that there are three basic skills needed to purposefully design and use programme.[21]

- Assessment
- Activity selection
- Intervention

ASSESSMENT

There are three components in assessment:

- An individual assessment of the needs of each group member
- An assessment of the stage of development of the group
- Identifying the objectives to be achieved

Chapter 3 contains a detailed account of how to identify individual needs and the stage of group development. All that requires to be said here is that assessment enables the leader to penetrate the welter of needs and problems thrown up by a group and its members, and pinpoint specific and strategic objectives. The important point to remember is that unless compelled to do so members will only attend a group if their expectations and needs are being met. Programme must arise from the needs of members and must be related to their mental and physical capacities as well as the group goals. Clear and accurate assessment, therefore, is the first key to creative programme design. In the early stage of a group I worked with, I asked adolescent boys and girls to engage in a written exercise to rate and prioritize certain desirable personal attributes. To my surprise and frustration they refused to co-operate with my carefully prepared exercise and would proffer no reason other than it was 'stupid' and 'boring'. They would not discuss the matter and got very disruptive when I pressed them. It was after another three or four sessions when I knew them better that they revealed to me that they had major difficulties with reading and writing and were fearful of exposing their impediments in front of relative strangers.

ACTIVITY SELECTION

Having identified individual and group needs and set targets the worker can begin to select or design programme activities which will achieve these targets. However, problems now arise which are familiar to many group leaders. How do you select activities from the vast array of resources available, which will have maximum impact in the desired direction? How do you identify the particular attributes of an activity that will be relevant to you? How do you then create consciousness among members as to the purpose of the activity?

Robert Vinter has looked at some of these questions and presents a formulation which I find very valuable in analysing, choosing, and modifying programme activities as diverse as football or group discussion.[22] He states that all activities have three elements:

- *A physical field* which is the territory or space, the people, and equipment associated with the activity, e.g. pitch, players, and ball in football.
- *Performance behaviours* which are basic and essential to the activity, e.g. kicking the ball, no handling, tackling opponents.
- *Respondent behaviours* which are evoked by the activity but not essential to it, e.g. hugging and kissing a goal-scorer, cheering, and arguing.

Vinter believes that performance and respondent behaviours can be achieved or modified by informed selection or modification of particular activities. He suggests six features of all activity that are open to modification.

- The rules or procedures for the activity
- The sources of agents of activity control such as referees, umpires, team captains
- The degree of physical movement involved
- Competence levels required to participate
- The degree of interaction with other people
- The types of reward associated with the activity

By altering or fine-tuning these variables, decreasing the level of competence, increasing the degree of physical movement, streamlining the rules, and so on, a group leader can achieve different effects for different members or for the group at critical stages in its development. (See Chapter 10 for suggestions about activities and their appropriateness in group settings.)

INTERVENTION

Intervention is a constellation of skills which requires the leader to make ongoing assessment and decisions about how to act in order to encourage, modify, or control behaviour of the group or individuals. This is a very creative and flexible part of the programming process because the leader may need to fine-tune any or all of the activity variables at any stage in the activity.

An important part of the intervention strategy is working out how to create consciousness for group members about the activity and its relevance to their lives. I try to do this by having a review of the activity after it has finished. In the review the group and I evaluate:

- The quality of group and member experience
- Levels of satisfaction
- Interactions between members
- What occurred in activity and why
- What was the purpose of the activity and whether it was accomplished?
- Relevance and significance of activity for individuals and the group
- What could be improved, modified?
- Where do we go from here?

A review like this need not take very long and can usually be talked through although there are times when it is good to do a written evaluation.

EXAMPLE OF PROGRAMME DESIGN USING THESE VARIABLES

- *Assessment.* I had been working with a group of eight 11- to 13-year-old boys and girls. We were about two months through a nine-month therapy group. Members tended to be quite defensive and solitary. They did not mix well, trust each other, or share much about themselves. I decided to focus on two objectives.

    o   To encourage and develop trust
    o   To encourage the children to co-operate and share.

- *Programme selection and design.* I chose guided imaging, drawing, and drama as the components of my programme.
- *Guided imaging.* Conducting the children on a fantasy journey meant I could start with an activity which required no equipment, no performance behaviour, no inter-action or movement. I controlled the pace and flow of the activity, there were mini-mal rules (eyes closed, no noise), and the children did not have to be competent at anything other than making pictures in their imagination in response to prompts from me. The exercise was one which was done alone which meant I started 'where the children were at'.
- I chose *drawing* to follow up the fantasy work. Drawing the journey meant that the children would make visible as much as they wished to reveal of their inner activity. The crayons were restricted in number and colour to ensure that the children would have to borrow and share with each other, thereby encouraging interaction.

    Depending on the interest generated by the first two stages of the programme I would suggest that we *acted out* one of the children's journeys. This would continue to stimulate the imagination and involve the children in communicating, building action sequences, casting characters, and acting out the final work – all cooperative and shared experience.

- *Intervention.* I settled and relaxed the children and then asked them to mentally choose three members of their group to accompany them on a perilous journey to rescue a fairy princess held in a castle owned by a fierce giant.

Choosing three members of their group, ostensibly to guide and advise on dealing with dragons, magic forests, and various hazards:

- Created a (mental) basis for interaction
- Stressed a positive and helping interaction
- Created a basis for interaction in actual group reality
- Provided an experience that the children could share

After we had completed the fantasy journey I suggested to the children that we should draw details of the experience. I decided to let the children do this individually rather than do a group drawing – the jump from individual imaging to group drawing would have been too big a transition. As the children were drawing I went around looking at the different drawings. I made public comments on the various group members who appeared in the drawings as a way of attracting their attention and generally applauded their exploits, bravery, and wisdom, generating much excitement and interest. The restriction in number and colour of crayons had the desired effect of ensuring that the children talked to each other, negotiated, borrowed, and shared.

It was an easy matter to introduce the idea of acting out a journey and involving group members as themselves, the dragon, the forest, the princess, the hero, and the giant. The drama involved the children in literal performance behaviours but also evoked respondent behaviours in applause, cheering, jeers, and so on. The children were all included in the one activity either as audience or actors. In the short review session afterwards the whole programme was seen as very attractive and popular and, it was felt, had drawn the group closer together. I subsequently repeated the session, building up a more solid foundation upon which the children could communicate and interact more naturally and informally. The whole sequence took two hours.

It is important in the early stages of a group that the leader knows what he is doing and has a programme that can convey this. The scheme we have looked at offers the leader a framework for designing a relevant programme of activities to manage and guide individual and group behaviour irrespective of whether the group is composed of stroke patients, elderly ladies, children, or adults.

Common mistakes in programming

1 Failure to base programme on identified individual or group need.
2 Failure to link programme and group objectives.
3 Programme content or objectives unrealistic (see 1, 2).
4 Programme is too rigid due to over-planning and failure to allow for spontaneous and unexpected incidents and events.

5   Inability to use the unexpected incident to develop programme objectives or take an entirely new course (see 2, 12, 15).

6   Not enough balance between the needs of the person and the requirements of the task (see page 70).
    Programme too little/too much task centred; too little/too much person centred.

7   Programme above or below the mental and physical capacities of members. May show them in a weak or unfavourable light (see 6).

8   Skill and competence levels may be too high or too low, creating frustration, boredom, competition.

9   Programme separates people because of a division of labour, skill, aptitude, interest.

10 Programme may be unimaginative, repetitious, not stimulating (see Chapter 10).

11 Poor or inappropriate selection of activity.

12 Activity becomes an end rather than a means of heightening awareness or experience (see 4, 5, 15).

13 Failure to create consciousness for members around the programme (see 2, 5, 12, 14, 15).

14 Failure to review, evaluate as a way of fine-tuning or redesigning the programme (see 2, 4, 13, 15).

15 Programme can become a way of avoiding work with the group while giving the appearance of industry and business.

References

1   Whitaker, D.S. (1976) 'Some conditions for effective work in groups', *British Journal of Social Work*, 5, 4: 249.

2   Douglas, T. (1976) *Groupwork Practice*: 41, London: Tavistock.

3   Douglas, T. (1976) op. cit., p. 41.

4   Lowy, L. (1972) 'Goal formulation in social work with groups', in S. Bernstein (ed) *Further Explorations in Group Work*: 128, London: Bookstall.

5   Whitaker, D.S. (1976) op. cit., p. 426.

6   Parsloe, P. (1971) 'What social workers say in groups of clients', *British Journal of Social Work*, 1, 1: 39.

7   Whitaker, D.S. (1976) op. cit., p. 423.

8   Behr. H. and Hearst. L. (2005) Group=Analytic Psychotherapy. London and Philadelphia: Whurr, p. 29.

9   Paradise, R. and Daniels, R. (1972) 'Group composition as a treatment tool with children', in S. Bernstein (ed) *Further Explorations in Group Work*, London: Bookstall.

10 Bertcher, H.J. and Maple, F. (1974) 'Elements and issues in group composition', in P. Glasser, R. Sarri, and R. Vinter, *Individual Change through Small Groups*, New York: Free Press.

11 Rutan, J.S. and Stone, W.N. (1984). *Psychodynamic Group Psychotherapy*, London: Macmillan, p. 99.

12 Paradise, R. and Daniels, R. (1972) op. cit.

13 Tropp, E. (1976) 'A developmental theory', in R. Roberts and H. Northen (eds) *Theories for Social Work with Groups*: 217, New York: Columbia University Press.

14 Ibid., p. 217.

15 Ibid., p. 217.

16 McCullough, M.K. and Ely, P.J. (1971) *Social Work with Groups*: 6, London: Routledge & Kegan Paul.

17 Berelson, B. and Steiner, G.A. (1964) *Human Behaviour: An Inventory of Scientific Findings*: 360, New York: Harcourt.

18 Parad, H.J., Selby, L., and Quinlan, J. (1976) 'Crisis intervention with families and groups', in R. Roberts and H. Northen (eds), op. cit.

19 Behr, H. and Hearst, L. (2005) op. cit., p. 29.

20 Vinter, R.D. (1974) 'Program activities: an analysis of their effects on participant behaviour', *Individual Change through Small Groups*, op. cit., p. 233.

21 Ross, A.L. and Bernstein, N.D. (1976) 'A framework for the therapeutic use of group activities', *Child Welfare*, LV, 9: 627–39.

22 Vinter, R.D. (1974) op. cit.

Chapter 2

Leading and setting up the group

There is no single, universally applicable style or method of working in a group. Different groups demand different leadership styles and each group will require a variety of behaviours and responses from the leader as it moves through its phases of development towards greater capability and maturity.

Leadership in the group setting is determined by:

- Agency requirements of the worker and group
- Group purpose
- Individual and group needs
- Personality and worldview of the worker
- Role of the worker in the group

What distinguishes the leader is the authority given or ascribed to her to influence the group in certain ways, to achieve agreed goals. The employing or funding agency delegates authority to the leader to act on its behalf with a particular group of people. It substantiates this delegated authority with resource, time, and money and in return expects her to behave in certain ways. The group members invest the leader with authority by virtue of her position, skill, or expert knowledge and expect her to be able to move the group to perform the tasks it was called together to do. Whether the leader likes it or not she is required by her agency and perceived by her group to be a person who has authority and power to reward, induce, be an 'expert', be a model, inform, and empower (see page 103).

The first step in working with a group or in preparation for such work is full acceptance by the worker of the fact of her authority to influence and intervene in group experience. There should be no attempt to deny or fudge this. The group worker must claim her authority! Unfortunately many workers have not resolved their own feelings and attitudes to authority and send out conflicting or ambivalent messages about themselves as leaders. The result is to confuse group members, generate insecurity, suspicion, and fear that the worker cannot be relied on in a crisis.

Reluctance or refusal by the group worker to provide leadership to act on her authority can be very damaging at critical stages of transition when the group rightfully look to the worker for guidance, reassurance, and structure. Very often when looking back at why a particular group came to be a conflictual or apathetic experience for people, I have found that the roots lie in the vacuum created by a group worker not facing up to the responsibility and obligations of her authority and failing to provide the group with leadership when it needs boundary and direction.

To determine the nature of her authority base the worker needs to be clear about the requirements and expectations the agency has of her:

- What goals does the agency have for this group?
- What roles and tasks are the worker required to perform with this group?
- What accountability is required of the worker and to whom? (see page 45)
- Are these expectations and requirements compatible with the group goals?

The worker also needs to accept that group members have a right to expect from her:

- Consistency, fairness, honesty
- Recognition of worth, respect, and consideration
- That the worker develops and creates new experiences
- Structure, direction, boundary
- Protection of standards, norms, and values
- Feedback, advice, suggestion
- An increasing and proportionate role in making decisions
- That she act as a model of legitimate and compassionate authority

The next step is for the worker to select a model of groupwork which will guide her thinking and understanding of group behaviour, offer suggestions as to leadership style, interventions, and programme. Usually the model of groupwork is based on the worker's professional training so a social worker or youth worker might use a social groupwork approach whilst a psychologist or community psychiatric nurse might find a cognitive behavioural model of groupwork more familiar. Selection of a groupwork model should be related to the goals of the group, member needs, and the worker's personality and worldview. At this stage it is then possible to begin to determine a style of leadership which will accommodate member needs, group goals, and the worker's personal and theoretical perspectives.

We can identify four broad styles of leadership:[1]

- *Directive*: Leader assumes major responsibilities for organizing, convening, guiding, identifying tasks, maintaining flow of ideas and emotions.
- *Permissive*: Leader is non-directive and assumes that if purpose is clear and acceptable, group members can accomplish their goals. The leader does not abdicate her authority but tries to allow the group to determine its own behaviour incentives and strategy.
- *Facilitating*: Leader sees herself as a member of the group but with expertise, role, and function which is different from other members. She places major responsibilities for group process and task accomplishment on the group and its members and tries to be supportive, encouraging, and involved.

- *Flexible*: Leader adapts her position and behaviour in response to her assessment of group functioning, needs of members, and the task and will take up any of the other three leadership styles if it appears appropriate to do so.

In some situations an exclusive or predominant style of leadership may be indicated; disturbed children may require the structure and containment of the more directive stance; a facilitative style of leadership would suit a therapeutic group whereas a community group would benefit from the permissive approach. The style of leadership should be flexible and tailored to the needs and functioning of the individual and the group. For further discussion on this see Chapters 4–7. Also have a look at Chapter 8 for a full discussion on the dilemmas and challenges which confront the group worker.

Co-leading

The issues of co-leading with more than one worker should be considered carefully in the planning stage. Many group workers start their career co-leading with at least one other worker – very often from a different agency and sometimes from a different professional background! I have found that lack of preparation and consideration of the nature of the co-leading relationship is a major source of distortion and restriction of the group process. My own position is that joint or co-leading is a very sophisticated way of working and not one that I would recommend to the beginner.

For co-leading to be a productive and creative experience:

- Each worker needs to be aware of the contribution of the other, value this, and believe in it.
- Each worker needs to be very clear about her own role and contribution.
- All workers should be clear and in agreement about the purpose of the group.
- Each worker should be clear why their agency wants them present and what the agency hopes to contribute to and get from the group project.
- All workers should be prepared to fully discuss the conflicts, tensions, and feelings aroused in them by joint work and group experience.
- All workers should be willing to permit and invite differences in perception, style, and approach as long as there is agreement about purpose.
- All workers need to collaborate, share, trust, talk to each other, in and out of the group. The ability of the group to share, and deal with conflict and interpersonal issues is directly related to how effective co-leaders are at this.
- This requires that all workers have negotiated agency agreement that sufficient time can be set aside for preparation and debriefing and that adequate supervision of practice is available.

Let's consider some of the rationales advanced for co-leading the group

(a)   in terms of the group workers:

- The workers are co-equals from the same agency.
- One worker is a novice/apprentice/student learning about groupwork alongside a more knowledgeable colleague.

- The workers are from different agencies that wish to co-operate on a particular project.
- The workers have different professional backgrounds that are deemed helpful for the group.
- The workers can support each other with the difficult and fast-moving dynamics in a group.

(b) in terms of the group members:

- Group members have disabilities that require the presence and attention of more than one worker.
- Group members are younger children who require boundaries and containment.
- Group members are learning new life skills and behaviours that require the input and knowledge of different professionals.
- Group members are psychologically vulnerable or disturbed or dealing with a trauma such as sexual abuse and more than one group worker provides a sense of safety and secure boundaries.
- Group members are suffering with life impacting medical conditions such as cancer, diabetes, and other illnesses that require the input of different professionals.

We can distinguish between at least three styles of co-leading:

- *Supportive co-leading* is where one member of the team takes the lead role and the other member rotates among group members to provide support, assistance, and clarification. This is a good model for a pair of workers from different disciplines working with say a psychoeducational group or an activity group (see Chapter 13). Which worker is in the lead and who provides support may change during the session or from one session to the next depending on particular programme objectives. It is important that the role and skill contribution of the supportive co-leader is clearly valued by the pair so that the lead worker does not feel an unequal burden of responsibility and the support leader does not feel less important and that their expertise is ineffectively used. This means the pair must continually discuss their experience of their roles and interactions and consider how this may be affecting the group process.

  A variant of this style of co-leading is to be found where one worker is a novice/ apprentice/student learning about groupwork alongside a more knowledgeable colleague. While this is a perfectly acceptable rationale I would prefer if the novice or apprentice was given their own group to operate under the regular supervision of the more experienced colleague. This is because the novice would then undertake responsibility for the group from the start and get to grips with group process and dynamics rather than often sit marvelling at the superior technique of the senior leader and feeling useless and ignorant. The beginner can all too readily idealize the senior worker and devalue their own contribution and decide that this work is not for them. In a worse scenario the beginner may feel compelled to prove their worth and compete with the senior worker. The senior worker may find themselves wanting to impress the novice with their expertise and forget the need of the group members in the desire to make exciting and spectacular interventions.

  Groups are very good at picking up on the variety of tensions and power differentials between workers and may repeat earlier unhealthy experiences of parental couples and family dynamics. If it is deemed suitable for a senior and novice to co-lead the group they must make time to discuss the difference in power, authority, and experience between them and be constantly vigilant for how this affects their partnership and the group. This is an additional and onerous responsibility for the senior worker as she must be alert to the dynamics of the co-leading mini-group of which she is a part as well as manage the group dynamics and be mindful how the co-leading pair affects the group. It would be very helpful if the pair could have some supervision from a neutral third party to keep these rivalries and idealizations under scrutiny, manage the potentials for shame and blame, and promote the professional development and learning contract that underpins the nature of this form of co-leading.

- *Collaborative co-leading* is where the members of the team have taken a decision to equally co-work alongside one another and jointly share responsibility for planning, intervening, and assessing the progress of all members in the group. This is a more advanced and mature facilitative style that requires more time, co-ordination, and knowledge of and trust in one another's skills. The collaborative co-leaders need not necessarily share the same theoretical or professional backgrounds although this is of course very helpful if they share some commonality, but they do need to have a real regard for each other's contributions and be very comfortable with different perspectives and orientations. Such group workers are skilled in exploiting their different styles and perspectives in service of the group members. A male and female pair or a same sex pair can provide healthy and alternative couple role models and identifications in a psychotherapy group. They can model healthy difference and disagreement about what they observe in the group and can talk to each other about this as a means of promoting effective communication about events and incidents in relationships that can take into account different perspectives without the need to resort to an either/or, right and wrong, or black and white approach.

- *Specialized co-leading* is usually found in a psychoeducational group that is set up to help members deal with the effects of an illness like diabetes or cancer or help promote healthier lifestyles for obesity or post-operative conditions or a host of group interventions. Each worker may be from a different professional background and is specifically present to bring their particular expertise to educate, inform, and develop coping strategies. This requires time for planning contributions, roles, and interventions between the principals and cannot be condensed or glossed over. The professional and theoretical base and orientation of a social worker or youth worker or health visitor, or physiotherapist, nurse, or other clinician must be considered and respected and their particular contribution must be valued and discussed in terms of the group objectives and desired member outcomes if the multidisciplinary input is to be effective and not blur or collapse. If each professional cannot explain to themselves or the other workers or the group what their role and contribution is they should not be in the team.

Typical problems in co-leading

- *Misunderstanding of the nature of co-leading.* I have all too often found over the years when supervising co-leaders that they misunderstand or are unaware of the essential nature and potential of co-leadership. Co-leaders tell me that they will provide mutual support for each other, model co-operative leadership, provide feedback for each other and so on. But when I press a little an astonishing fear emerges. The pair are afraid of the group. If asked to reveal their worst fear, it is that the group will suddenly fly out of their control and break down with members refusing to return. Their unconscious fantasy is that the darker side of human nature will escape in the group, overwhelm them, and cause others to act in a destructive way. They dread being flooded with unbearable feelings. They are frightened by the number of people in the group, feel alone, and threatened by the spontaneity and unpredictability of group members. So co-leading in this scenario is really an attempt to protect the pair against the imminent chaos and provide company for each other, security, and predictability. The idea is that two heads are better than one to ensure that the group is successful, well-attended, and orderly. This fear is not confined to the actual co-leaders but may also reflect an agency fear of litigation and of being blamed if the group does not work out in some way, and so an insistence on two or more workers is a means of maintaining constant vigilance in order to avert failure.

In reality the whole point of co-leading is to expose group members to different perspectives, thoughts, and ideas. The real advantage of co-leading is in the willingness of the leaders to exploit and explore their differences in perception of the group experience for the benefit of the individuals and the group.

Group members learn that other people think differently from them; they come to understand why others think that way, and it shows them that their way is not the only way. Healthy and creative difference becomes the lived experience and reality for the group modelled initially by the co-leaders.

Co-leaders who understand the true nature of co-leading do not act as a benevolent authority imparting knowledge and skills to a compliant and receptive group. The co-leaders recognize that they themselves are a mini-group whose core project is to engage members in mutually agreed, self-generated, and internalized controls and values rather than complying and acquiescing to externally asserted norms and values. By initially embodying this with each other co-leaders engage the group to move closer to the ideal of a community as increasingly autonomous members re-choose to be in the group and come together to express and fulfil their purpose. Co-leaders who understand the real nature of co-leading understand that power and authority are not invested in them but are functions and rights of group membership and the inner experience of the individual. They make room for another co-leader. They make the group their co-worker! They look for every opportunity to work alongside their group. 'What does the group think about this incident?' 'What does the group make of this?' 'What does this mean for the group?'

• *Rivalries*. Co-leading involves taking turns to intervene as the group will not function if both leaders are speaking at the the same time and this can create problems for the workers. If the pair is not mature the co-leaders may become resentful and jealous of each other. One worker may be more active or vociferous. One may feel left out or that her partner is more popular, or does the more glamorous work. There may be competition for who makes more interesting interventions. Differences in attitude particularly in the sensitive areas of discipline and control can create conflict which is amplified and exacerbated by the presence of group members. The group is quick to spot the presence of latent or explicit conflict, split the workers, and play one off against the other. It is important for the team to recognize the potential for disruptive rivalries when discussing co-leadership at the group planning stage particularly when there are different professional disciplines and theoretical bases to be co-ordinated. The co-leaders should talk together about their different perspectives and differing leadership styles as well as personality styles and consider how these can mesh, and think also about how they can conflict. If this is honestly done they will be alert to how rivalries can develop and be well placed to minimize this.

- *Shame.* Because the group is a public arena where everyone can see everyone else all the time co-leaders and members can find themselves compelled to behave in ways that avoid a loss of face and demotion of status and prestige. Co-leaders may present a particular face or image that protects their professional competence and self-esteem. They may find themselves overly sensitive to the possibility of making a mistake or being seen to be less efficient than their partner and so may work harder than required to present a 'perfect' front. Novice workers in particular but also more senior workers can come to believe that silent attention may be seen by group members as inexperience or ignorance and that active intervention is more valuable and evidence of great experience, and so may intrude unnecessarily. This can excite shame and rivalry in a pair and create unhealthy patterns of co-leading. The potential for shame between the workers should be acknowledged at the group planning stage and strategies developed to minimize it. Ensuring that each co-leader has a clear role and is comfortable with it can go a long way to promoting co-operation and a sense of contributing to the working of the group. For example, in a particular session the co-leaders can determine that one leader will concentrate on what is happening at an individual level and make appropriate comments and the other co-leader will focus on what is occurring at the group process level and intervene accordingly. In the next session the pair can swap over roles thus ensuring that each participates equally and neither is privileged. In time the pair will come to feel more comfortable with each other and a respectful co-leading style develops.

- *Fear of difference.* One often finds that there are co-leaders who believe it is important to present a united front at all times, irrespective of whatever division there may be in the team. Sometimes this is due to a fear or avoidance of conflict, sometimes to a belief that leader disagreement will have a damaging effect on the group. This avoidance of different perspectives between the workers in my view nullifies the reason for co-leadership.

It is absolutely essential for co-leaders to talk to each other, all the time, in and out of the group, about their different perceptions, insights, feelings if they are to exploit co-leading to the full. Reasons put forward in the literature for using co-leaders include the advantages of support, sharing, feedback on each other's performance, time to observe more closely, modelling co-operative leadership, and so on. For me, the real advantage of co-leading is in the willingness of the leaders to exploit and explore their differences in perception of the group experience for the benefit of the individuals and the group.

Differences in perception and response, even lack of agreement, if handled creatively can be an exciting and enhancing experience for group members providing more information, contrasts, and alternatives, offering opportunities for giving opinions, sharing, taking stands, assessment, consideration, and decision making. In certain situations lack of agreement between co-leaders may be inevitable. If the relation-ship is to work the co-leaders must be able to publicly permit and allow the other's understanding of the situation and value it as a contribution in its own right to the total experience. When this occurs there need be no conflict or necessity to force one viewpoint on the other. Each leader builds on the experience of the other to help the group and its members. Ability to tolerate differing perspectives creates the pos-sibility of synthesis and a new understanding of any and every situation. The fear and misunderstanding of difference is minimized if the co-leaders take some time before the group session begins to talk about how things might go and then take time after the session to debrief. This is essential and should be agreed at the planning stage and with agency approval and support. I have been astonished to find that on occasions co-leaders have not met until the first session and do not meet with each other after the session pleading pressures of other work commitments. In such situations it is not surprising that confusion and anxiety is the common experience of co-leaders as they struggle to implement some manualized and digitalized approach to groupwork.

- *Illness, holidays, and breaks.* I have seen situations where illness for one co-leader can prompt the other to cancel a session or suspend or even terminate the group prema-turely as they do not feel able to continue without their partner. The group may be similarly cancelled if one or both co-leaders has leave or is on holiday. The remaining co-leader often does not have the confidence to continue the group or may suffer from some of the fears discussed above. The disruption caused to the group can be alleviated if the co-leaders have understood the nature of co-leading. The remain-ing co-leader can easily continue with the group as their co-worker! They do not need to cancel or suspend the group. In the case of holidays it would be better if co-leaders considered this at the planning stage and tried to ensure that holiday leave will minimally impact the group. This seems rather obvious but too often co-leaders start a group and then find that one of them has to take leave during the life of the group. A little bit of foresight can be helpful and the group can be prepared for the absence of a worker. The group can be tasked with telling the returning co-leader of their activity and progress in her absence. The co-leaders need to discuss the planned absence thoroughly so that feelings of rivalry do not get stirred up as one co-leader has the group attention while the other is away. Illness cannot be predicted and can strike at any time. The co-leaders can determine if this is a temporary event or more significant and decide how to manage the group in this light. It is important to be straight with the group and give some time and space to talk over their concerns and fears if illness for one co-leader is to last more than a session or two.

- *Lack of thinking time for the co-leaders.* It is essential that the co-leaders have planned thinking time and supervision for their work. They need to be able to think about how they are impacting on each other and on the group and how the group is stir-ring up uncomfortable feelings in them. Co-leaders should meet before and after the group session to reflect on what has happened in the group and consider how things might be improved or changed for the better of all. The co-leaders are a couple or mini-group and can be sensitive to unspoken or unconscious group dynamics being lodged in them. Recognizing that they have this resonant capacity is an important part of effective leadership and facilitation. I have seen situations where co-leaders are expected by their agency to undertake groupwork in addition to their normal duties and have not been allocated time for reflection and supervision let alone compensatory time off in lieu. Not only is this woeful agency management and ignorance of the complexity of groupwork it is also unprofessional of the workers to comply with this and not assert their need for adequate thinking time. I always encourage co-leaders in such a situation to go back and renegotiate a more professional contract with their agency or talk with the agency myself and encourage a more realistic understanding of what is involved in working with groups.

Some examples of co-leading in practice

(i)   A therapeutic group for eight adolescent girls aged 14–17 years was co-led by a male and female social worker. The group had been set up to address difficult behaviours that the girls were experiencing at home and at school and that had resulted in some girls being suspended from school while some others were in social work care homes. The group was a prestige project, well funded and had a lot of agency expectations riding on it. The male worker was experienced in this work while the female worker was working in this type of group for the first time. The group was frequently turbulent and only contained by ongoing exploration of the behavioural choices of the members and consequences of these choices for the continuation of the group. A lot of the co-leaders' time was spent looking at how the group contract was frequently broken and patiently examining the reasons for this and putting things back together again.

The male co-leader was frequently verbally and emotionally attacked because the girls' experience of males was so negative and the female co-leader was encouraged to join with the girls in these assaults. When she did not join in she often became the object of rejection. The constant splitting activity was recognized by the co-leaders and they were able to support each other and offer a different and more mature response than the girls had experienced with their own parents. The emotional demands on the co-leaders were great but not overwhelming. They were both parents themselves and could see the obvious childlike quality of many of the group interactions. At other times the members competed with each other and with each co-leader for attention and to be favoured. They would envy the relationship between the co-leaders and seek to undermine it. Again the co-leaders could recognize what was happening and could support and protect each other. Meeting before the group sessions and debriefing afterwards was very important in helping the co-leaders think about what was happening in the group and how the group was using them.

As part of the programme two residential weekends were planned. The first residential took place after 12 sessions and was carefully planned and agreed with the members. A contract was agreed in which the members promised to comply with reasonable boundaries around behaviours and to refrain from alcohol and drugs. The co-leaders and the group considered potential boundary infractions and thought about a range of consequences including terminating the residential and returning home in the event of extreme behaviours. As might be expected on the first night of the residential extreme behaviour occurred as a consequence of smuggled in alcohol – a clear and flagrant breach of the previously agreed group contract! The co-leaders got little sleep that night as they struggled to contain the group. The next morning obviously demanded an examination of the breached contract and while the co-leaders were minded to terminate the residential as agreed they allowed themselves to be persuaded by the apparently contrite members that they had learned from this and it would not happen again. The co-leaders wanted to maintain a therapeutic stance and were unwilling to be seen as punitive by ending the residential. Much of the day was taken up with group examination of what had occurred and it appeared that some positive work was done. That night proved however to be a repeat of the previous evening and again the following and final morning was given over to an exploration of the deliberate breaching of the group contract. The group residential ended as planned and the group returned home. A number of the following group sessions were given over to discussion of the unruly residential and the co-leaders believed that the members made some progress in taking responsibility for their behaviour despite the obvious fact that there had been no consequences for the members.

A second residential had been planned for 15 sessions later and was to go ahead. There was much discussion about potential breaches and infractions of the contract and the group were fully a part of the negotiated contract and aware of the consequences for unacceptable behaviours. This residential was scheduled for a hotel in a city 100 miles away. The evening programme went as planned on the first night and all seemed well until the hotel reception woke the co-leaders at 2am to inform them that the girls were drunk and shouting out of their bedroom windows at passers-by in the street. The co-leaders immediately rounded up the group and drove them straight back home, delivering subdued girls to their angry parents at 6am! The co-leaders refused to listen to the pleas of the members to discuss their behaviour and enforced the sanction of early termination as agreed. They supported each other in this difficult decision.

The co-leaders met with the girls and their parents over the following days before the next planned session and agreed with them that the group must continue and that it was the business of the group to decide how to manage what had happened. This time the members did take responsibility for their behaviour and were able to connect consequences to the choices they did and didn't make in their lives. The rest of the group programme was given over to examining how members' lives were blighted and restricted by thoughtless and impulsive behaviours. The group ended as planned some months later and was deemed by the members and the co-leaders to have been successful.

This was a good co-leader pair who supported and protected each other and could understand and usually manage the testing and difficult behaviour of disadvantaged adolescents, but they made life difficult for themselves by not enforcing the group contract when it was breached in the first residential. They believed in a therapeutic stance but failed at that time to realize that a therapeutic stance also means protecting the group boundaries and making firm interventions and being willing to become an object of anger and resentment and even hatred in service of the group well-being. They were not embodying this group's desired learning outcome that choices have consequences and members should consider their actions in that light. By the time of the second residential the co-leaders had realized their mistake and were able to act decisively and demonstrate that the continuation and well-being of the group was their primary concern. The result was that the group survived a difficult experience and matured from it.

(ii) Two male co-leaders facilitated a psychotherapy group containing five females and three male members. The two co-leaders were experienced group psychotherapists and had worked successfully together for a number of years. John was the elder of the pair by 20 years and had a more formal groupwork style while Peter was a more active and informal worker. In a particular session Susan described feeling worthless, without value and wept bitterly. It emerged that her marriage was under severe stress and that her husband bullied and dominated her. She told the group that her husband was monitoring her and would determine in three months' time if the marriage was viable and that he might leave her. The group was very supportive of her and Edith tried to reassure Susan that her husband had an investment in maintaining the marriage. John asked Edith how she could be sure of this and perhaps she was supporting a relationship that needed to end. Edith had a similar bullying relationship with a man that she had finally terminated after a lot of exploration with the group. At this Peter intervened to comment that Susan's husband like Edith's partner might not want to give up a slave! John turned to his co-leader and asked him who did he think was the slave in Susan's marriage since he thought the pair were co-dependent. Susan challenged this fiercely and John said to her that while he thought that there was something authentic trying to emerge in her recognition of her marital difficulties she also struggled hugely with dependence which he believed she saw as weak and contemptible. The co-leader said that there was a bit of her like a barnacle clinging onto the marriage because the other side of her fear of dependence and the pain of loss was her fear of separation and isolation. This infuriated Susan and she attacked John telling him that he was just like her husband calling her a parasite and humiliating her. The other group members jumped in to refute that John had said anything like that and to try to point out what had really been said to her but Susan couldn't hear this for her rage and tears.

Peter then came in to gently point out that it was good that she could get angry with his co-leader as she could then practise arguing with a male here in the group and develop more effective ways of asserting herself that might help in her marriage. He also pointed out that the thing to remember with John was that he might get things wrong sometimes: he would do anything to make a connection with her. This intervention served to calm Susan and Peter continued to encourage her to carefully explore why she thought John might want to belittle her and to begin to consider whether his message about her ambivalent feelings about dependency might actually be worth thinking about. The ensuing discussion expanded to involve the other group members in examining their own difficulties in their own relationships and provide a more inclusive context for Susan to think about her role in her marriage.

What this vignette demonstrates is how two co-leaders are able to talk to each other and think together in a fraught group session. John had attempted to show how Edith's assumption about Susan's husband was based on her own unhappy experience and might actually not be helpful to Susan. His comments to Susan, while correct, unconsciously carried some of the dynamics of her marriage with his use of the image of the clinging barnacle. When she exploded in rage with John she was seeing him as her dominating and humiliating husband and he was no longer able to engage with her. Peter recognized this and his intervention aimed at supporting her wounded self while also keeping her connected with his co-leader and available to work on her problem. He was able to soothe her by implicitly acknowledging that John's image of the barnacle was not helpful to her but was an attempt on his part to make a connection. Peter knew that John would not be shamed by this and could trust that his co-leader would not feel put down by him. The two co-leaders could see that the dynamics of Susan's marriage was being enacted in the relationship with John and that Peter had to be the neutral party who could get them to think about this and help Susan develop more mental space to reflect on what was being said to her. The co-leaders were able to respond to each other and take turns to work on the individual and group preoccupations. They were able to exploit and explore their differences in response and perception of the group experience and permit and allow the other's understanding of the situation and value it as a contribution in its own right to the total experience. They were mature co-leaders who did not need to rival or to force one viewpoint on the other. The co-facilitators knew that their relationship could catch and resonate with the group's unspoken and unthought emotional preoccupations and were willing to talk to each other about their internal experience of the group with this perspective in mind. They were able to harness their emotions and apply them to tasks like thinking and problem solving for the benefit of the group. The group members were then able to internalize the co-facilitators in their mind as a more mature and less critical model of authority and interpersonal relationship.

(iii) A psychotherapy group had lost its original leader due to his premature death and two new co-leaders stepped in to take over the running of the group. The male co-leader Jim was an experienced group worker and the younger female leader Donna had not worked in this type of group before. Much of their work with the group in their first year was helping the group deal with the trauma of the loss of their previous worker and they were very successful as a pair with this difficult work. Jim was idealized by members for stepping in to 'save' the group whereas Donna was viewed as a 'loyal acolyte' whose job was to support and protect Jim from any stress in the group. After the first year Jim decided that the time was right to introduce a new member and wanted to inform the group. Donna thought that the announcement might be delayed for a few weeks as Jim was due to go on leave and they could talk to the group together. When the new member turned up after Jim returned from leave he realized that he had given her a date for starting but had 'forgotten' to inform the group and had to ask the new member to come back when he had told the group and given them some time to think about this.

The group were very angry with Jim over the next three sessions and couldn't understand how a good facilitator 'had allowed bad things to happen'. Jim tried to get the group to think if they might have a role in his 'forgetting' but they insisted it was his error alone. Jim then accepted it was his mistake but wondered if there might be an unconscious influence at work. When questioned as to what this might be Jim said that perhaps he had wanted to make the group special because of the trauma of the loss of its original leader and rescue them by providing an ideal experience this time around.

After some consideration of this Roberta then said that the group was giving Jim a bad time and maybe they should think about Donna's role in this. She tried to get Donna to say what she knew about the starting date of the new member but Donna sidestepped this to Roberta's disgust. Roberta said that Jim and Donna were like 'good cop and bad cop'. She said that Donna was given to observations and was detached and looked down at the group from a lofty height whereas Jim was more hands-on and interacted with members and encouraged group responsibility. This led to discussion of Donna's role as a junior and trainee and that the group had come to not expect much of her anyway.

When the session ended the co-leaders reflected on how the 'mistakes' in the group administration might reflect some dynamics in their relationship around power and authority and also resonate with group preoccupations. Donna pointed out that Jim had not included her in the decision to bring in a new member and had acted unilaterally. Jim asserted that she needed to take more power in the group and she pointed out that when she did try to be more active in the group he ignored her which the group had recognized in their discussion of her role as a detached junior. She pointed out that she had found herself having to be sensitive to the possibility that Jim might not cope well if she asserted herself more powerfully in the group. The pair were able to have a forthright discussion about the quality of their communication and how they managed power and authority and what this might mean for the group. They considered how Roberta's desire to protect Jim and see what Donna knew about the starting date of the new member might be a way of finding out what power Donna had and whether she would be able to take care of Jim if he continued making mistakes and whether she could then take care of the group. This helped them understand Jim's desire to provide an ideal experience for this traumatized group and his unconscious presumption that he had to take care of the group by himself. They were able to agree that actually they both could and should take care of the group together. This was a watershed for their co-leading relationship and they were able to return to the group and work much more effectively as a pair.

What this vignette demonstrates is how these co-leaders were initially caught up in a traumatized group's desire for perfect care and how this issue permeated their working together. Jim unconsciously assumed the role of the good cop and unwittingly cast his co-leader in a less important role with the group's collusion. When Donna insisted that the notice to the group of the entry of a new member be delayed she was asserting her power and this caused Jim to make a 'mistake'. She was puncturing his omnipotence and insisting that she could also take care of the group. They were able to reflect on their rivalry and think about this in terms of the group dynamics. The group had matured under their watch and no longer needed a saviour and Donna no longer needed to prop up Jim and could now insist on a meaningful and co-equal partnership. They were able to talk honestly about their co-leadership dynamics and reflect on the implications for them and the group. The co-facilitators knew that their relationship could catch and resonate with the group's unspoken and unthought emotional preoccupations and were willing to talk to each other about their internal experience of the group with this perspective in mind. They were able to harness their emotions and apply them to tasks like thinking and problem solving for the benefit of the group.

We can see from this case study how effective and powerful co-leadership can be when both partners are professionally mature enough to be able and willing to exploit and explore their differences in perception of the group experience for the benefit of the individuals and the group.

Accountability

Much of this will have been worked out when the leader examines the requirements of the agency around the group. Some of the important issues to be clarified here are:

- To whom is the worker accountable?
- Who will guide, monitor, or supervise the worker's practice?
- Who needs to be informed about what is going on in the group?
- How much do they need to know?
- What kind of recording is required?
- Where will it be kept and who will have access to it?

It is important to have clear and explicit agreements or contracts governing these issues, particularly in the sensitive areas relating to communication with colleagues and other agencies interested in the group.

Presenting the group

There are two aspects to presenting the group:

- Presentation of the group to agency for validation, acceptance, permission to proceed, and release of resource
- Presentation of the group to potential members

The group should be presented to the agency in planned form. It should consist of a clear, simple, well written proposal containing your thoughts, intentions, and requirements in these areas:

- Background history to proposal
- Definition of problems to be tackled
- Purpose, goals, and objectives for the group:
  1   Agency perception
  2   Member perception

- Role of worker/s
- Proposed methodology and programme details
- Expenditure, resource, transport, equipment required

- Size of membership, time, date, venue, duration of group, length and frequency of session
- How you intend to evaluate and assess the value of the group (see page 333)
- Relationships with colleagues or other parties
- Try to anticipate any possible difficulties that may arise

Evaluation

An important area to cover in your presentation concerns how you intend to assess and evaluate the success, or otherwise, of the group.[2]

Try to be clear about your reasons for evaluation:

- To improve the overall functioning of the group
- To determine if objectives and goals have been achieved
- To assess whether the group is tackling priority needs and has relevant goals
- To ensure the group is using resources effectively
- To identify necessary skills and facilities
- To improve workers' practice
- To provide material for supervision
- To influence policy making
- To validate the group and ensure its survival and funding

Consider whether you intend to evaluate:

- *Outcomes*: The extent to which the group achieved its goals in producing change in the targets of intervention.
- *Service delivery*: The types of service offered, their relevance, quality, acceptance, characteristics.
- *Structure and process of the group*: What actually occurred in the group, the quality of work, how it was organized, how resources were used.

Some of the issues you need to think about and a guide to evaluate them are contained in Chapter 17. I raise the subject of evaluation here to remind you that even at the planning stage you should be considering how you intend to assess the effectiveness of the group. The clearer and more specific you are now about what you intend to assess, the easier will be your evaluation at the end of the group. Agencies like to have value for money and indicating to your agency that you fully intend to assess the worth of the group can create a lot of sympathy and goodwill for your proposal.

Presenting the group to potential members

Having presented the group proposal to your agency and obtained approval to start the group, the next step is to meet with potential group members. When I am forming a group I try as far as possible to meet with prospective members before the first session. If I am recruiting for a psychotherapy group I will meet with potential members for three preparation sessions before they enter the group. Referrals will often indicate that a particular person will make a suitable candidate for the group but meeting with them is really important because it may show that they are patently not suitable for the group: they thought the group was something different; they are only proposing to attend to please the referring agent; or they are only mildly interested in the group. Without pre-group interviews people can come along to the first two or three sessions in a frame of mind that is unsettling for the group and can be damaging.

I have a number of objectives for the pre-group interview:

- *To introduce myself (group leader)*, explain my role in the group, and get a sense of who the prospective member is. While this will not determine the person's behaviour in the group, after interviewing several prospective members I have an impression of how people will get on with each other and have some ideas about what I need to do in the first session with this particular group.
- *To provide information about the group and its objectives.* I try to be very clear about how I see the group and what it is about. It sometimes happens that at this early stage the prospective member can decide that the group is not for them or not what they thought it was. Usually people want to know what we will actually do in the group and seek information about the other members, who they are, what they will be like, will they accept the new member?, etc.
- *To relate the group objectives to the prospective member's perception of need.* Without each member being motivated to attend and committed to the group objectives, the group will not work. So it is important to help the prospective member examine his reasons for wanting to join and determine the relevance of the group to his needs. This is a crucial stage because it is easy for the worker to get into 'selling' the group in order to make up the numbers, and not be rigorous about matching member need to group goals. Some prospects can feel intimidated by the worker and against their inclinations may go along with his enthusiasm and conviction. The worker also has to guard against potential members creating unrealistic expectations about the group; there are people who expect immediate 'cures' or deep, intimate relationships by the end of the first session. It is important to short-circuit this by helping the prospect identify specific features or themes in his life which can be worked on in the group, rather than permit global aspirations or expectations. It is easier to use the group 'to obtain feedback on interpersonal behaviour', than it is to use the group 'to become a happier person'.
- *Negotiate an individual contract with the prospect.* By contract I mean a clear agreement between the prospect and the worker about:

  o   The purposes and objectives of the group
  o   The tasks to be undertaken by the prospect in the group
  o   The prospect's expectations of the worker and the group
  o   The worker's expectations of the prospect
  o   The prospect's willingness to attend the group

The particular clauses in the contract are determined very much by the prospective member's acceptance of the legitimacy and relevance of the group for him. One prospect may wish to attend the group for a few sessions to see if it is appropriate for him, so a 'try it and see' clause is more important to him than working out specific tasks to be undertaken in the group. Another prospect may be very willing to accept the group and more energy will go into how he can use the group to achieve certain desired goals.

By making an individual contract with the prospect before the group starts I try to:

- Motivate, engage, and encourage the prospect
- Define what it is that he wants in the group
- Clarify expectations about what is possible, what is not, what is required, what is not
- Emphasize that the prospect is responsible for his use of the group experience
- Show the prospect that he has rights and he will not be used against his will
- Demonstrate that the group is designed to be a caring and compassionate experience

---

The individual contract will be augmented in the first session by a group contract, made with the other members, but since the prospect only has a contract at this stage with the group worker, it is important to make these agreements as a way of substantiating the idea of the group and engaging the potential member. Individual contracts can be written or verbal; the clauses relating to members' needs and goals can be renegotiated throughout the group experience. Here is a short example of some of the clauses governing expectations that worker and member may have of each other and which can be included in the contract either at pre-group or first session stage.

Our expectations of each other

What you can expect of me	*What I expect of you*
1 To make available my skills, knowledge, and concern to help you make best use of this situation.	1 To help me create a situation where you can develop, learn, and grow. This means you choose to use me and others appropriately.
2 To be as honest in everything I do with you as I can. I will take risks with you and others in saying what I really think and feel.	2 To be as honest in your dealings with me as you can, take appropriate risks with your thoughts and feelings.
3 To be accepting and supportive of you and ready to clear the air through discussion with you.	3 To take responsibility for yourself, your being here, your growth and learning.
4 To allow and assist you to develop your own potential, satisfy your needs for growth and esteem.	4 To be accepting and supportive towards me and the others and ready to clear the air when necessary. Our growth is your growth.

Perhaps you would like to delete some of the clauses and add others of your own.

1 ——————————————   2 ——————————————

A friendly group experience or a threatening encounter? Dealing with potential members' anxieties

It really is important for you to keep constantly in mind that you are bringing people into a work group who may have had traumatic experiences in previous groups or may have social problems which can make group membership difficult or threatening. They are being asked to participate and get involved in a group that can stir up a whole range of anxieties and interpersonal tensions. The group is a very public space with multiple opportunities for blaming and shaming to take place and that this can agitate and trigger anxieties and concerns to do with loss of face, criticism, rejection, scapegoating, competition, rivalry, envy, and a plethora of social tensions and emotions. Take a look at Chapter 8 to explore this more fully.

For now be aware that the invitation to join to the group and make a commitment to attend and not to flee the threatening relationships, as previously they might have done, activates members' anxieties and sets off their typical devices for avoiding intimacy and sabotaging relationships.

John Hodge suggests that an important part of the pre-group interview is to *anticipate the fears and anxieties that the prospect may have* about the group experience and work out ways of acknowledging or resolving these.[3] He suggests that potential members may:

- Wonder what a short-term group can achieve when a problem has existed for years
- Be fearful that group discussion will undermine their method of coping with problems
- Be anxious that sessions will be depressing or morbid
- Worry that sessions will activate feelings and memories they would rather leave undisturbed
- Be concerned that they will be exposed or may have to give more than they wish

I find that by bringing these fears and anxieties out into daylight, I give the prospective member permission to have them, can identify potential obstacles to the prospect's participation in the group, and can begin to dispel the more groundless of them. Acknowledgement of the validity of some of these fears, common sense, and compassion, as well as emphasizing the prospect's own power through the contract, all helps to reassure people who have not been a member of a formal group before and who are worried about what they may be letting themselves in for. I have found that prospective members often express the following fears:

- Fear of contamination and contagion
- Fear of being flooded
- Fear of being engulfed by others

- Fear of being blamed or shamed
- Fear of being rejected
- Fear of disclosure
- Fear of intimacy
- Fear of conflict
- Fear of change
- Fear of being stuck

Let's see what is at the bottom of these fears and consider how you might neutralize or defuse them.

Fear of contamination and contagion. Frequently I have had prospects tell me that they couldn't possibly join the group when they hear that there are going to be other depressed people or delinquents or lonely people with social problems like them in the group. They fear that being in the presence of people like themselves will only worsen their problems. They are afraid of being contaminated or catching some emotional disease from these unknown but feared others. Such prospects are projecting unacceptable and unwanted aspects of themselves onto others and treating these disowned parts of themselves with aggression and contempt.

The key to minimizing and possibly neutralizing this anxiety is to stress the solidarity that can be derived from meeting and working with fellow sufferers. Try to highlight the relief and support that can be gained from connecting to others who have experienced similar life events or circumstances which may be by their nature isolating.

Some prospects are wary of groups because they are afraid of being flooded by over-whelming internal feelings. They are often unconsciously afraid of their own rage swell-ing up and damaging themselves or others. Such individuals may have a history of poor impulse control and may mistrust emotions. They will seek to avoid situations and inter-personal relationships that threaten expression of feeling. Since groups can in fact amplify feelings, prospective members may well have had previous experiences in groups that they will cite as proof that groups are dangerous places. Alternatively they may also scoff at the 'luxury' nature of 'California-style' therapeutic or personal growth type groups and be derisive about 'touchy-feely' groups but again be aware that this contempt is masking fear of being flooded by unwelcome feelings.

The best way of approaching this prospective member is to emphasize the containing and supportive nature of the group. Acknowledge that there are emotional energies and currents in groups but point out how the prospect's relationship with their emotional life is problematic and alienating them from people and that membership of the group while challenging can offer opportunities to learn how to cope more creatively with feelings.

Some potential members may be put off the group by their fear of being engulfed by other people. They may not have a very secure sense of their own self and may have a history of finding it difficult to assert themselves and are easily exploitable. Consequently the idea of joining a group becomes threatening and anxiety-making as they may fear that their history could repeat itself. They may agree reluctantly to attend the group but then worry about a possible tendency to be silent or shy or withdrawn and how others might react to this.

With these prospective members it often proves helpful to work out an individual contract which offers a trial basis for membership and can be reviewed (see p. 48). In this individual contract include some clause about how the prospect might alert you and the group if they are starting to feel overwhelmed. Ensure that you have agreed this alternative to walking out of the session or not returning. Point out that everyone in the group will also be negotiating a core dilemma which involves how to get close to others but not too close while being separate but not too separate and that this is a central task for the group but which can also benefit the leery prospect (see.p. 203).

Probably the commonest anxiety has to do with the fear of being blamed or shamed in the group. It is part of everyone's social conditioning, starting in the family and continuing through school, one's peer group, workplace, and so on. It has its roots in one of the oldest forms of social control and is at the emotional centre of the scapegoat phenomenon (see p. 69 and 203). The very public nature of the group means that members fear loss of face and demotion of status and prestige and so they will go to great lengths to protect their social standing and self-esteem. Members are alert to criticism and depreciation from the leader and peers and so are sensitive to the possibility of being made out to be in the wrong or somehow mocked and made to feel contemptible.

Based on their previous experiences potential members may raise objections to joining the group. They may voice their concerns about being found out or stripped bare by the others. They may fear disclosing personal material about themselves as this runs a considerable risk of them being found wanting or stigmatized in some way. They are afraid of something being discovered or revealed about them that could lead to being shamed or rejected and may worry about the consequent damage to their self-esteem. Deeper feelings of being unloveable or unworthy may surface at this time and it is vital to take time and explore and soothe these fears if possible. The anxiety to do with somehow being unacceptable and the dread of rejection is at the basis of much initial resistance to joining the group. Voluntarily making oneself vulnerable to the reaction and control of others can be a terrifying and extremely off-putting fantasy.

The best way of dealing with these core anxieties is to remind the worried prospect that everyone else is in the same situation and that getting to know other people and how they might respond is going to take time, and until they feel comfortable they should not take unnecessary risks. It is important to emphasize the generally supportive nature of groups and highlight the benefits of belonging to a group whose members take seriously their responsibility and obligation to one another. Be clear with the prospect that if anything like their fear of being blamed or shamed or rejected occurs that you will support them and require the group to explore what is going on and not just behave according to the member's past experience. Point out how important these opportunities are for personal growth and development and that you will protect such possibilities to the best of your ability. Don't be afraid to meet with such an anxious prospect a number of times if necessary to appropriately allay their worries. By showing willingness to take seriously the prospect's fears you can encourage an emotional bonding that can be helpful for the member in the early stages of the group's life and you will find that as the member grows in confidence with the group they will naturally reduce their dependence on you.

The fear of intimacy is a worry for some potential group members. All humans desire contact and connection but many people have found this to be a traumatizing and debilitating experience. Some prospects have personal biographies in which instances of physical or sexual abuse or emotional neglect may make them suspicious, withdrawn, and aloof.

Others may have been so damaged by these experiences that this becomes their normal style of relating and they may find themselves currently repeating original wounding and frustrating relationships. The thought of joining a group with all its attendant risks may excite fears about managing personal boundaries, negotiating relationships with unknown others, and being able to assert oneself.

It is important to point out how dissatisfying is the prospect's current mode of relationships and pattern of managing intimacy and emphasize the opportunity in a well-regulated group to learn new relational styles and a strategy for negotiating personal and emotional proximity and distance. I have found that linking this with the need to acquire appropriate skills of self-assertion and will training is helpful for a vacillating prospect. I highlight the capacity of the group to promote an ability to learn to be a self-directing and responsible agent (see p. 216 for a useful discussion of the importance of developing one's capacity for agency and intentionality).

Most prospective members report their fear of conflict occurring in the group. They may have personal histories replete with negative experiences of the effects of excessive competitiveness, aggression, violence or frightening argumentativeness. The idea of joining a group and having to manage the inevitable competition and sibling rivalry, subgrouping, and power issues may prove too daunting for some. Your own attitude to conflict in groups is important in terms of whether you secretly and gloomily agree with the prospect that groups are fearful, hostile places or whether you can convincingly reframe this fear of conflict as a central energy in the group which can be creatively managed for the benefit of all. It might be important to turn at this point to the section in Chapter 4 which explores the nature of conflict in the group. Chapter 5 also contains a full discussion of the worker's management of conflict in the group's life cycle.

It is important to draw out and explore the prospective member's catastrophic fears and fantasies about what will happen in the group and to them in situations of conflict. Anxieties ranging from those to do with fragmentation, chaos, and annihilation to those to do with being personally attacked, mocked, or ridiculed can be ventilated and tested against a reasonable expectation. Remind the prospect that they also have power to act and assert their rights and boundaries in any situation and that you will support them in that. Emphasize the capacity of the group to provide opportunities to develop skills of self-assertion and personal agency and assure the prospect that you see the healthy and creative management of conflict as a therapeutic feature of the group and that part of your role is to help the group take collective responsibility for actions and communications in the group.

Some potential members will surprisingly report in the pre-group interview that they are afraid of change as it might make them unlike themselves or disturb their existing relationships. They are afraid that they will not know who they are or dislike themselves. They may discover terrible secrets they have kept from themselves and have to live with disappointing new truths about significant and loved relationships. Others may describe a fear of becoming ill or not being able to cope with unexpected difficulties. It is important to take seriously these fears about the future unknown because people do frequently change as a consequence of their participation in a group and that is not always initially welcome.

It is best to acknowledge that change may occur which has repercussions for one's view of oneself and implications for current and past relationships, but that ultimately this will produce a more authentic expression and way of living in the world. Consider if necessary with the prospect strategies to be activated such as individual sessions or telephone support between sessions if the group does stir up unwanted or difficult side effects. Again you should emphasize the power of the group to accompany and support the prospect on a journey of change and growth.

More common is the expressed fear that the prospect cannot change and will remain stuck in some debilitating pattern of behaviour. This may mask an underlying depression or sense of meaninglessness or may be a defensive posture against the imagined cost of making certain required changes in the prospect's life circumstances. The sense of futility must be sensitively confronted and it may be worthwhile spending some time articulating realistic and achievable goals and targets. Making an individual contract which can be periodically reviewed with the group is a good strategy to promote.

Promote the therapeutic characteristics of the group

With all these fears and anxieties it is important for you to constantly look for opportunities to promote the therapeutic and positive characteristics of the group as a way of helping the potential member understand the value of the group in coping with their particular worries. You are the first embodiment of the group and the representative of its efficacy at this point. Look at Chapter 8 for a fuller discussion of these therapeutic features. In your preliminary discussions at this pre-group stage emphasize:

- The normalizing quality of group participation
- The universalizing nature of group involvement as a way of dissolving isolation
- The capacity of the group to generate, contain, and change powerful emotions
- The value and relief of peer support and solidarity

My final objective is to *prepare potential members for meeting with the others* in the first session. Typically the prospective member is anxious about speaking in public, revealing his needs or problems, his fears and fantasies about the other members, and generally wonders what it will be like. Explaining the intended format of the first session and reassuring the potential member that everyone else will feel the same as he does can be very comforting. In extreme cases of anxiety I may ask the group member to close his eyes and visually rehearse the whole experience of the first session, preparing him mentally for it and desensitizing the situation of its fear. It is also important to arrange details about transport, time, date, and venue of group sessions as this can be easily forgotten.

The first session

The first session and indeed the early phase of any group is a crucial time for individual members and is critical in determining how subsequent patterns of interaction and communication unfold within the group. Each individual brings to the group his life experience of membership in previous groups and relationships established at earlier stages of his existence.

These experiences will colour his perceptions of and reactions to other group members and the worker. How each member of the group initially presents himself, communicates, behaves, and interacts with the others has enormous repercussions for how the other members will react to him, then and subsequently. Initial impressions can determine how much freedom within the group individuals have to experiment with different aspects of self. Often in the opening sessions group members can become stereotyped and trapped in roles and behaviours that are difficult if not impossible to escape later. For these reasons, it is vital to consider the importance of the first session for individual and group behaviour.

Importance of the first session

- First experience of the group
- First contact with other members in group context
- First contact with worker in group context
- First opportunity to reveal self, behaviour, attitudes, etc.
- First opportunity to hurt or be hurt
- First opportunity to enjoy the group
- First opportunity for worker to establish climate, and engage members in work

With a little reflection, you can extend this list. The important point to grasp is that the *first session is the moment of social and psychological birth for the group*. It is the beginning of familiarization, association, and commitment by individuals to the group life.

Role of the worker in first session

How each individual manages his entry to the group and is facilitated by the other members is crucial if the group is to be seen as a place where persons are valued, and are worthwhile. Central to the whole process at this stage is the worker, and his activity in the first session can go a long way towards inhibiting or facilitating group experience. I believe the group worker should try to convey three simple messages to the group in this first session:

The three Cs

- *Competency*: The worker should know what he is doing, be sure about group objectives, his authority, have planned the session thoroughly, and be able to convey to group members that he can be relied on. This does not mean that the worker should cover up his own tension or hide his own natural anxiety. I will share my feelings of tension with the group if it is appropriate, but I am very careful to demonstrate that I am not overwhelmed or incapacitated by them, and that I am competent to work with the group. In this way I normalize feelings of anxiety and act as a role model by showing that I have the power to determine my response to a situation and can think and talk about it without becoming overwhelmed.
- *Compassion*: It is important for the worker to display consideration, concern, care, and compassion for members from the start as a way of setting the tone for group interaction, and helping people feel safe and included. This does not mean that the

worker engages in unctuous protestations of care to a group of people he barely knows. Compassion can be easily demonstrated by ensuring that everyone knows and agrees with what is going on, breaking things down and waiting for slower or more defensive members, clearing expectations, making contracts with members, and generally showing that you want to understand and be involved with each member.

- *Commitment*: The worker should display a commitment to and belief in the efficacy and power of the group. Schwarz talks about the worker sharing, 'his own vision of the work' with group members and this is essential at the beginning of the group when members cannot be expected to have a sense of community or even understanding of the power and value of the group experience.[4] If you do not believe in what you are doing or have reservations, you cannot expect members to believe in the group and they will very quickly discern your ambivalence. This applies particularly to those situations where you are thinking of using 'trust games', ice-breakers, and warm-ups (see page 189). Frequently I find group workers using trust games and exercises with people in a group when they readily admit they do not themselves like to be in groups where they are used. Trust games are okay for clients but not for workers! This sort of double standard suggests to me a contempt and lack of understanding of the nature of working with people in group situations. As a basic rule of thumb you should endeavour never to try anything in a group that you are not committed to or believe sincerely to be valuable. And never take a group or its members into any experience you would not be prepared to go into yourself.

Some tips for the first session

- *Try to sit with people in the group.*
- *Use first names if possible*: Use a person's name each time you speak to them. Don't be afraid to ask if you forget. Names are so important as a way of drawing people into the session.
- *Try to link people together*. If a member makes a point, try to link him with those others in the group who feel or think similarly. You are a *weaver* in this first session, trying to intermesh and link people together. Look for the common ground and shared experience between people. Look for themes and patterns that you can reflect. One of the notions I bring into this first session is the idea that we *build on* and add to each other's contributions in order to get a fuller picture. So I'll say things like, 'Let's see if we can build on what Mary is saying,' or 'Let's add to John's point.' The idea here is of the different parts coming together to form a higher-level whole. Each part has an important contribution to make and initially the worker must facilitate the synthesis of the parts.
- *Expect to be understood*: I go into the group clearly expecting to be understood. I also expect members to signal that they don't understand me or each other. To do this I continually ask, 'Does this make sense to you?' 'What is this like for you?' By drawing attention in this way to the need for clarity and comprehension I find that I can encourage more risk-taking, more inquiry, and that members soon learn to feel more confident about stopping the content to share confusion or look for help. I am also

clearly stating to the group that I expect them to talk to me in a two-way fashion. I expect group members to reply, question, give their own opinions.

- *Use plain language and keep your sentences short*: Talk to the group members as if you were talking to a friend. Avoid jargon and long-winded descriptions and monologues. Speak simply and briefly and expect a response.
- *Make your voice, tone, body communicate warmth and interest*: Be aware of what you are communicating by your posture, gestures, facial expression. Arms hugging your tummy or your hand around your throat communicate tension and give the lie to your words of calm. Adopt an open, relaxed posture which is comfortable and conveys warmth and attention.
- *Try to find out what people expect of you, the group, and each other*: This is called 'clearing expectations' and is something I believe is essential if you are going to be sensitive to the needs and wants of members. Shortly after introductions I build in a space where group members and I can share and discuss our expectations and begin to agree what is realistic, possible, and desirable.
- *Make a contract with your group and keep it simple*: A contract is important for group members. It outlines the rights and responsibilities of worker and member and gives a mark against which all behaviour in the group can be measured and valued (see p. 94). The group contract is vital to ensure that members understand what is being asked of them and can agree to pursue particular agreed objectives. Conditions of the contract will vary according to the group but generally you should include clauses about:

  o   Purpose, objectives of the group
  o   Members' choice to be in the group
  o   Confidentiality – what can and cannot be taken out of the group
  o   Time-keeping, breaks, starting times
  o   Participation

We can summarize the role of the worker in the first session:

- To introduce members to each other, the group worker himself, and the group
- To provide information on group objectives and operation
- To check expectations and perceptions of the group by members
- To negotiate a contract with members in terms of worker's and members' roles, expectations of each other, purpose of group, etc.
- To minimize frustration and reduce competition and tension
- To ensure fast satisfaction and success in activity and relationships
- To facilitate and promote flow of communication between members
- To invite trust in worker, members, group
- To encourage exploration
- To establish the psychological climate of the group and begin to teach the language and procedures for work
- To engage members in work

Typical behaviour in the first session

Most groups start cold, shy, and awkward. They most likely do not know each other or the worker and are unsure how to behave. This may be expressed in the following behaviour: milling around; tension due to unfamiliarity; overdependence on leader; avoidance of each other; silence; superficiality; talking too much; ambivalence and vacillation, etc. (see page 86).

It is essential for the worker to allow what is happening in the group to happen and to help members see group experience as natural, normal, and workable. Thus the worker might decide to reflect what is happening to the group and ask for comment from members. He may point out that it is natural for people meeting for the first time to feel shy and awkward. In this way the worker removes the need for group members to defend and maintain their positions. He accepts the normality of their feeling and draws attention to how members have power to select and determine their responses to situations.

Another way of dealing with the emotional content of the first session is to encourage group members to think about and discuss other first-time experiences, job interviews, what it felt like the first day at a new school or job, moving to live in a new neighbourhood, making new friends, and joining new groups.

How to plan the first session

Clarify

- What are your reasons for working with this group?
- What are you expected to do?
- What sort of group is it?
- What is the purpose of the group?
- What are your objectives for the first session?

Consider

- What do you know about the members: their needs, interests, backgrounds, age, sex?
- How much experience or knowledge do they have about purpose of group or subject of the first session?
- What do they expect of you?
- Try to tune in and anticipate how they may be feeling
- Spend some time in quiet reflection and meditation to centre yourself

Context

Try to identify one theme/topic or subject for this session, e.g.:

- Introducing yourself
- Meeting new people
- My feelings about beginnings, etc.

This theme is your central thesis for the session, will guide your interventions, enable you to structure feedback, and make sense of group behaviour. The theme gives you a *context* for the session.

Presentation

- Choose methods of presentation which are most appropriate to objectives for the session
- How do you intend to create the context for this session?
- Design a programme of activity or presentation which is related to abilities and needs of members and session objectives
- If you decide that you want to reduce tension or facilitate communication think about specific exercises, warm-ups, activities to look at themes like shyness, who I am, meeting and talking to people for the first time
- Consider how you create consciousness about your theme: debriefs, discussion evaluations, feedback, questionnaires

---

Anticipate

Anticipate as many behavioural outcomes as possible but do not be rigid about it. Consider how to acknowledge and what to do if:

- Members are fearful or unwilling to participate
- There are long silences
- Anger or aggression is expressed
- Members ignore each other and relate only to you

Ensure

> • Co-leaders and special personnel (guest speakers, video operatives, etc.) clearly know what their role is, what is expected of them, and will be there on time
> • Make sure group members know where to come to, what time, what room, are picked up if necessary

Relax

Enjoy the session. Remember, while it is nice to get everything right in the first session it is not always possible and you will have plenty of opportunities in subsequent sessions to redeem and salvage lost ground. Since most first sessions are carefully planned, they tend to exceed the expectations of workers, so do try to relax!

Some examples of first-session planning

The therapeutic group

- *Time*: One and a half to three hours.
- *Setting*: A weekly group to explore specific personal problems.
- *Objectives*:
    o   To introduce people
    o   To provide information about the group
    o   To help people say why they have come
    o   To build trust and intimacy
    o   To promote self-disclosure

- *Theme*: Being together for the first time.
- *Plan*:
    o   Arrange group seating in small circle to facilitate communication and interaction.
    o   Provide (optional) soft music to relax, tea, and biscuits.
    o   Welcome members, start, explain objectives for session.
    o   Self-introductions (leader directed):
        •   Who I am
        •   How I'm feeling right now
        •   Why I'm here tonight
        •   My fantasy, expectations, fears about the group. (These statements can be made separately in rounds or all together in one round.)

- *Leader*: Decide whether to evaluate or pass on. If evaluate, decide:
    o   To give feedback to group on your impressions, feelings
    o   To give feedback on themes: common problems, shared expectations, mutual fears, fantasies, or

- o   To ask group to evaluate self-introductions, or
- o   Use themes as basis of discussion, e.g. being together for the first time; how we are feeling, or
- o   Use themes as context for your selection of trust exercises, ice-breakers (see p. 189)

- *Link relevant themes* expressed by members to your (leader's) understanding of group purpose and negotiate a group contract

  - o   Contextualize group (background and history) purposes, aims
  - o   Indicate how you see the role of leader
  - o   State your expectations and requirements of members
  - o   Check and clear expectations and negotiate with members
  - o   Negotiate a group contract (see p. 93). Clauses to include:

    - Purpose of the group
    - Choice to be here
    - Taking responsibility for self
    - Attendance
    - What I want for myself in this group
    - Confidentiality

- *Share time out between members to focus on*:

  - o   What they want from the group
  - o   Why they are here
  - o   What it is like for them to be here for the first time

  Do self-disclosure exercises, or a selection of trust exercises, ice-breakers.
- *Process this work* (evaluate it, discuss, share feelings, impressions) in the group with each person or in pairs, threes. Does anyone need anything at this time?
- *Review the session*: Comments, reflections, feelings:

  - o   What I liked about the session
  - o   What I didn't like
  - o   How I'm feeling now
  - o   What it was like for me to be here
  - o   Booking time on next session's agenda

- *Check out* (see p. 167).

Running a training workshop

- *Time: Two and a half hours.*
- *Setting*: A weekly group to study leadership behaviour in groups.
- *Objectives*:

  - o   To introduce people
  - o   To provide information about group purpose
  - o   To determine people's needs and interests
  - o   To plan a relevant programme

- o   To develop cohesion and team spirit
- o   To model leadership behaviour

- *Theme*: Leadership is the process of creating a flexible structure within which people can achieve their goals.
- *Plan*:

    - o   Arrange seating as required. Check equipment.
    - o   Welcome members. Start.
    - o   *General introduction* (leader). Explain: purpose of group, objectives for this session.
    - o   Self-introductions:

        - •   Who I am
        - •   Why I am here
        - •   The type of group I lead
        - •   My expectations of the group

- *Negotiate a group contract:* Provide a short summary of need for contract, link this to leadership. Work out clauses.
- *Exercise* to identify member's needs: Reflective meditation and writing. Themes to be explored might include:

    - o   What are my work needs as a group leader?
    - o   How do I deal with problem behaviours in the group?
    - o   What are my weaknesses as a leader?
    - o   What are the qualities and characteristics of the ideal leader?

- Find a partner and share, develop, and expand ideas (15 to 20 minutes).
- *Brainstorm* collective needs and interests onto flipchart.
- Categorize areas of need and interest. Prioritize.
- Identify programme units. Discuss and get agreement on an agenda for following sessions.
- Check if group needs a break.
- *Discuss* ways of implementing programme: role play, exercises, case study group discussions. Get agreement on procedures.
- *Select* one theme from checklist for group to work on for remainder of session, e.g. 'My weakness as a leader' or 'My leadership style'. Brainstorm ideas on it to stimulate group discussion, or
Split into small groups to explore and discuss a particular feature of the theme. Feedback to larger group, or
Is theme amenable to role-playing? Set up short scene. Use observers, doubles, and alter-egos to stimulate involvement (see p. 180). Finish with group discussion.
- *Review session* (see p. 167).
- *Check out.*

Making a presentation

- *Time:* Two hours.
- *Setting:* A talk on the relevance of groupwork, to an audience made up of colleagues.

- *Objectives*:

  o   To stress the universality of group experience
  o   To identify the positives in group situations
  o   To point out the relevance of groupwork to a particular clientele
  o   To allow colleagues to air their views and feelings
  o   To persuade them groupwork is worth considering

- *Theme:* Group membership is a natural human experience and one that can be used to help people.
- *Plan:*

  o   Welcome. Start. Indicate your objectives and expectations for session.
  o   *Brief introduction* to topic covering some of the major issues to be explored.
  o   *Brainstorm exercise*

     - Ask members to identify groups they have belonged to since childhood
     - Pick out four groups. Ask members to identify various benefits of membership
     - Ask members to find a partner. Ask them to assess 'Why do people join groups?' Feedback to group after ten minutes and large group discussion on the three exercises

- Leader. Short talk
- Group *discussion*. Leader: focus discussion on relevance of groupwork to one or two client groups of interest to audience.
- Leader: *summarize themes*, views, feelings of the meeting. Ask for final comments, questions. Make your final statement (see thesis). Thank people for their participation.

Checklist for planning a group

RESEARCH AND JUSTIFY THE NEED FOR GROUPWORK

> - How does the demand for group come to your attention? Who makes application, why, for whom, what do they want, what do beneficiaries of the group service actually need?
> - What are your reasons for responding to request or requirement to provide a service?
> - Gather preliminary information about group (see page 12 and 17)
> - Decide that groupwork is appropriate for this client or group
> - Identify a general aim
> - Inform colleagues and superiors of your proposal. Request co-operation. Clear lines of communication. Submit a preliminary proposal if possible
> - Gather referrals
> - From referrals establish common needs, problems, themes. Begin to identify goals
> - Check goals are consistent with objectives of employing or funding agency. Identify contribution of group to agency service delivery
> - If considering inter-agency work establish each agency objectives, areas of work. Anticipate grey areas or possible difficulties

ATTENDING TO MEMBERSHIP

- Decide to select, recruit (page 17), work with existing group membership.
- If select:

  o   Decide what information you want
  o   Gather referrals
  o   Assess referrals on descriptive and behavioural attributes (see page 19), common themes, motivation to work

- If recruit:

  o   Decide group purpose and goals
  o   Advertise – posters, press, word of mouth, clinics, youth clubs, community centres

- If working with existing group membership:

  o   Consider what you know of their needs, interests, age, sex, backgrounds
  o   Knowledge or experience of group purpose/subject

- Decide on size, frequency, and number of meetings, open or closed groups, duration, length of session

PROGRAMMING THE GROUP

- Decide why you are going to use a programme
- Consider needs of members, stage of group development
- Identify clear objectives
- Consider how to achieve objectives using activity:

  o   Determine rules, controls, competence, degree of movement, interaction, rewards associated with different activities, personal and task requirements of group
  o   Consider physical limitations of premises, materials, tools required; how much they cost; where you get the money to pay for them
  o   Design a relevant programme on basis of all these considerations

- Build review slots into programme

LEADING THE GROUP

- Analyse and investigate authority base of leader
- Determine goals of agency:

  o   Required roles and tasks of worker
  o   Accountability of worker
  o   Needs of members

- Consider available models of groupwork. Select an appropriate model to guide thinking and intervention
- Decide on a style of leadership
- Decide how many workers
- What are their roles, tasks, functions?
- Anticipate differences, conflicts, and ambiguities between workers
- Ensure appropriate time for preparation and debrief
- Identify to whom worker is accountable (see page 45). Supervision, record keeping, confidentiality

PRESENTING THE GROUP:

- Write up the group in detail (page 15)
- Present and clear proposals with colleagues and superiors
- Arrange funding, provision of resource, time, etc.
- Work out how you intend to evaluate the group
- Present the group to prospective members. Pre-group interviews (see page 46)

PLAN THE FIRST SESSION

- Identify objectives for the session
- Consider members' needs, interests, backgrounds
- Select one topic as a context for session
- Design an appropriate programme of activity
- Check co-workers, resources, equipment, transport, etc.

References

1 For more detailed discussion on styles of leadership see Hartford, N.E. (1976) 'Group methods and generic practice', in R.W. Roberts and H. Northen (eds) *Theories for Social Work with Groups*, New York: Columbia University Press.
2 For a detailed account of evaluation approaches and techniques see Thomas, J. *et al.* (1981) 'Goal-setting and evaluation', in M.R. Whitlam (ed) *Practice Development Papers*, National Intermediate Treatment Federation.
3 Hodge, J. (1977) 'Social groupwork: rules for establishing the group', *Social Work Today*, 8, 17: 110.
4 Schwarz, W. (1976) 'Between client and system: the mediating approach', in *Theories for Social Work with Groups*, op. cit.

Chapter 3

An introduction to group dynamics and process

In the Eastern martial art of aikido, the warrior learns 'never to go against the opponent's strength', but rather to blend with and redirect the energy of his attacker.[1] The aikido master knows how to 'touch softly and gently' in order to use the power already generated by his adversary. In the midst of motion and conflict there is an exact point to apply pressure and a precise intervention that will subdue the attack. In contrast to this 'way of gentle harmony', the Western disciplines of boxing and wrestling are characterized by collision and force overwhelming force.

The aikido master is a metaphor for the effective group worker who rather than fight or wrestle knows how to be in harmony with his group. He can utilize the pressure points and redirect and employ collective energy and power to take the simplest path towards the desired goal. The simplest path is revealed by awareness and understanding of the meaning of individual and group needs, behaviour, and interaction. Unless he is attentive to and knowledgeable about what is happening inside the system in which he operates an effective group worker cannot adequately determine what is the most appropriate way to intervene or respond.

Unfortunately the study of group dynamics and processes can, at the beginning, be very off-putting and intimidating to the group worker. There are three main problems.

- *Mystique*: At first sight there seems to be so much to assimilate and digest. This is not helped by the impenetrability of much of the language of group dynamics and the reverential attitude of some group workers and the intellectual snobbery of others.
- *Problems of recognition*: Very often the clearly delineated models of group process and development do not match the confusion of the worker's experience, resulting in frustration, disappointment, and a sense of inadequacy.
- *Problems of application*: Even where certain processes can be identified and recognized many workers are unsure how to use them in order to create particular effects. In this chapter we will look in detail at how to use group processes to facilitate experience. For now it is enough to clearly and simply identify and present the essential pressure points or group processes which will inform the worker's actions and interventions, and suggest that they are natural and organic events which occur wherever groups of people meet and interact.

Some basic features of group life

Needs and wants of members

A group comes into being to satisfy the needs and wants of its members and unless compelled to do so members will only attend if their needs and expectations are met. In order to understand the behaviour of a group in various circumstances it is important to have firstly a picture of the needs of individuals, and secondly knowledge of how group membership serves each individual. Abraham Maslow offers us an insight into people's needs which we can present as in Figure 3.1.[2]

Maslow suggests that the basic needs for survival and safety have to be met and satisfied if an individual is to progress to the next level of need. Only an unsatisfied need can motivate behaviour and the need which is dominant in an individual is the prime motivator. People deprived of the basic needs abandon higher needs in order to satisfy the lower. If a man's head is held under water for a time he forgets about aesthetic values, social needs, and prestige. He devotes his energy to getting air. Having achieved this he may then move up the scale and feel outraged at this attack on his dignity and act to express this.

The implications of this work are very important for the group worker:

- Behaviour in the group can be construed as the interplay of one or more members' identification with certain needs
- Recognition of the need motivating behaviour can indicate the appropriate type of intervention (see page 27)
- Recognition of needs is important if you are to successfully develop motivation (see pages 86, 102 and 116)
- Programme planning must be based on the needs of individuals and the group if it is to be relevant and satisfying (see Chapter 1).

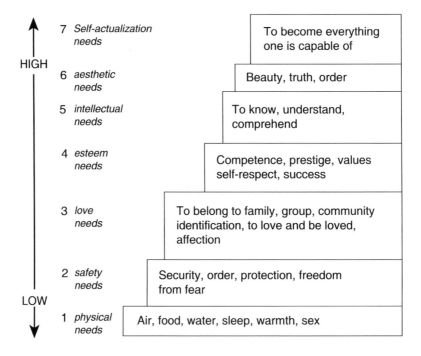

Figure 3.1 Diagram of needs hierachy

Needs determine goals

No matter how *similar* or *disparate* the needs of individual members, there must be agreement on the *goals* they will strive for while they are in association if the group is to survive and be effective. As the group develops, it continuously works on two levels at once: towards the achievement of group goals and towards the satisfaction of individual members' goals and motives (see page 70). Sometimes individual goals are not shared with other members and may be at cross purposes with the group goals. These *hidden agendas* can be very destructive to the effectiveness of the group and are often the source of conflict in the group. It is important to look for hidden agendas that may be present in the group and encourage their surfacing if appropriate.

Members' commitment to group goals is influenced by:

- How attractive the goal is
- How realistic it is
- How challenging and stimulating it is
- How much satisfaction it represents

A *goal structure* develops in groups, which indicates the quality of interaction among members. A co-operative goal structure develops when the individual goals of members are visible and similar, e.g. if a member of a quiz team answers correctly, all team members benefit. A competitive goal structure emerges where the individual goals of members are hidden or seen as different or opposed, e.g. in an adolescent group if one member wins the swimming competition, all the other members lose. Some of the effects of co-operation and competition on groups are identified below.

Co-operation	*Competition*
• Promotes helping, sharing trust	• Decreases helping, sharing trust
• Promotes effective communication	• Makes for ineffective and incomplete communication
• Promotes positive self-image	• Reduces group cohesion, encourages splitting and subgroups
• Promotes group cohesion	• Decreases creativity
• Encourages creativity and permits divergence	• Promotes personal skill acquisition at expense of group interaction
• Develops interaction and acquisition of skill and desirable attitudes	• Develops loser's and winner's mentality, hostility, distrust, and suspicion

For suggestions on how to develop a co-operative goal structure see page 14.

Goals lead to values

In the course of interacting with each other to achieve personal and group goals members develop a *value system* which refers to beliefs about which objects and behaviours are good and bad, desirable and undesirable. In a therapeutic group whose goal is relief of personal distress, values will emerge which will include an emphasis on honesty, trust, confidentiality, caring, and respect. In an activity group values might include fair play, team spirit, commitment, and sacrifice. The values of a group reflect its goals and purposes, and play an important and often decisive part in determining individual behaviour.

Values make rules

In order to ensure that members behave in accordance with agreed group values and goals, certain rules or *norms* are established which prescribe those actions in particular circumstances which are correct and proper, and those behaviours which are improper. Norms are values expressed in behavioural terms. The acceptance of norms by members depends upon their appropriateness to individual and group concerns, the cohesiveness of the group, and the nature of norm enforcement.

Norms are enforced by *sanctions* which will require or persuade individuals to *conform* to group values and beliefs. These sanctions will punish members who fail to conform to group norms or reward them if they do so adequately. In our example of the therapeutic group, violation of the norm of confidentiality might be met with demands for removal or 'expulsion' of the offender. In the activity group conspicuous adherence to the norm of fair play could result in an individual being rewarded with the rank of team captain or arbiter of standards.

The group's impulse to create norms and behavioural controls can be of great benefit to you when working with the group. Most beginning workers seek to establish *personal control* over the group fairly early on. They fail to realize that the most effective means of control within any group is that based on establishing norms of behaviour which are acceptable to all and identifying and using those norms which already exist. By trying to develop and make satisfying and rewarding existent norms, you will find that you are likely to be more successful than trying to control the group externally (see page 90).

Rules lead to roles

The emergence of group goals, values, and norms requires the members to behave in a co-ordinated and standardized way if group discussion, planning together, or participating in a particular activity are to occur. However, even within the standardized action patterns of a group, a wide range of behaviours and operations may be necessary in order to achieve the task or goal. Group discussion for example can be broken down into a set of sub-tasks: someone has to select or offer a theme, other members are required to give opinions, listen, share views, suggest alternatives, and engage in the repertoire of behaviours which will facilitate group discussion.

A division of labour begins to develop with individuals allocated certain tasks and functions. Over time these become institutionalized as *roles* in the group. The term 'role' derives from the theatre where an actor may perform in the role of Hamlet or Basil Fawlty or a king. A role is a series of actions which guide and determine our behaviour according to what is expected of us in a certain situation. Roles generate the consistency and predictability of behaviour, which we have seen is so important in group life, and create expectations about how members will behave in relation to each other and the group goals.

Throughout life we perform many roles as son/daughter, friend/lover, employer/ employee and so in groups we engage in role behaviour as member, follower, and leader amongst others. This information is vital to the group worker because now any behaviour of any member can be questioned: 'What role do these actions represent and is it appropriate?' Let's see how this can be developed.

All roles are functional in that they serve individual and group interests in some way. But problems can arise.

People are induced to occupy certain roles because of group pressure to *conform* to expectations and norms. Sometimes group pressure to conform can be very intense and individuals outwardly conform to the norm out of fear while inwardly disagreeing. This can have disastrous results for the group, ranging from apathy and impotence to sabotage and acts of defiance.

Each role carries a measurement of worth. Some roles are more valuable and sought after by members than others, because they have more *status.* The role of leader usually carries high status while the *scapegoat* denotes low status and may be ascribed to a member of the group who is unpopular or disagreeable. Role status can be used as a reward or punishment and leads to the development of a social structure, usually hierarchical, which can stratify members, reduce mobility and cohesion, and create subgroups.

Because of a lack of flexibility and role fluidity individuals can come to be *locked* into a role. *Role lock* limits the opportunities and options in interpersonal relationships and creates rigid and stereotyped behaviour. This fixed position may be chosen by an individual or ascribed to him but either way is used to prevent change, remain static, and avoid responsibility.

Role conflict can develop because:

- Members are obliged to occupy roles which carry expectations and instructions for behaviour which are incompatible or disagreeable to them
- Two people may make opposing or conflicting demands on the role holder. This happens frequently in groups where the leader wants a member to behave in a way which will alienate him from his peers, e.g., 'Tell me who stole the biscuits!'
- Often we fill so many different roles in rapid succession and the demands of one may conflict with the demands of another, e.g. my role as group leader conflicts with my role as husband when I have to work yet another weekend group

Group performance and effectiveness can be seen as the interplay of three main sets of needs and behaviours each of which gives rise to a series of formal and informal roles

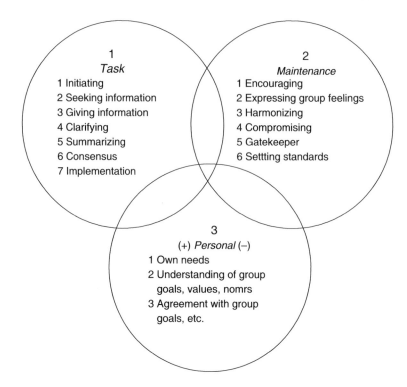

Figure 3.2 Task, maintenance, and personal functions in the group

(Figure 3.2). These functional roles of group members were first described by Benne and Sheats in 1948 and have been used continuously since then.[3,4,5]

The first circle refers to those needs, behaviours, and roles that are required to help the group achieve its goals. The second circle encompasses those behaviours and roles that help the group look after its emotional and interpersonal well-being. The third circle is concerned with the purely personal motives of each individual. The circles overlap because some behaviours are task- and maintenance-oriented at the same time, and because all task and maintenance behaviours are mediated by personal motivations which can result in positive or anti-group behaviours and roles. We can begin to identify members' behaviours, and the roles with which they are associated over time, in terms of whether they impede or facilitate the group.

Behaviours and roles related to members' needs rather than the task

In each of the behaviours and roles listed on page 71, personal need is taking precedence over collective need. A group member may not be able to adequately listen to others because he desperately needs listening to himself. Try to identify the need motivating behaviour and role in order to make your intervention and responses more relevant and sensitive (see page 67).

Anti-group behaviours	Anti-group roles
• Not listening • Cutting people short • Deflating people • Picking on people • Nit-picking on details • Refusing to yield • Messing about • Inappropriate joking, sarcasm, black humour • Inappropriate aggression, anger, arguments • Self-pity	• Blocker • Avoider • Saboteur • Critic • Dominator • Martyr • Scapegoat • Isolate • Double/cynic • Persecutor

Behaviours and roles aimed at helping members interact more effectively

Pro-group behaviours	Pro-group roles
• Involving other members • Reconciling disagreements • Praising people • Communicating • Relieving tension • Co-operating • Encouraging and exhorting people • Listening to others	• Encourager • Harmonizer • Gatekeeper • Standard setter • Mediator

Behaviours and roles focused on accomplishing the group goal

In the behaviours and roles listed below the group member is not feeling deprived or deficient but is focusing on other people or the task from his own needs to contribute to the group, be a part of what is happening, join in. Your response in this situation might be more to permit this, facilitate, and acknowledge individual efforts.

Pro-group behaviours	Pro-group roles
• Starting things • Sharing information and resources • Organizing activity and members • Giving opinions • Asking opinions • Elaborating and explaining • Looking for agreement • Summarizing	• Initiator • Orienter • Co-ordinator • Evaluator

Questions to ask yourself about role-behaviour in the group

- Is this behaviour recurrent enough to be called a role?
- How would I describe this role? What is this person saying to me and the group through the role?
- Does the individual seem happy with this role?
- Is he trapped in this role?
- Is he experiencing role conflict?
- What status or position in the group accrues to this person as a result of this role?
- What are the gains and losses to the group of this person conforming in his role?
- What is the individual's perception of his role?
- Is this role related to task, maintenance, or personal needs?
- What does the individual need or want in order to change, develop, be more included in the group?

Group process

These aspects of group culture that we have been looking at are outward manifestations of the group process. Group process is one of the most hallowed dogmas in the modern groupwork liturgy, and to beginners one of the most confusing. We are going to look in detail at what group process is and why it is so important, but first it is necessary to distinguish between the content and the process of a group.

- Content refers to the *what* of group experience – what is being talked about, what activity is taking place, what the group members are going to do next
- Process refers to the *how* of group experience, the *way* in which a group discusses or acts together and is reflected in the quality of group experience
- Content is the substance of group activity which can be clearly seen on the surface and gives the members a *social* context within which they can interact. It is usually manifest and *seen*
- In contrast, process is what happens underneath the surface on the psychological level of group operations. It is usually latent and *felt*

Group process as a frame of reference

From this perspective group process is 'a frame of reference which limits, focuses and directs the worker's efforts in a group'.[6] It is based on the assumption that group process can be 'controlled and influenced by the worker's actions'. Group process can be defined as changes over time in the internal structure, organization, and culture of the:

- Whole group
- Part of the group
- Individual member

and expressed

1   *Structurally* in the:

  - Effectiveness of communication
  - Quality of decision making
  - Allocation of roles
  - Quality of power and authority in group
  - Calibre of group culture, norms, values, goals

2   *Behaviourally* in the:

  - Quality of interaction
  - Silence, anger, tears, avoidance
  - Lateness, absenteeism, getting stuck
  - Gesture, posture
  - Seating arrangements

3   *Psychologically* in the:

  - Degree of trust, cohesion, intimacy
  - Extent to which the individual feels:

    o   Valued
    o   Included
    o   Able to contribute
    o   Defensive versus open
    o   Split or integrated

Let me draw attention to a number of important principles in this process approach to working with a group:

- Individual and group experience and interaction *change condition* over time. There is movement, flux, and process. This flux and change is not random or chaotic but is *organic* and natural. There is an ebb and flow, a development and decline that we can call process. It is possible to discern themes and patterns in this movement (see page 77).

- Individual and group experience has distinct *energetic* manifestations:

  o   The tension of strangeness and embarrassment
  o   The cold of silence and indifference
  o   The heat and rush of anger
  o   The warmth of companionship and co-operation

  The fact that group experience and interaction can be emotionally and physically felt means we can quite easily develop skills of working with process by becoming more receptive and open to what is occurring.

- Like the aikido master who used the energy and momentum of his adversary's attack to subdue him, the group worker can influence, alter, and control the energy manifested at any stage of the group process. For example, knowing that a group of people are meeting for the first time we can design a programme in the opening sessions which is nurturing and warm and helps people with the business of inclusion (see pages 85–90); or seeing that members keep getting stuck at a particular point we can intervene from a number of angles to help people with the experience (see page 28).

- Individual and group experience and interaction is continuously unfolding in the present tense of group life. Because of the 'nowness' of process every experience is open to change. Attending to individual and group phenomena as they occur right here and now gives members the potential and opportunity to change direction and devise new strategies. Each member can learn to become a participant observer because he is in the events that concern him, and making them happen at the same time that he is watching them. This can be a difficult experience for members at first, and methods for process analysis may have to be built in so that group members come to learn that it can be productive to take time out from *what* is happening to look at *how* it is happening.

  For the leader, working with group process can at times be like a canoeist negotiating tumultuous white water rapids – you have to roll under this wave, block that one, switch direction suddenly, be swept along by the river for a time, then head for the bank, swerve, sway, lean, and pray!

Love and will polarities in the group

In the introduction we identified the drive mechanism for movement and growth in groups as deriving from the tension generated between two poles of human psychology – the urge to be attached and the urge to separate. Being a member of a group requires an individual to surrender part of their autonomy in service of the whole but not to surrender so much that they merge with or are overwhelmed by the group, whilst at the same time asserting their individuality but not in such a way that they are alienated from the group or narcissistically preoccupied with themselves at the expense of group involvement (see page 203). That human experience can be considered as the manifestation of two opposing but complementary polarities requires to be demonstrated and in order to do this we need to examine the quality, nature, and direction of the opposing tendencies. For convenience I shall call the urge to be attached, the love principle and designate the urge to be separate as the will principle.

I do not mean that the love principle is simply a matter of feeling or affect. Assagioli asserts that the varied manifestations of the love principle 'express the law of attraction, of the tendency towards approach, contact, unification and fusion'.[7] Andreas Angyal calls it the 'trend towards homonymy' and describes it as the tendency by which 'a person seeks union with larger units and wishes to share and participate in something which he regards as being greater than his individual self'.[8] We can state some of its functions and qualities:

Functions	Qualities
• Relating	• Nurturance
• Uniting	• Sensitivity
• Fusing	• Reciprocity
• Connecting	• Identification
• Attachment	• Intimacy
• Possession	• Compassion
• Understanding	• Support

The love principle manifests in human behaviour which is magnetic, connective, and inclusive:

Behaviours	Distortions
• Making friends	• Shyness
• Joining in	• Embarrassment
• Taking sides	• Fear of rejection
• Conversation	• Superficiality
• Sharing	• Silence
• Trusting	• Jealousy
• Co-operating	• Suspicion
• Encouraging	• Hostility

The will principle is characterized by its tendency to separate, initiate, and dominate. Angyal sees the will as an expression of 'autonomy', the capacity of an organism to operate according to its own nature rather than under the control of external forces.[9] Evolution can be understood in terms of this energy, as the graduations from vegetable kingdom to man are characterized by an increasing ability to differentiate and self-determine.

Assagioli states that 'The most important personal characteristic of the will type is the will to power.'[10] This is expressed in the desire to lead or dominate. Degenerate forms of the will to power result in selfishness, stubbornness, and contempt. We can think about the will principle like this:

Functions	Qualities
• Separate	• Vision
• Differentiate	• Purpose
• Lead	• Persistence
• Govern	• Independence
• Determine	• Self-reliance
• Action	• Courage
• Judge	• Control
• Complete	• Power

The will principle manifests itself in human behaviour which is separative, exclusive, and concerned with mobilizing power and energy. It has positive and negative implications dependent on the individual, the group, and circumstances:

Behaviours	Distortions
• Starting things	• Rivalry
• Organizing activity	• Stubbornness
• Leading	• Selfishness
• Subgrouping	• Powerlessness
• Problem solving	• Apathy
• Decision making	• Restlessness
• Concentration	• Violence
• Confrontation	

It should be clear now that psychological and interpersonal life is the consequence and manifestation of the tension generated by love and will polarities in the group. Each individual and the group as a whole has to reconcile these opposites if the experience is to be productive and worthwhile. The recurring dilemma is to be close but not too close – separate but not too separate!

Each reconciliation of the opposite is a synthesis of the essential elements in each. Synthesis differentiates new behaviour and experience and produces an upwardly spiralling effect. This makes for an intensification and a refining of the quality of experience at different levels and at different stages in the development of the group. It is through this upwardly spiralling synthesis that the group grows and matures.

Sometimes the process is characterized by a protracted series of conflicts, crises, approaches, and avoidances, as group members oscillate between the two extremes. At other times the process is more harmonious and members are able to synthesize and transmute the polar energies. In the next section we will look at some of the typical patterns in the process and in Chapters 4 to 7 suggest ways in which the worker can work with and facilitate group development.

Patterns and stages in group process

It is apparent that group conditions change over time as a consequence of the energy generated by love and will polarities in the group. Observing and understanding the change in conditions is a basic skill of groupwork practice. By analyzing the oscillation in condition and discerning the themes and patterns of interaction, relationship, and behaviour, it is possible to determine what needs prevail in the group at any given time, and permit intervention to emerge out of the particular group situation.

Most writers describe a series of phases or stages in the developmental patterns of the group. Schutz for example has suggested a three-stage scheme of (1) inclusion, (2) control, (3) affection.[11] Tuckman describes four stages in group development: (1) forming, (2) storming, (3) norming, (4) performing.[12] Garland, Jones, and Kolodny insist there are five stages: (1) pre-affiliation, (2) power and control, (3) intimacy, (4) differentiation, and (5) separation.[13] If we ignore the number of stages, what emerges from these writings is a description of the interplay of love and will energies in the group. Although they use different words each writer is clearly talking about the effect of these two principles on group interaction and development.

Tuckman, and Garland and his colleagues, in common with many writers assume a linear or sequential progression in group development. As we observed earlier (page 65) this academic and orderly delineation of group process can be alien to the experience of many beginning group workers as they survey the apparent chaos and confusion of their own groups. Groups clearly do not only move sequentially through neat phases, but also move backwards and sideways as well as forwards. Again, each group differs in the amount of time it spends in a particular stage of growth and some groups can get stuck and never progress beyond a certain stage.

The three-stage formulation of Schutz goes some way towards allowing for lateral and retrograde mobility. Schutz hypothesizes three linear phases but he does suggest the notion of circularity and spiralling. In other words a group can reverse and repeat sequences and can move forward by apparently going back through stages and even by going around in circles.

The first stage of group development is, according to Schutz, the *inclusion phase*. Inclusion behaviour refers to the desire to connect to and associate with other people, to want interaction and relationship. This is a period when group members are acclimatizing to the group and becoming familiar with each other though they have not yet formed close ties. There is a lot of restlessness, tension, and mobility. Members are evaluating and probing each other for mutual or complementary interests, exploring possibilities and beginning some preliminary pairing. (For a detailed description of typical behaviours at this stage see page 86.) Tuckman sees orientation, testing, and the establishment of dependency relationships by group members as the chief characteristic of this phase.

The central issue for members at this stage is to belong to the group or not, to be in or out. Garland and his colleagues highlight the ambivalence experienced by members. They identify two divergent tendencies operating in the individual, 'the tendency to approach and involve himself', and 'the tendency to avoid the situation because of the demands, the frustrations and even the pain which he may anticipate'.[14] As we shall see in Chapter 4 there is a great deal that the worker can do to help members recognize and resolve their inclusion issues and establish a sense of belonging.

Once the problem of inclusion has been satisfactorily resolved, Schutz suggests that *control* issues become prominent. Control behaviour is the independent and assertive activity of group members in the areas of power, authority, status, influence, decision making, and communication and would be equivalent to our will principle in operation.

Once the group has begun to form it starts to differentiate and develop a social structure. People assume or are ascribed roles and functions, positions and ranks. Cliques form and alliances are made as members jockey for status and power. There are two central issues for members at this stage:

- How much influence can they exercise in the group?
- How much personal autonomy do they have to surrender in order to be part of the group?

Members want to know where they are in status and hierarchy. Top or bottom? Members often compete against the formal authority vested in the group worker. At times this is an attempt to determine how much control they have and how much the worker has over events in the group. At other times the testing of the worker is a boundary-setting exercise, an attempt to determine what is and what is not permissible in the group. Members also conflict with the worker as a way of establishing his competency, ascertaining that he can be depended on, that he can maintain control, and can be trusted.

The struggle between members is, according to Garland and his colleagues, 'an attempt to define and formalize relationships and create a status hierarchy'.[15] Members come to this new group from other settings and have to renegotiate and establish their positions and identities. The discomfort of creating and adjusting to a new social structure can manifest itself in a variety of behaviours such as hostility, scapegoating, withdrawal, subgrouping, power struggles, and deviance which take members *away* from each other and pit them *against* each other (see page 102).

In my experience this is the phase of group development least understood and most threatening to the beginning group worker. A previously docile or compliant group can suddenly erupt into conflict, bickering, and apparent mutiny. A therapy group may turn on the leader, a work group may split into factions. It is a tempestuous time for worker and group alike as can be seen by Tuckman's description of this phase of development as '*storming*'. Hartford calls it a period of 'disintegration followed by rapid termination or reintegration'.[16]

While groups can get stuck in this phase, the flux and dynamism of the turmoil brings with it much potential for reconstituting the group relationships on a higher level of involvement. Confirmation of this, and for the worker – words of comfort – can be found in the *I Ching* or *Chinese Book of Changes* which makes change itself the purpose and meaning of life. In a commentary on '*Chen*', the Chinese word for 'thunder' (Hexagram 51) the *I Ching* asserts that 'Thunder indicates success,' and goes on to say that, ' . . . it laughs and shouts in fearful glee, yet afterwards everything is in order.'[17] And anticipating Hartford by some 3,500 years in a commentary on '*Huan*' meaning 'disintegration' (Hexagram 59) the *I Ching* states that 'Dispersion leads to accumulation, but this is not something that ordinary people understand.'[18]

In accordance with these laws of transformation the will energies of the group give way and love energies begin to predominate. These love energies operate on a higher level than the love energies of the earlier inclusion stage. Whereas the inclusion stage is about the decision to belong or not, this *affection* stage, as Schutz calls it, is about building emotional ties and deciding on the degree of intimacy to be developed with the other group members. Garland and his colleagues in fact call this the stage of *intimacy*. More prosaically, Tuckman calls it *norming* although he emphasizes, 'intimate, personal opinions are expressed'.[19]

In this period the group assumes an importance for members. There is a sense of identity and pulling together. Participation and involvement increase and members are more sensitive to each other. The interpersonal relationships stabilize and it is possible to observe the heightened emotional feeling between pairs of members, triads, and subgroups. The group is increasingly experienced as a trustworthy supportive environment. This leads to more genuine encounter and interaction.

Tuckman and Garland now see the group move up another level under the influx of more integrative will energies. In what Tuckman calls the *performing* stage the structure of the group has evolved to the point where it is 'supportive of task performance'. Roles have become flexible and functional 'and group energy is channelled into the task'.[20] Garland and his colleagues call this fourth progression, *differentiation*. People begin to acknowledge each other's uniqueness and permit individual differences to emerge. The standards and norms of behaviour are established and increasing reference is made to the internal mores rather than to external values and associations.

Increasing differentiation in the group finds its natural expression in the ultimate *separation* of group members, although Garland and his colleagues see separation as a distinct phase. However, they do agree with Schutz that separation involves 'regression and recapitulation', a spiralling back through earlier phases. Schutz suggests that as groups terminate they deal firstly with the personal feelings of members about closure (affection) then decide to comply or rebel against the leader's wishes (control), before finally discussing the possibilities of continuing the group, assessing the original commitment of members, and preparing for entry into the outside world (inclusion). In Chapter 4 we will come back to explore these patterns in group process in more detail as a way of suggesting how you can co-operate with, influence, and intervene in group process in a relaxed and organic fashion.

The anti-group phenomenon

The oscillating tension between the approach-avoid, attachment-separation dynamics of the love and will polarities in human interaction means that groups can sometimes create more problems than they alleviate. Nitsun warns against an over-optimistic and idealizing view of groupwork with the formulation of his concept of the 'anti-group'.[21] He asserts the anti-group is a broad term 'describing the destructive aspects of groups that threatens the integrity of the group and its therapeutic development'.[22] The anti-group phenomenon is really 'a set of attitudes and impulses conscious and unconscious that manifest themselves differently in different groups' and has three main sources:

- Resistance to participation in groups stemming from distrust, fear, anxiety and dislike of groups
- Aggression and hostility arising in the group that not only threatens interpersonal cohesion but is aimed destructively at the ongoing life of the group itself
- Accelerating destructive processes that could not be contained in the usual way

I have described a psychotherapy group meeting in Belfast at the height of the 'Troubles' that was composed of several disturbed and aggressive individuals who believed that the group opportunity was a substandard form of help and continually agitated for individual treatment.[23] Their hatred and contempt for the group was hard for the beginning and untrained therapist to bear and when the premises in which the group met was destroyed by a fatal bomb explosion a spiral of destructive forces was unleashed in the group that led ultimately to the complete breakdown and dissolution of the group. While the therapist could just manage the hostility of the group before the bomb explosion, the massive disintegration of the external environment seemed to activate an equally massive disintegration and fragmentation in the internal and interpersonal world of the group. The implosion of the group was an inevitable consequence of destructive anti-group forces amplified by the environmental trauma. In this example we can identify several determinants of anti-group behaviour:

- Poor selection of members – too many highly aggressive members
- Poor preparation for group – not enough attention paid to members' anxieties and distrust of the group modality including the misconception that group treatment is second best to individual work
- Flawed development of the group
- The group therapist's lack of training and lack of support
- Group operating in a situation of civic conflict
- A sudden group crisis that could not be managed

An anti-group dimension is a natural part of the development of all groups (see Chapter 2) and can be understood and managed and even transformed. The group worker who accepts that conflict is a central feature of group life and is attuned to aggressive and destructive forces is much more likely to be able to manage and channel these processes than a worker who is frightened of conflict and seeks to avoid or deny their presence. Rather than endeavouring to inhibit the expression of conflict the creative group worker realizes that hostility is a sign of hope and anger, often initiates change, and prepares the way for forgiveness and reparation. The following chapters all contain useful suggestions and strategies for contextualizing aggression and utilizing and reframing the positive value of hostility.

Stages theory is a map, not the territory

It is important to recognize that like human fingerprints, no two groups are identical in their development. Every group experience is unique and will not strictly adhere to a neat model of sequential phases. Groups are in motion all the time and there is overlap, spiralling, regression, and continual oscillation between the polarities of love and will in the group. At times both energies are clearly operative in the group, particularly at transition points, and the group has the option of staying put, regressing, or going forward. There is no guarantee that the group will automatically progress and because of this it is essential that the worker is attentive to what is actually happening in the group in terms of members' love and will needs and issues, rather than looking for confirmation of a favourite model.

Many workers in my experience come unstuck, become frustrated, and even doubt their own competence when their groups do not appear to follow the neat schemata outlined in the groupwork texts. It is important to remember that stages theory is only a map. It is *not* the actual territory. The territory must be negotiated as it is being traversed. The map can offer pointers and markers but only if it is intelligently used and not slavishly followed.

Review

- While every group is unique there are certain basic features of culture and structure
- Behaviour is not random
- Behaviour is comprehensible
- Behaviour can be anticipated
- Behaviour in the group is best understood at the level of group process, rather than solely in terms of individual personality
- The drive mechanism in group process is the tension generated by the archetypal urge to attach and its opposite, the urge to separate
- Group process is organic and displays unfolding themes and patterns of growth and development:

    o It is possible to recognize these themes and patterns and influence them
    o Groups naturally contain regressive and destructive forces. These antigroup forces can be understood and transformed

References

1 Lerner, I. (1976) *Diary of the Way: Three Paths to Enlightenment*: 26, New York: Ridge Press.
2 Maslow, A. (1954) *Motivation and Personality*, New York: Harper & Row.
3 Benne, K.D. and Sheats, P. (1948) 'Functional roles of group members', *Journal of Social Issues*, 4, 2: 41–9.
4 Underwood, W. (1970) 'Roles that facilitate and inhibit group development', in R.T. Golembiewski and A. Blumberg (eds) *Sensitivity Training and the Laboratory Approach: Readings about Concepts and Applications*, Itasca, IL: Peacock.
5 Bogdanoff, M. and Elbaum, O.L. (1978) 'Role lock . . . monopolisers, mistrusters, isolates, Helpful Hannahs, and other assorted characters in group psychotherapy', *International Journal of Group Psychotherapy*, 28, 2: 247–62.

6   Sarri, R.C. and Galinsky, M.J. (1974) 'A conceptual framework for group development', in P. Glasser, R.C. Sarri, and R.Vinter, *Individual Change through Small Groups*: 71–86, New York: Free Press.

7   Assagioli, R. (1983) *Psychosynthesis Typology: Psychosynthesis Monograph*: 27, London: Institute of Psychosynthesis.

8   Angyal, A. (1969) *Foundations for a Science of Personality*: 172, New York: Viking Compass.

9   Ibid.

10 Assagioli, R. (1983) op. cit., p. 21.

11 Schutz, W. (1979) *Profound Simplicity*: 111–37, London: Turnstone.

12 Tuckman, B.W. (1965) 'Developmental sequence in small groups', *Psychological Bulletin*, 63, 6: 384–99.

13 Garland, J., Jones, H., and Kolodny, K. (1965) 'A model for stages in the development of social work groups', in S. Bernstein (ed) *Explorations in Group Work*, London: Bookstall.

14 Ibid., p. 35.

15 Ibid., p. 43.

16 Hartford, M.E. (1972) 'Phases in group development', *Groups in Social Work: Application of Small Group Theory and Research to Social Work Practice*: 63–93, New York: Columbia University Press.

17 Blofeld, J. (1968) *I Ching: The Chinese Book of Changes*: 185, London: Allen & Unwin.

18 Ibid., p. 201.

19 Tuckman, B.W. (1965) op. cit., p. 396.

20 Ibid., p. 396.

21 Nitsun, M. (1996) *The Anti-Group: Destructive forces in the group and their creative potential*, London & New York: Routledge.

22 Nitsun, M. (1996) op. cit., p. 44.

23 Benson, J.F. (2005) 'Management of intense countertransference in group psychotherapy conducted in situations of civic conflict', *International Journal of Group Psychotherapy*, 55, 1: 63–86.

Chapter 4

Work at the beginning stages of the group

Inclusion issues

In the last chapter I said that it was possible for the worker to consciously co-operate with the organic processes of growth and development in the group in order to liberate and utilize its creative energy and resource. A statement like this immediately raises questions about what precisely it is that the group worker co-operates with and how he goes about it.

The answer is quite simple when one remembers that movement and change occur as a consequence of the energy generated by the tension between the love and will polarities which are always present in the group.

However, in the volatile, rowdy, and often apparently chaotic atmosphere of many groups the beginning group worker can find that he lacks the expertise and confidence which would help him understand and feel competent to deal with what is happening. With this thought in mind I have written this chapter to help you recognize what these love and will energies actually look like in the group and how they influence behaviour. I have also included specific instructions on how to use these energies to enhance the process of the group. Before moving to this let me mention three basic principles that will recur.

The group is organic and capable of evolving

What I mean by this is that group experience is an organic and unfolding process in which behaviour is neither random nor illogical but can be discerned as comprehensible themes and patterns of experience and need. The group is not in its essential nature a chaotic, static, or inert phenomenon. Groups are energetically dynamic and tend to develop in an increasingly inclusive and more organized manner.

Behaviour reveals its meaning when seen in context

Following on from this is my belief that observing and understanding these themes and patterns is the first and most basic skill for groupwork practice. You will not know how to respond, how to intervene, or help your group if you cannot see and accurately understand what is happening between people.

How are you to make sense of the events that you are experiencing in a group situation? When two people argue, for example, are they merely expressing differing viewpoints? Do they not like each other? Could it be that they feel unsafe in the group? Do they not understand what they are supposed to do? And how are you to intervene? How can you know what exactly is taking place?

What I am pointing to here is the *meaning* that we attribute to a particular interaction or event; the real nature of what it is that you are looking at, hearing, or attending to. An organism and its actions are not independent of its environment. There is a clear relationship between the whole and its parts and when we blur or avoid this relationship we often cannot see the wood for the trees. Unfortunately many new group workers have a tendency to respond to events in the group at an immediate and surface level, failing or forgetting to see these events in the context of group life. They can experience group behaviour as random, illogical, and meaningless and often find their interventions are uninformed, lacking in precision, and too emotive.

The meaning or nature of an event or interaction can only be fully understood when it is seen against the background or in the context in which it occurs. Nothing exists without a context or ground. Clouds are seen against the background of the sky, waves against the sea, and you are able to recognize these words because they are set against the whiteness of the page. So the meaning of a specific behaviour or interaction in a group should always be seen in the context of that particular stage of group unfolding.

The importance of love and will energies

The third theme which we will explore is concerned with how the leader uses the love and will energies in her own psyche as well as in the group, to relate to members individually and collectively. The point here is that whilst everyone has available to them the love and will energies, men and women are traditionally cast in typical sex roles which tend to overdevelop certain energies and qualities of the self at the expense of underdeveloping others. For example, men are expected to be more concerned with the will and assertion energies in everyday life and women are required to operate more under the influence of the love principle. I am not saying by this that men are unable to be caring or sensitive or that women cannot be assertive or competitive. I am pointing to common attitudes and experiences which I believe have important implications for working with groups. What I am saying is that when working with a group, leaders should be careful not to operate solely out of their usual sex-role identifications or the group will tend to develop in a one-sided way. Following the example of the leader, members may avoid conflict, scorn the expression of feelings, be overly competitive, or uncomfortable with vulnerability.

Irrespective of gender the group worker needs to use both the masculine and feminine energies in the self if the group experience is not to be impoverished. Workers should give careful thought to ways in which they might transcend stereotyped sex roles at important stages in the group life. A male worker could consider how to more consciously use the love energies available to him in order to meet group needs for reassurance, protection, and sympathy. A female worker could consider how to employ her will energies to provide the group with an experience of boundary, consistency, and order.

The importance of the worker being able to use the love and will energies in himself is underscored if we consider the group as a representation of the archetypal family. Irrespective of age or ability and despite the purpose or task for which the group was set up there is a level at which individuals can come into relationship with the leader and the other members as if with the parent and siblings in the archetypal family. This can be readily seen in any group at different stages of its life where individual members act towards each other and particularly the leader in a dependent, aggressive, rebellious, or jealous manner.

On these occasions the worker and his colleagues in the group come to embody for individuals the love and will energies involved in parenting – the mother and father aspects of the archetypal parent. So at different times in the group members will look to the worker for certain parenting responses. This is important in all groups but particularly in psychotherapy groups where there is an emphasis on correcting or making repair of impoverished or deficient ego development. As we shall see, in the inclusion period of the group members are dependent and anxious and will look for a nurturing or positive mothering approach from the worker. As the group successfully resolves its ambivalence about inclusion, the mothering side of the worker has to be experienced as negative so that members can separate from him and begin to explore relationships with each other.

There ensues a time of conflict and aggression; of seeking after power and challenging authority. The group now looks to the worker to use the will energies of the archetypal father to model leadership, give structure, and permit appropriate rebellion. In time the group passes through the 'control' stage to the more mature and interdependent relationships of the 'affection' stage of group life. Here members are able to transcend the love and will issues of the two previous stages and relate to the leader and each other in a more adult manner. It is as if members have used the maternal and paternal qualities of the earlier stages to create the atmosphere in which they can now begin to individuate and use the group reciprocally to benefit themselves and each other.

From this brief discussion it is clear that the worker needs to recognize and be able to use both the love and will/assertion energies in himself as well as in the group. A negative and often destructive spiral can easily develop if the worker does not realize what is taking place and makes an inappropriate will or love type intervention. Just as with parents, group members will react against the inappropriate response with all the old stereotyped strategies of childhood.

Inclusion issues

Recognition

Whether the group is a counselling, work, educational, or recreational experience, the first issue that emerges as soon as people come together is about belonging. From the start each individual has to decide to be part of the group or not; to be *in* or *out*. At the same time each individual has to decide his degree of commitment to and inclusion in the group. How much or how little contact, interaction, and communication does he wish to engage in?

At the inclusion stage group members may engage in a wide variety of behaviours as a way of resolving their anxieties and preoccupations. These anxieties result from the conflict and demands of two divergent tendencies operating in the mind of uncertain members. On the one hand the momentum of the love principle generates a concern to attach, belong, relate, connect with other people (see page 74). The impulse to belong is further enhanced by the strength of the individual's desire for *this* group experience; for the gratifications promised in *this* group opportunity. On the other hand the will principle generates an impulse to separate and be independent (see page 75). This is partly because of the demands, frustrations, and anxieties that may be anticipated and is often fuelled by memories and experiences of previous groups (see boxes below and page 74).

These opposing tendencies create tension and ambivalence and cause the potential member to ask himself questions such as:

- What will the other members be like? What will they think of me? Will I fit in? Can I trust them? Will I like them?
- What kind of group is this? Can I get what I need in this group? What do I have to do here? Can I cope in this group? Will it be a good group?
- What is the leader going to be like? Can I trust him? Is he dependable? Will he like me? Whom will he like best? Will he be strict?

Moving towards other group members (Love principle)	Underlying needs and motives
<ul><li>Introductions</li><li>Initiating conversations 'cocktail party talk' *Themes*: weather, football, government, people we know</li><li>Sharing of similar/previous experiences</li><li>Establishing mutuality</li><li>Joining in activities</li><li>Exploring/examining environment, equipment</li><li>Sharing space, material, food, equipment, conversation, self</li><li>Establishing rules, procedures</li><li>Humour, joking, teasing</li><li>Depending on the leader</li><li>Beginning relationships</li></ul>	<ul><li>To approach, connect, belong, be part of, interact</li><li>To be protected, feel secure, have order, system, rule</li><li>To encounter other members, know them, assess them</li><li>To be regarded as worthwhile, significant, valuable</li><li>To determine possibilities offered by the group</li></ul>

Moving away from or against other group members (Will principle)	Underlying needs and motives
<ul><li>Absenteeism</li><li>Lateness</li><li>Silence</li><li>Halting/sporadic conversations</li><li>Talking too much/chattering</li></ul>	<ul><li>Fear of being rejected, attacked, ridiculed, making a mistake</li><li>Need to assert self as competent and significant, valuable, worthwhile</li></ul>

Moving away from or against other group members (Will principle)	Underlying needs and motives
• Repetitiveness/asking for instructions, information previously given, going over ground again • Superficiality, skimming/glossing over issues • Preoccupation with tasks, procedures, and rules • Refusing to join in activities, withdrawal, self-sufficiency • Expressions of boredom, contempt, indifference • Hovering, hesitation, fence-sitting, edge of group activity, distancing, suggestions for separative activity, e.g. hide and go seek • Impulsive behaviour, greed, aggression, random activity • Vandalism of furniture, equipment, environment • Exhibitionistic behaviour, attention-seeking, showing off, boasting • Overdependence on the leader	• Fear of being taken over by group, of being obligated, committed, coerced • Fear of being dependent, needy, vulnerable • Need to avoid close association • Need to defend and maintain a separative self • Unwillingness to trust others • Need to 'wait and see' • Need for order, direction, security, protection, safety

Anxiety about these issues is expressed in this opening phase of group life in the form of individual-centred behaviour which satisfies both the love and the will impulses simultaneously, in behaviour which facilitates involvement, exploration, and self-disclosure while at the same time permits some distance and protection from too much encounter too soon.

It is possible to identify some of the more usual patterns of behaviour in the opening sessions of the group. Remember that there is no clear-cut sequence in which one behaviour follows from another! Each group is unique and depending on its goals and the nature and motivations of the people who make it up, one, some, or all of these behaviours may be apparent on different occasions in the beginning.

Mothering: nurturing the group at the inclusion stage

Guiding the group through the inclusion stage demands a great deal of awareness and sensitivity from the worker. The prime requirement is to 'see' behaviour in the opening sessions as the expression of a very natural 'approach-avoid' ambivalence; as the way in which potential members struggle with and reconcile the tensions and implications of beginning group membership.

A perspective like this shapes the way a worker relates to the group. Now, interventions are made not so much to correct or proscribe behaviour, but rather to positively respond to and use the love and will needs being expressed in particular behaviours.

Knowing how people are likely to feel and behave the worker can conduct himself in such a way, and provide a programme which minimizes anxiety and frustration and reinforces the desire of members to join in. Similarly, instead of getting exasperated or feeling inadequate about members' unwillingness to participate in activity, their silence, or superficiality, a worker might decide to go beneath the behaviour to *acknowledge* and *permit* people's fears in new situations. By involving members in discussion about their anxieties and their needs the worker communicates a clear message that it is alright to be anxious and that something can be done about it. The worker also begins to create an environment which values and facilitates awareness and choice rather than compulsive and fear-determined behaviour.

But what precisely, does the worker do at this stage? I would suggest that the worker's operations derive from the fact that the group is a multidimensional experience. There are layers or levels of experience mediated by the love–will polarity, which influence and determine individual and group behaviour. These layers or levels of experience can operate simultaneously as well as hierarchically and will usually produce some confusion for members.

There is a *physical* level at which members need and want to interact but may worry perhaps about how touching each other will be construed. People get tired, restless, and want to move. They react to noise, cold, distractions in the environment, the size of the room, and seating arrangements (see pages 202 and 217).

At the *feeling level* members can be anxious, fearful, shy, and embarrassed. At other times they may be eager, excited, or impulsive. On an *intellectual level* members usually have questions about the group, its objectives, purposes, methods of working and are curious about each other's background and reasons for being in the group.

The range of behaviours which may manifest on these different levels of group experience suggest four major tasks for the worker at this stage:

* Fostering members' attraction to the group
* Establishing structure and control
* Developing trust and cohesion
* Negotiating agreement on the work of the group

In practice, I find that these tasks tend not to be very separate and discrete but rather form a continuum of worker activity that is distinctly 'nurturing' in style and effect. When I talk about 'nurturing the group' I mean that I try to nourish and reassure members at the physical, emotional, and intellectual levels of group experience. In other words I attempt to create an atmosphere which is warm, gentle, and friendly, accepting but purposeful, and which inspires trust. A metaphor which I consciously employ here is of the '*worker as group mother*'.

I believe that the opening sequence of the group calls for a gentle, nurturing approach irrespective of the worker's sex, an approach which tends to be associated with females and mother. Earlier I said that the first session was the moment of social and psychological birth (page 54) and so the inclusion stage of group life can be likened to the time of infancy and childhood.

There is a certain level at which, regardless of age, each prospective member relates to the leader and the other group members as might a child. This can be seen in the kind of questions the member brings to the group (see page 86). This does not mean that the individual is childish but rather that the prospective member comes to group sessions new, uncertain, and ambivalent. Such a member is dependent particularly on the leader and then on the other people for the warmth, acceptance, experiences, opportunities, guidance, and information which will help him use the group.

While each individual comes to the group with a 'transference' potential towards the other members (see pages 201 and 222) the first relationship is with the leader. Because of the transference potential in the situation this tends to evoke the dependency of the earlier mother–child relationship. The mother is usually the first adult that the infant connects with and the quality of relationship established with 'mother' can be powerful in determining the quality of subsequent relationships. So from the start I accept the role of the 'mothering one' since I will usually be cast in a 'parenting' role anyway, and concern myself with the physical, emotional, and intellectual needs of the members in order to 'bond' with them. In this way I try to establish a firm and secure basis upon which each member can begin to move out into the group and engage with the other members.

I want to look at this now in relation to practice in the opening sessions of the group.

Nurturing at the physical level of group inclusion

Where possible I would suggest that you try to consider in advance how the environment will affect or constrain the group. Try to inspect and, if necessary, arrange the room you will work in so that it looks attractive and friendly. Consider: Is the room too big, too small? Will it permit people to move about during the course of their work? Is it warm and airy? How will people sound in this room? Can you be heard outside? Are you likely to be disturbed by external noises? Do you have to be careful with room furnishings or particular materials? Where are the toilets and kitchens?

Music, food, and names

As the group gathers for the first session I often play some suitable music in the background as I have found this a good way of 'warming' people and it creates a friendly and welcoming atmosphere. I may also provide tea and biscuits as a traditional and sometimes practical method of nourishing people as well as giving them a means of gently easing into the group. Where possible try to seat the group comfortably in a circle as this allows each member to view the others and be seen. It also promotes optimum conversation and communication. Always greet people as they enter the room, go forward to welcome them, shake their hand and say their name if you know it, or ask them if you don't.

Exercise and games to break the ice

Think about using games or physical activity if appropriate as a way of relieving tension, getting people to contact each other, and facilitating interaction and communication. In the early sessions group members can be anxious, withdrawn, and wary of contact with each other. This can result in members blushing, inhibiting their breathing, and stiffening their posture in order to separate and defend themselves. The energy in the group can feel cold, staccato, and introverted. Well thought-out physical activity can be useful, therefore, in releasing some of this inert energy and breaking the ice. It is important that any programme of activity at this stage is kept simple. A minimum of clear instructions will indicate what is expected of members and a minimal demand for skill competence will be more likely to engage members and promote success. There is a wide range of games and exercises specifically designed to 'accelerate' the process of inclusion and Chapter 10 contains a selection of activities and suggestions on how to use them.

Nurturing at the emotional level of group inclusion

Try to foster group cohesion and the development of trust from the start.

Group cohesion and the building of trust is a dynamic process which can be altered or changed by particular incidents, the strength of members' attraction to the group, and its relevance to their lives. Cohesion is a primary factor in keeping a group together and a major determinant of the quality of the climate and the effectiveness of the group. Cohesion develops through the acknowledgement of common elements so look for emotional themes and patterns in the early stages of the group. In this way you help people begin to see that they are not alone in feeling anxious or shy and they have more in common with other people than they at first realize. Concentrate on linking and connecting people by encouraging them to discuss and share whatever experiences they are having here and now in the group. Reward and reinforce any attempts by members to reach out towards each other. A way of doing this is to begin to develop desirable norms of behaviour.

Building group norms

Try to establish and promote those norms and values which will foster group cohesion. Here are some examples of relevant norms:

> - Everybody is important and worthwhile in this group
> - As far as possible only one person at a time should speak
> - It is important that other members pay attention and listen
> - Do not judge people's behaviour: try to discover the need behind or meaning of the behaviour
> - Group members will try to help each other sort out problems and difficulties
> - The sessions are to be kept confidential

An easy way of developing positive norms in the beginning is to give the group permission to behave or feel in a certain way. A technique that I often use is to write certain permissions on sheets around the room such as:

> - It's OK to make mistakes here
> - It's OK not to know here
> - I can ask for help here

I then ask members to select one or two from the dozen or so cards, which they can use as their 'motto' for the session. You can also ask members to discuss why they chose a particular permission.

Another way of fostering desirable norms is to reinforce statements by members which will help the group accomplish its goals or maintain its emotional well-being such as, 'I think we should be honest about how we feel,' or 'I think it would show commitment if we all agreed to come on time.'

Members will be more accepting of norms that they have set up so pay close attention to what people say they want and what they say will make them do certain things. When you know *what* will move people then you know *how* to move them.

Permit what is happening and acknowledge the real issues of concern

Allow whatever is happening to happen. Permit people to be silent or passive or shy. Do not force them into discussion or activity in order to fill up spaces or give the impression that this is a busy and therefore successful group. You may feel that you want to avoid embarrassing pauses and silences but by 'filling in' you may miss an opportunity to focus on what is really bothering people.

I have found that members are generally relieved and appreciative when I acknowledge how difficult it is to talk with people we hardly know. By drawing attention to those gaps in conversation in a warm and nurturing way you can make them normal and legitimate, and you can demonstrate to members that you understand and care about their ambivalence and tension about inclusion. It is then much easier than you would think to get people talking about their anxieties about speaking in public or fears about revealing too much of themselves.

In other situations members may talk too much; there may be a lot of repetitiveness or showing off. I will endeavour to point out how these behaviours may be a way of avoiding contact with other people, dealing with threatening silences, or forcing the leader to provide more structure. I take care to acknowledge the needs and fears as natural and only to be expected whenever people come together initially. I then try to help members explore why they feel like this in this particular group and look at what they can do about it.

Put events in context and make connections

Try to refer members to previous experiences of 'beginning' such as the first day in a new school or job, moving to a new neighbourhood, or making new friends. By '*contextualizing*' beginnings in this way you can help group members see their current inclusion experiences from a wider life perspective and this can desensitize the situation a great deal. Themes which often emerge at this stage include how people present themselves, poor self-image, fear of rejection, lack of confidence, fear of forming relationships with the opposite sex, and inadequacy in basic social skills. The purpose of the particular group will determine how much time you will spend discussing these themes. The important point to remember is that emotional needs and concerns about inclusion must be acknowledged and worked with if they are not to sabotage and undermine the group endeavour.

Do not force or insist on trust

Many group workers like to develop cohesion and trust in the group through the use of 'trust-games'. I do use these games but have sometimes seen them used in a way which can be injurious to the development of healthy group trust. Cohesion and trust develop in a group through members' unfolding experiences and encounters with each other. This takes time and it is in the nature of things that trust should unfold, should be earned. Overemphasis and insistence that group members *should* trust each other or *must* be more trusting can often indicate insecurity on the part of the worker, may come across as insincere and fraudulent, and can actually produce the opposite outcome. It is much better to establish cohesion and trust in the manner I have suggested – working directly out of members' behavioural and emotional expressions in a gentle, nurturing, and accepting way.

Establishing structure: the check-in

Gradually members come to see that there is a structure emerging in the group; that it is alright to have these feelings of anxiety or helplessness or ambivalence and that there exist ways of dealing with them. This gives a sense of definition and control which is reassuring and actually enhances conditions for increased risk-taking, disclosure, and the development of trust.

From the start of the group I try to develop a sense of structure and foster the emergence of consistency and predictability by assuming a firm and 'directive' stance which is compatible with and supplements my nurturing of the group. I will indicate when the sessions start, usually by asking people to 'check in'. This involves members individually connecting to the group by verbalizing how they are feeling, what they have done since last session, what they are anxious about or looking forward to in this session. The check-in acknowledges the need to 'include' at the start of each session and builds in a structured nurturing and orienting period. It also gets each member to speak for a short time in a low stress situation since each individual can decide the length and content of their contribution.

Clearing expectations, contracting, routines

In the early sessions I will find out from each member what expectations they have of the group, what they want from the group, and why they have come. People tend to expect this and are usually happy to supply this information. Another method of establishing structure and control in these opening sessions is to negotiate a contract with members about what is and is not permissible (see page 48). Throughout the early sessions of the group I attempt to build a safe and stable context within which members can participate and interact successfully and with satisfaction. I am not afraid to arbitrate and make decisions, since members expect this of me. I do try to explain why I have chosen a particular course and look for comment and feedback on this, if appropriate.

Consistent patterns are important in building a sense of structure and orthodoxy and so I establish regular routines such as meal breaks, activities, check-ins, reviews, and planning periods which can be easily formalized and structured into group experience.

Do not be afraid to lead

I should emphasize that I am directing the group in a light and sensitive manner as a way of acknowledging and responding to people's need for structure and boundary. This directing is more in the sense of guiding or showing the way rather than imposing arbitrary rules on group members. I think it is very important that from the outset members can see that the leader is willing and confident in his ability to lead and guide the group. This instils confidence and trust in the leader and makes it easier to explore what the group has to offer.

Some group workers seem to expect members to 'take responsibility' for the structure of the group from the start, refusing to guide and direct on the grounds that 'it's your group'. In some instances this is to misunderstand the responsibility and nature of the authority vested in the group worker, seeing only the negative aspects of power and control; and worse, ignoring members' legitimate needs for direction from the group leader. The consequence can be to unwittingly turn the group into an unsafe and random experience where a form of jungle law predominates in the absence of a carefully designed boundary and structure.

Nurturing at the intellectual level of group inclusion

At the level of members' intellectual needs there are a number of issues to be aware of. Members will be curious about you and about each other, so creating space to satisfy this curiosity is essential. Because personal information and reasons for being in the group are often vague, superficial, or not fully absorbed in the tension and anxiety of having to speak publicly, I tend to use pairing-type exercises as a way of deepening and obtaining knowledge about each other. Making a short statement about myself from a more personal angle is a useful way of dispelling any reasonable curiosity about me and can always be augmented by allowing members to ask questions.

Clarifying purpose and making a group contract

It is important that members focus on the purpose of the group, think about why they are here, and reflect on their commitment to the group goals. A way of doing this is to set aside time right from the start to clarify expectations. Do not be afraid to ask lots of questions in order to help people identify and make explicit their expectations, fantasies, and apprehensions about the group's purpose, its way of working, and their role in it:

- What do you think this group is for?
- Why have you come?
- What do you want for yourself from the group experience?
- What are you worried about?
- What do you need in order to be here?

This process can be enhanced by encouraging individuals to make personal contracts with you or the group. These personal contracts can range from how people intend to use the group, to telling you before they run out of the session. Make *lots* of these contracts. They are a very powerful way of clarifying people's desires and fears and eliciting and engaging their ability to determine for themselves.

Aim also to arrive at a statement of what is realistic, possible, and desirable in this group which can be put to members in the form of a group contract. This group contract is vital to ensure that members understand what is being asked of them and can agree to pursue particular objectives. Without an explicit agreement which members consider binding it is just not possible for you as the group leader to work effectively or creatively. Let's pause for a moment to consider in more detail why the group contract is so essential.

The group contract as a way of managing conflict

I have come to believe that when working with groups the key problem for the worker is managing the inevitable conflict that appears to be the life and nature of the group. This conflict simply arises because of the very presence of the individuals who constitute the membership. You bring a number of people together on a regular basis and you will inevitably have diverging and contradictory perspectives and opinions. The multiple membership of the group makes for a very complex experience and this can be confusing and disturbing. The central feature of this complicated experience has to do with managing difference and is a manifestation of the will principle as a part of the drive mechanism for movement and growth in groups that we talked about earlier (see page 74).

No member experiences the group exactly as the others or sees events as the others do. Everybody has a unique perspective on group life and member presentations and interactions.

> - Different perceptions
> - Differerent expectations
> - Different experiences

These differences can initially cause friction and friction can cause conflict. If this conflict can be understood as a normal and natural phenomenon and is well managed by the worker, the group modality is a powerful change agent. However, each member still has to manage a complex and sometimes unpredictable variety of interactions and communications that can generate anxiety and fearful and regressive behaviour. Particularly with a new group whose members may not know each other, the centrality of their experience of difference may well feel more threatening and can activate unhelpful and unhealthy coping mechanisms and defence strategies. So, before the group can coalesce it has to negotiate its inclusion issues and that means learning how difference can be creative rather than disintegrative and separating. The attitude and activity of the group worker at this crucial time can contribute hugely to the development of a growing atmosphere of trust and safety.

The central task for the group worker is to recognize and accept the natural conflict state of the group for what it is and not be afraid of it. Conflict in the group is a manifestation of the will principle. It is the psychological and social dimension of a fundamental impulse towards differentiation and lies at the heart of group life even in the most successful groups.

These different perspectives and experiences of members that threaten to pull the group in irreconcilable directions can be metabolized and managed by a skilful and creative worker utilizing the love principle in activities which are connective, magnetic, and inclusive (see page 74). This is where the group contract comes in because in order for any group to work its members are going to have to make agreements together.

I like to think of the contract as a psychological skin that contains natural conflict within the group and prevents it spilling over into chaos. Just as an actual human skin contains our inner organs and allows heat to escape while minimizing intrusion from the environment so the group contract performs similar psychological functions for the group:

- The group contract regulates what stays in the group and what can go outside
- The contract asserts how members will interact with each other
- The contract determines what is permissible and unacceptable behaviour
- The contract is clear about the purpose of the group
- The contract emphasizes that members are responsible for themselves
- The contracts asserts the primacy of communal life and action
- The contract affirms the group is designed to be a caring and compassionate experience
- The contract manages the tension between closeness and separateness (see page 203)

The group contract can contain as many or as few clauses as is helpful for you and the group. My own contracts are sparse and usually contain three apparently simple clauses or conditions. The first clause of the contract is invariably a statement about the purpose for the group. This is important as it states clear boundaries as to how group experience and material will be managed by the worker and clarifies what can reasonably be expected of group members, so that for example a group which is met for educational purposes will not expect group experience to be processed as in a psychotherapy group.

A second condition of my usual contract governs individual members' choice to attend the group. I make a distinction between volunteers and conscripts in which volunteers have a degree of self-determination denied to conscripts who are required to attend the group by a court order or psychiatric or educational injunction.

Even where members are conscripted into the group I assert their individual choice to make the experience as useful and enjoyable as possible. What I am going for in this second clause of the group contract is to engage each member's will and agency. I am attempting to evoke each member's capacity to be self-determining agent and to encourage them to be responsible for the quality of the group experience rather than expecting me to be the sole responsible one. This emphasis on will and choice at the beginning of the group carries on throughout the life of the group with an insistence on the sorts of consequences that attend the choices we make (see page 216).

The third condition of my group contract asks individual members to take care of themselves. The symbol that underpins my thinking here is of the chain that is as strong as its weakest link. In other words a group at its beginning is simply a collection of individuals. It is not yet a group but may become a group in time.

Members are more aware of their differences and distinctions at the start than they are of their samenesses and connections and as we have seen above this can generate suspicion and anxiety which may slow down or disrupt the development of mutual and collaborative bonds. So I find it best in the beginning to normalize this difference and the sorts of feelings that come with it and encourage members to find appropriate ways and means to make themselves as comfortable as possible with others. In other words I start from the fact of the individuals present in front of me and each other and proceed to work towards becoming a group. I recognize and accept as normal the idea that making this group requires individuals to participate in and get involved in an arrangement that might reawaken fears and anxieties about groups and since this is going to take time it is important for members to look out for themselves.

This may seem to you counter-intuitive but my experience has been that supporting the individual to take responsibility for their own safety promotes a willingness to move towards group collaboration more quickly than being required to surrender a fragile or threatened individuality too quickly in service of group objectives.

Many group workers have been surprised that a group which at first seemed so compliant and easy to work with can quickly come to seem fractious and hostile. While the next chapter explores this phenomenon in depth it is worthwhile saying here that *often workers are mistaken in supposing a group to exist in their minds when in fact members may see and experience themselves more as individuals or possibly subgroups than as the group the worker imagines.* Those members who may hide behind a premature group association with the unwitting complicity of the worker may very well need later to attack the group more robustly as a means of asserting their identity and individuality than if they and the worker had allowed more time in the contract at the beginning for individuals to experience their separateness and growing desire to form a group.

These three conditions are the basis of any contract that I make with a group. Members may wish to add conditions of their own but in practice these are variations of the core principles.

If we continue with the analogy of the group contract as a kind of skin then it becomes apparent that just as we have to constantly maintain our physical skin in order for it to perform its functions so we have to monitor and maintain the effectiveness of the group contract as a psychological skin. In other words the group contract is not a one-off activity that the group worker engages in at the beginning of the group and then forgets about or takes for granted.

The group contract is an ongoing and organic aspect of the group's evolution. I cannot state the organic and continuous nature of the group contract enough. The group contract becomes the rationale for exploring the process issues that dominate so much of the time and attention of the group as well as being the primary vehicle for teaching the group how it will learn from its own experience. Utilizing this idea of viewing the group contract as a psychological skin makes it possible to consider every event, phenomenon, and communication in the group in terms of whether it facilitates the purpose of the group or disrupts it. From this perspective the worker can now monitor and evaluate any group activity and make it a basis for intervention or not.

Example of worker's use of group contract as an intervention

A psychotherapy group had been meeting weekly for some three months and began to turn its attention to a member, John, who had been turning up late for the sessions. When challenged by the other members of the group about this behaviour the latecomer insisted that he had to come a long way to attend the group; that traffic conditions determined his lateness; and refused to see that there was anything untoward in his behaviour. The group backed off and John continued in the following sessions to come late. When it appeared that there was going to be no further consideration of the matter the group worker intervened to remind people that they had agreed to attend the group in order to think psychologically about their personal behaviours and interactions and it appeared that both the group and John were unwilling to really take this latecoming event in the group life seriously and this seemed to be limiting real communication in the group. The worker also reminded John that he had made a choice to attend the group but seemed in two minds now about this and this also needed looking at. It was clear that John's way of taking care of himself was antagonising the group and preventing genuine communication.

By drawing attention to the purpose of the group meeting and the quality of members choosing to be in the group the worker was endeavouring to demonstrate that the basic group contract was being breached in a number of ways and that this was a matter that demanded group attention. The members slowly began to address their feelings about John's lateness and this caused a deal of hostility with John feeling attacked and in turn attacking the others. For a few sessions there were sharp exchanges but gradually John and the other members came to get a feel for each other's points of view and John stopped coming late. He showed that he could be responsive to others' needs and the group was confirmed in the belief that thinking about things and talking about things, no matter how painful initially, could produce change. By highlighting the nature of the contract that members had agreed to and how it was being frustrated the worker was able to develop a benign therapeutic environment and promote an effective therapeutic group.

Example of worker's use of group contract as a basis for experiential learning

A therapeutic group for 14–17-year-old adolescents with emotional and behavioural difficulties was exploring the theme of self-assertion through the medium of a particular game when things got a bit heated between two members and resulted in some rough pushing and shoving. The worker immediately stopped the activity and asked the two members what had happened. Each blamed the other for being overly aggressive. The worker asked the other group members for their reactions but they said that talking was boring and that the two members should be sidelined to allow the group to continue with the game. The worker responded by querying who would want to come to a group where people got shoved around and there was no attempt to deal with things in a less aggressive way. He pointed out that the game was meant to explore how one asserted oneself in situations but the theme had become a real issue in the group now and had to be explored here if this group was to work. Members quickly vented their frustration at the disruptive members and it was some time before the worker could engage the group in a less emotional examination of what had happened. Gradually a theme emerged to do

with the importance of respect and how members felt obliged to respond disproportion-
ately if they felt they were being disrespected. The worker intervened to say that the initial
dispute between the two members and the group's response to the stopping of the activity
suggested that people did not believe that their anger would be taken seriously unless it
was demonstrated in action and wondered if the group could come up with another way
of managing personal and collective boundaries. Through a series of role plays the group
then considered a variety of ways in which members might assert themselves in threatening situations, using words to articulate their needs rather than acting out their feelings. It
was possible to come up with an agreed formula that members promised to try out before
the next session and then report back to the group on its merits. In the next session some
time was set aside for this discussion and the varying reports were refined to come up with
a more appropriate and helpful tool for self assertion.

In this example the worker uses the breakdown of an activity to draw attention to the
disruption of the group contract. The threat to the continuity of the group becomes the
rationale for a live opportunity to explore the group process in the context of broken
boundaries and the need for appropriate self care and assertion. Out of this the worker
enables the group to develop new and agreed ways or working and behaving which have
relevance inside and outside the group. This theme is developed more fully in Chapter 10.
One can see the organic nature of the group contract and the importance of maintaining
the psychological skin of the group.

It should be clear now that establishing a meaningful agreement with members and
between them is an essential and ongoing activity of the effective group worker. Articula-
tion of goals at the individual and collective level develops consensus, motivates behaviour,
and indicates tasks and performances as well as creating security and a sense of well-being.

It is important that the group contract is discussed fully and that members can interact
and share ideas about the proposed goals and programme. Obviously this will vary from
group to group. In one group there will be a clear and acceptable task and members will
get down to work immediately. In another group, particularly those that emphasize more
personal work, it may take several sessions to successfully negotiate why it is that people
have come and what they expect and agree to do together.

Share your vision of the group

You can help a good deal by joining in and stating how you would like to see the group
developing. Some workers see this stance as too directive or manipulative and prefer to
withdraw to the sidelines to let the group decide its own purpose and direction. My own
position is that since I am in the group for a particular reason and have an investment in it
by virtue of my time, resource, and energy I have a professional right, if not an obligation
on behalf of a funding agency, to seek a preferred and agreed purpose and direction. My
experience is that people appear relieved, respond better, remain committed to the group
task, and are more motivated when I am explicit and unambiguous about my wishes for
the group and maintain no secret ambitions or hidden agendas.

In carefully putting out my vision of how the group might operate I aim to not only
declare what I am unwilling or not prepared to undertake but also to stimulate discussion and begin to develop consensus as to what we are here for. If you decide to suggest
possibilities and options for the group in order to help people identify their needs or
make up their minds the important point to remember is that you must always allow

individuals the space and respect to consider and decide for themselves how they will meet their needs.

You can promote respect, develop consensus, and facilitate the emergence of a healthy task and goal structure by ensuring that:

- Individuals understand your purpose in setting up the group/working with the group
- Can discuss this if necessary
- Individuals can identify particular personal needs or problems that the group can help with
- Individuals can see how other people can contribute to their circumstance and can see how they can reciprocate
- There is minimum competition and maximum co-operation
- Group goals are clear, feasible, and attractive
- Group goals are relevant to individual needs
- Individuals feel valued, significant, and listened to
- You approach the business of goal-setting, group contracting, formulating pro-gramme, establishing rules and procedures with humour, common sense, and a willingness to negotiate with and involve people

If you have been effective in working with the group at the levels of physical, emotional, and intellectual inclusion members will have been helped to make a decision to belong to the group and the group will feel as if it has an existence of its own. You will be able to tell if members have included themselves and whether or not the group is developing satisfactory levels of cohesion and trust because:

A high degree of cohesion is indicated by:	*A low degree of cohesion is indicated by:*
- Good attendance - Frequent meetings - Punctuality - Stable membership - Members like each other, are friendly, trusting, supportive, open - Members work well on tasks and goals - Group feels warm, humorous, and fun - Members adhere to group norms	- Absenteeism, poor or erratic attendance - Infrequent meetings, postponement, cancellations - Lateness, bad time-keeping - Turnover, loss or change of members - Members unfriendly, guarded, suspicious - Members compete with each other on tasks and goals - Group feels cold, strained, anxious - Members disregard group norms

Review

- Behaviour in the opening sessions of the group can be construed as the interplay of the love and will energies expressed individually and collectively in terms of basic needs for survival, safety, and membership. (Look at Maslow's hierarchy of needs on page 66 to see how his first three levels of need correspond to the inclusion stage.)
- Recurrent behaviour can indicate that individuals are assuming or are being assigned to roles which may be related more to personal need than to the task or goals of the group (see page 69).
- Recognition of the need motivating the behaviour or role is essential if intervention is to be appropriate.
- The group cannot evolve to its next stage of development until its basic needs have been met.
- This requires the leader to work with the group on the physical, emotional, and intellectual levels of its being.
- The leader assumes a nurturing and guiding stance in relation to group members.
- Irrespective of gender the leader assumes the role of the mothering one – the group mother.
- The leader fosters the development of trust and group cohesion.
- The leader seeks to establish structure and consistency within the group.
- The leader negotiates a contract with members that is explicit about the purpose of the group and the ways in which it will work.

  o This group contract functions like a psychological skin to contain conflict and prevent it spilling into chaos.
  o The contract is not a one-off activity but is an organic and continuous task for the leader to maintain.

Chapter 5

Work at the middle stages of the group
Control issues

Just when members seem to have decided to invest in the group a change in atmosphere may occur which can at first be confusing and alarming to the more inexperienced group worker. Previously friendly or helpful individuals may suddenly reveal a less attractive side to their personality. Without warning the worker can find himself under attack, may be sabotaged, flouted, or even rejected; members start to fight with each other and everywhere there seems to be competition, conflict, and rebellion.

Despite the evidence to the contrary, what is happening in the group is in fact quite natural. The seeming chaos is simply another manifestation of the dynamic tension between the love and will energies which are always present in the group. The successful resolution of the inclusion stage has come about because the love principle has prevailed over the individuals' need to pull away from the group. Now the will principle begins to eclipse its twin as members get to grips with what it means to be in this group. The love principle begins to wane as members increasingly adjust to new roles and ways of functioning and start to explore and test collective, personal, and worker limitations and potentials. In other words the group is beginning to differentiate. Having made the decision to join in the group, people are now trying to define and formalize relationships, mark out boundaries, and create a social structure.

This period is called the *control stage* because the problems of status, rank, competition, power, influence, and authority become dominant issues. The control stage represents a crucial period of transition from a less intimate to a more intimate system of relationships within the group and, strange as it may seem, the way in which intimacy is established is through competition and the struggle for leadership.

Underlying interaction at this stage are two central issues which each individual eventually has to confront:

- How much influence can I exercise in this group?
- How much personal autonomy do I have to give up to be in this group?

These two concerns generate the following types of questions in the minds of members:

- *The others*: Who are the influential and powerful members? Who is the most powerful? Where do I fit in? How much power have I got? Can I get more? What is the currency or medium for power and influence? Do I have to fight anyone here? How can I get on the winning side? Who should I support here?
- *The limits*: What are the rules in this group? Do I agree with them? Can I change them? Who makes the rules? What will happen if I break them? What sanctions and

penalties are there? Who makes the decisions in this group? Will I be involved? How much will I be involved?

- *The leader.* Can I trust him? Is he dependable, reliable? Can he maintain control in the group? How will he handle conflict? Is he strong or weak? What will he do if I break the rules? Does he have favourites? Does he like me? Will he intervene in time?

During this stage of group life each group member experiences anxiety and tension about whether they have too much or not enough power and influence and whether they have too much or not enough personal freedom. In order to minimize this anxiety each group member behaves in a way which will create the degree of influence and autonomy that is most comfortable for him. This behaviour tends to be directed towards the leader and other group members, who can often experience these actions as skewed and distorted if not openly destructive.

The inexperienced group leader and members may react to attack or threat by fighting back or fleeing from the scene, succeeding often only in exacerbating the situation. The more experienced leader comprehends the 'fight or flight' nature of group behaviour and intervenes appropriately.

In some groups the actual period of disintegration may be slight and after spending some time exploring its functioning a group may make the necessary adjustments to its structure or goals and move on with its work. In other situations the struggle may be protracted or unresolved and the group can get stuck at this stage, regress to the previous stage, or in some extreme instances terminate. Before we go on to examine ways in which the worker can facilitate the group let us identify some of the more typical behaviours to be found at the control stage:

Moving away from or against other members (Will principle)	*Underlying needs and motives*
• Absences, lateness • Silence • Avoidance of issues/members • Selfishness, refusal to share, compromise • Walking out of group • Drop-outs, ending of membership • Verbal or physical violence • Scapegoating, blaming others, excluding • Emergence of powerful or aggressive members • Monopolizing, dominating, character assassination • Development of subgroups, cliques, alliances • Power struggles, jockeying for position, rivalry, competition, plots, conspiracies • Questioning, belittling the group	• Need to be valued, esteemed • Fear of being rejected • Need to exercise power, influence • Fear of being dominated, attacked, oppressed • Need to be separate, autonomous, independent • Need to protect self from more powerful members • Need to run away – engage in flight activity • Need to attack as a way of asserting, maintaining, or defending self • Need to join with other more or less powerful members • Need to determine rank, status position within the group

Moving away from or against the leader (Will principle)	Underlying needs and motives
• Direct or indirect verbal attack • Sabotage, undermining authority, rebellion, flouting rules • Trying to provoke leader into anger, disapproval, rejection • Searching for evidence of inconsistent behaviour • Trying to get leader to side with an individual, subgroup • Looking for evidence of favouritism, special treatment • Testing leader's commitment to group goals, contracts, rules	• Need to know leader can be trusted, relied on for protection, is competent • Fear that leader will not be able to prevent group from disrupting completely • Is the leader strong or weak? • Is he clear about his values? • Need to know what the leader's limits are • How much rebellion will he permit? • How much control will he allow members over their own affairs? • Need to assert self and be independent of the leader • Need to 'kill the father' • Existence of positive or negative transference

Moving towards other group members (Love principle)	Underlying needs and motives
• Pairing behaviours • Expression of sexual attraction • Subgroup formation • Compromising, sharing, agreeing, rules and norms • Consensual decision making • Resolution of conflicts • Joining in activity	• To interact, be part of, connect • To be valued, affirmed, esteemed • To be protected, feel secure, have order, system, consistency, and predictability • To influence, exercise power in a positive way

Fathering: leading the group at the control stage

If the worker is to sensitively guide the group through the control stage it is essential that he adopt a stance which facilitates the needs and objectives manifesting in individual and collective behaviour at this time. Although the confusion and inconsistency of this stage can appear most bewildering to the beginning group worker it is in fact within certain bounds essential for group development as a way of establishing for group members:

- A sense of self-control and adequacy
- An ability to initiate one's own activity
- Competence in the physical, social, and intellectual requirements of the group
- Power, status, and the leadership in the group

The worker's ability to tolerate and permit a degree of rebellion is absolutely crucial if members are to successfully negotiate this stage. Unfortunately many workers do not fully understand what is happening in the group at this time and fiercely resist any attempts by members to diverge from the worker's wishes.

It is worth saying a little about this. In my experience of supervising workers, the control stage of group development causes most confusion, worry, and fear for the beginner and even for the not-so-new leader. The physical and emotional noise, violence, and hostility which can be met with at this stage is often quite frightening to the novice and almost always is construed as a reflection on his personal and professional competence.

Just why it is that a worker comes to see a group's behaviour as a threat to his image of himself as a worker is very interesting. One major factor is that most new workers would appear to have a fantasy of how a group should behave and how the ideal leader should operate. This fantasy has been built up from reading about the successful and glamorous interventions of accomplished group workers. Perhaps the worker has seen films of groups run in a children's home or an American drug addiction centre or has even had some positive experience himself in a professionally run group. When the worker's own ego needs, to be helpful, esteemed, and successful are added to this pastiche, the result can be to create quite definite impressions, assumptions, and expectations of how a group and its leader should behave. Very rarely is the worker able to acknowledge the unreality of the role he has mentally reserved for himself or for members.

Faced with the sometimes ugly and painful reality of the group they are working with, most leaders amazingly prefer to preserve their idealized image and conclude that either something is wrong with the group or that they are obviously inadequate as a leader! Both conclusions are usually gross distortions and most unhelpful to a group which is struggling with very real and substantive issues of power and autonomy.

Frequently I see a beginning worker make one of two decisions. Some workers decide that it is their *personal responsibility* to make the group succeed in spite of deviant members. Since their way of doing this is to make the group conform to rules and the leader's personal authority the result is to initiate a spiral of ever-increasing repression, counter-sabotage, and inhibition. Other workers decide that they are inadequate in the circumstances and not cut out to be a group worker. They may slide into a paralysis which frightens group members who behave even worse in a vain attempt to engage the leader in some effort to direct and control. When this is not forthcoming the group can degenerate into panic, chaos, and ultimately termination.

What these workers are failing to see is that the struggles between members or subgroups or with the leader are an expression of the way in which each member resolves the anxiety and tension generated in establishing the degree of influence and autonomy that is most comfortable for him. Inevitably the style of leading adopted by the worker is out of gear with the needs of members and only adds to the group's problems. What is actually needed is a philosophy and style of working with the group which provide clear direction and control and yet permit a degree of rebellion in which individual autonomy and influence can develop.

I believe this can be done only when the worker 'recognizes and accepts the members' need to see him as the group father'.

Earlier I likened the inclusion stage of group process to the stage of infancy and childhood watched over by the nurturing mother, and, developing the analogy, the control stage corresponds more to that period of adolescence which is characterized by the association and supremacy of the peer group and rebellion against the authority of the 'father', however actual or symbolic.

The world of the adolescent is increasingly the world of the 'father' – the external world of role and responsibility, power and influence, status and prestige. The adolescent is at once attracted to this world because of what it offers, and repelled because it threatens to curtail and inhibit him through the operation of the greater power of the father. And yet each individual finds himself moving away from dependence on the mother and a more introverted world and seeking an image of himself as a unique, autonomous, and influential person. Vital to this process is the way in which the individual manages the significant social relationships of the peer group and the model of authority and leadership presented to him initially through his struggles with the father.

What group members need from their leader at this stage is not repressive conformity to rules or the other extreme of paralysis but the understanding, permission, firmness, and protection that come from acknowledging their need to challenge and seek for power and discover their impact on authority. Put another way what members need from a leader at this stage is for him knowingly to take on their projections and become the 'group father'.

By taking on the role of group father the worker clearly signals to the members his willingness to be in an authority relationship with members – but one which has individual and collective interests at heart. The leader indicates that he will permit members to challenge him for a share in leadership but that he will not allow them to disrupt the group completely. He will not take total responsibility for the operation of the group because that would only foster an unnatural dependency; but he can be relied on and trusted in the struggle for self-sufficiency. As group father the leader will be available to support, encourage, and help each member, and he will agree to exercise restraint in the use of his power in order to help each member connect to their own authority.

There are a number of tasks that the group father must accomplish at this stage.

Role of the group father at the physical level

Using programme therapeutically

One prime way you can influence norms and encourage the behaviours you desire at this stage of group development is through the planning of programme activities (see page 24 and Chapter 10). With some individuals or groups, for example, you may need to provide opportunities to release aggression in a controlled way.

Individuals may need to attain a sense of mastery or control over their own bodies or the environment. Activities such as chess, dance, art, or craftwork can satisfy this need and prevent its manifesting in the form of bullying or vandalism. Members' needs to compete, test authority, or overwhelm can be carefully channelled with a little thought or simply by asking the group what they could do.

I have indicated in the previous section how you can promote problem-solving and decision-making skills by using simulations and exercises, and you can, for example, cultivate sharing or co-operation by increased use of teamwork or activities which directly reward shaping behaviours. In another situation you may decide that the conflict or chaos in the group is a result of poor or inadequate communication skills. You can then devise a sequence of activity which will aim to build up the required repertoire. This need not be as complicated as you may think. A game like mimes or charades can be very effective in developing attending and concentration skills and non-verbal ability in a fun way.

The worker's role in this phase is to help group members to begin to relate to each other in an increasingly sophisticated and considerate manner. Since members need assistance to do this in most groups you need to give time to planning how you will use the programme to deal with the particular problems or conflicts that crop up. But do not feel that this is *your* responsibility exclusively. It is also important to help members perceive that group experience is something which they can modify in some degree to achieve particular ends and outcomes.

Role of the group father at the emotional level

Permit what is happening to occur

We have seen this before (see page 91). Do not assume that you always have to intervene in an argument or fight between members or that you must always respond to provocative behaviour. It is vital that you are on guard against taking responsibility which belongs to the group, particularly when the limits and boundaries are being tested. Often members will attempt to induce you to act in an authoritarian way which will allow them to slide along relatively uninvolved or force you to structure or set the limits.

Acknowledge that you can see something happening. Let them know you have got the message but do not necessarily jump in. Let the situation develop a little if you can, in order to see what is really going on or to think about an appropriate response. By allowing what is happening, you encourage members to express themselves more freely and indicate that you expect them to begin assuming more responsibility for themselves and negotiate their own solutions.

Provide protection and support where necessary

Clearly there are times when what is occurring in the group is actually or potentially hazardous or injurious. In these instances you may decide that it is appropriate for you to intervene in order to assure the physical or emotional safety of an individual or the group. While you might attract ridicule or hostility for your intervention usually the group is secretly quite relieved and reassured that you are prepared to come to someone's aid.

When members know that you can be relied on in these times of crisis or emergency they are encouraged to be more open and take greater risks in relationship. This has major implications for the development of a more respectful and egalitarian structure in the group since the presence of appropriate protective controls tends to inhibit jungle law and the emergence of hierarchies.

A situation which often appears to demand the use of protective controls is the presence of a scapegoat in the group. Before rushing in to protect the scapegoat it is important to evaluate the situation thoroughly if you are not to actually make it worse.

Scapegoating usually involves the displacement or transfer of anger from its real object onto a weaker and more acceptable target. Much scapegoating occurs in groups where members do not feel able or safe to attack the leader and so they vent their anger on a weaker member. Certain members seem to be more likely to be scapegoated than others:

- Anyone who emphasizes their difference from other people whether it be through sickness, weakness, or superiority or because of gender, culture, religion or ethnicity
- Anyone who openly expresses what the group is trying to avoid
- Anyone who provokes in a manner inviting attack or victimization

While these people attract hostility in their own right they are often attacked only because members are reluctant to direct their anger to where it really belongs. So when preparing to protect or support a scapegoat check to see if you are in actuality the real target of aggression or whether anger should be redirected towards a very dominant or able group member. If this is the case it might be more appropriate to describe what you think is really happening. In this way you can help the group express itself more realistically and then begin to help the involved parties understand the curious and ambiguous relationship between victim and persecutor.

In other situations you can protect and support in subtle ways. Shy people or members who find it hard to speak up can be more easily encouraged if you sit facing them where you can give them non-verbal cues without interrupting the conversation. You can support those people who want to be thought of as leaders in the group by sitting close to them. Applaud and compliment people when they deserve it and try to praise the act rather than the person as this comes over much more sincerely and avoids embarrassment and confusion.

Members can very easily get depressed and discouraged at this stage and will often ask if they are the worst group you have ever worked with or whether you consider them bad or even mad! While they may or may not be the all-time low, it is important that you reassure them that their struggles and conflicts, questions and doubts are really quite natural at this period in a group's life. Only then can you begin to refocus their attention and get them to look at the underlying power issues which so strongly motivate their behaviour.

Role of the group father at the intellectual level

Clarify the issues when you intervene

In deciding whether to intervene in a particular situation try as far as possible to understand the needs and motives of the people concerned and the position of the group so that you can focus on what is really happening (see page 91). Much behaviour is an individual or collaborative manoeuvre to engage the leader, avoid involvement, or appear significant and it will be important to address the deeper meanings of these actions if members are to begin to express themselves more appropriately and articulately.

Whether you know what is happening or not you may sometimes feel that you just have to act immediately to prevent or proscribe behaviour but usually most situations will, on reflection, allow you several other choices.

- You can allow the situation to continue in the expectation that other members will eventually become so impatient, bored, or restless that they will deal with it. You can then intervene or not to examine what was taking place and promote insight and learning
- You can ask the group why they are letting this situation develop
- You can ask the people involved what it is that they really need in the group at this time
- You can ask the people involved and the group to help you look at what is happening

Any one of these choices will help to focus the group on the *process* of their interaction and begin to identify and articulate the real issues of concern for the group.

Although Chapter 9 contains suggestions on how you might teach a group to analyze its own process at any period of its life I think it would be valuable to look at a simple sequence which will help you clarify the various issues at the control stage. Obviously it will help if you have carefully cultivated throughout an attitude that difficulties and differences are natural and that group members should be concerned for each other and willing to stay with problems and work them out.

- A situation may recur or be identified which you believe needs to be properly explored. Try to identify a specific behaviour or pattern that you can focus on: a particular conflict; repeated avoidance and distraction by members when asked to concentrate on a topic; flouting of a certain rule, or belittling the purpose of the group.
- Identify who is involved and when:

  o One individual versus another
  o An individual versus you, the leader
  o An individual versus a subgroup/whole group
  o Subgroup/group versus you

- Identify the needs and the values *you* wish to preserve at this time. Here are some of them:

  o You need to provide good leadership
  o You need to maintain the group's well-being
  o You need to help the group be productive
  o You need to protect standards

- Try to identify the needs and values of the participants. They will centre upon:

  o Members' need to be affirmed as worthwhile
  o Members' need to be accepted and included
  o Members' need for influence
  o Members' need for autonomy

- Try to find some needs or values that you and the people concerned have in common.
- Decide if it is appropriate for you to intervene.
- Make a short statement about what you see happening. You might want to say how you feel about this, or what effect you see this behaviour having on the group. Talk about the values you have in common and say *why* you want to look at what is happening. Try to give people reasons to say *yes* to you – reasons that are to their or the group's advantage.
- Ask if people are prepared to look at the issues involved. When doing this try to ask questions which will engage people and elicit a 'yes' answer: 'You do want the group to work, don't you?' 'You want to get on with the activity, don't you?' 'You want to enjoy the group, don't you?' If people are unwilling to look at the issues don't push it at this stage because you might only exacerbate the situation or build opposition. Leave this responsibility with the group, knowing that they may change their mind or more likely the situation will recur again. Situations which are unfinished nearly always recur in the group and the next time you can legitimately put out some ultimatums.

If you decide to issue an ultimatum, place it firmly in the context of the group contract that everyone agreed to. I find this a very effective way of depersonalizing the situation and invoking powerful reasons why this episode should be concluded. People find it very difficult to keep avoiding when you balance the issue against the purpose of the group or a contract that they freely entered into.

- Assuming you have agreement to explore the issue, invite contributions towards a mutual definition of the problem. Avoid tendencies to make the issue personal, blame others, or seek revenge. Try to get people to make statements about what they really *need* in the situation and watch for openings that permit you to respond to people's needs.

- Help the group consider the consequences of the behaviour in terms of costs and gains. This is important if you are to encourage members to identify the desirable or undesirable outcomes and make agreements or decisions about what to do.

Do not be discouraged if you find that events occur too quickly or explosively in your group for you to use this model as you might like. Members may resist or you may find it nearly impossible to identify your own needs in the situation let alone theirs! With practice, and most importantly, by continually expecting group members to work on their problems you will find that you and the group are increasingly able to disengage from the struggle and begin to work more creatively on areas of common concern.

Encourage effective problem solving

Many groups founder at the control stage because they are unable or unwilling to resolve their problems.

Some of the reasons for this are:

- Lack of clarity in understanding the problem
- Lack of clarity in presenting the problem
- Not enough information
- A critical, overly evaluative, or competitive climate
- Interpersonal conflict or tension
- Pressures to conform
- Lack of motivation or interest
- Haste, urgency, or fear
- Ineffective or immature problem-solving skills
- Lack of leadership

Part of the role of the worker as group father is to inculcate in the group those norms and values which support the collaborative resolution of problems and difficulties. You must be explicit in your expectations that members will agree to seek solutions to their problems and will concur that a threat or difficulty for even one member immediately becomes a *community affair* involving the collective well-being. Only if these attitudes are present will the group be motivated enough to focus on their affairs.

Often I find that a group needs assistance or training in order to use inquiry and problem-solving methods to advantage. In these situations I use a simple five-stage model to teach the group the necessary processes:

1	Identifying the problem
2	Analysing the problem
3	Drawing up alternative strategies
4	Selecting a strategy
5	Evaluation

These stages can be very effectively taught by doing a 'force-field' analysis on a particular problem. Basically what this means is that most problem situations can be understood in terms of forces that push towards improvement and forces which hinder this movement. By identifying the 'helping' forces and the 'restraining' forces it is possible to generate a number of points which will permit intervention in order to produce change.

The most difficult part of the whole problem-solving process for the group is making a clear, reliable, and accurate statement of the problem. The discussion in the previous section on how to clarify the issues in a particular situation will help you negotiate an agreed definition of the problem and elicit a commitment to work on it.

The next step is to conduct the force-field analysis in order to determine the nature and magnitude of the various forces involved in the problem. To do this, involve the group in making lists of all the restraining forces and then all the helping forces. Try to do this without prejudice or criticism.

Review each list and rank the forces according to their importance in affecting the problem. Identify the more important restraining forces and list some possible methods of reducing or eliminating each one. Turn to the helping forces and make a list of ways in which the effect of each helping force could be increased.

The third step in problem solving is to draw up alternative strategies. Force-field analysis is a particularly useful way of drawing up alternative strategies for solving a problem because it gives three options:

1	Increase strength or number of helping forces
2	Decrease strength or number of restraining forces
3	Simultaneously increase helping forces while decreasing restraining forces

It is important to review the group problem in the light of each of these options and discuss which is most promising. Look for the positive and negative consequences of each option and add any new steps that will expand the alternative and make it more successful. Ensure that everyone participates and is listened to and that those who disagree are allowed to express themselves.

Once all the possible options have been drawn up and discussed, the group needs to select the strategy it will implement. This procedure involves the group in decision making which is fully explored in the next section. In selecting an appropriate strategy the following points might be helpful:

- Select the most promising alternatives and weigh up the positive advantages in adopting each one
- Cost each strategy in terms of time, resource, money, people, etc.
- Weigh up the likely benefits against the cost of implementation
- Try to anticipate possible obstacles and impediments
- Choose the most viable strategy
- Identify and assign roles and responsibilities for implementing the strategy
- Initiate the strategy

The final step in problem solving is to evaluate the success of the strategy in terms of bringing about the desired outcome. Sometimes solving one problem brings other problems into the open and the whole sequence has to be repeated for a new situation. Again the desired outcome may not be achieved and the group will have to develop and try new strategies until they find one that is effective. In evaluating these circumstances it is important to reinforce the idea of problem solving as a process which is continually evolving and unfolding rather than as a static, fixed point affair, if you are to help the group guard against depression, futility, and inadequacy.

I like to foster effective problem solving and provide the group with plenty of practice by combining exercises and simulations designed to develop problem-solving skills, with appropriate difficulties thrown up by their real-life interaction and attempts at achieving the group task. In this way members learn procedures and acquire confidence and dexterity in handling uncertainty, settling their own affairs, and dealing with problematic situations. If you wish to use an exercise or simulation to promote problem-solving skills with your group you can find some examples and suggestions in Chapter 10.

Here are ways to encourage effective problem solving.

- Make the problem specific, clear, and simple
- Make it to people's advantage to solve the problem
- Expect members to be involved
- Discourage defensiveness, blaming, criticism
- Make the problem a communal one
- Ensure everyone gets a fair hearing
- Discourage coalitions or alliances which block or stifle other members
- Focus on those aspects of the problem which can be solved
- Make space for members to express their feelings
- Bring conflicts and disagreements out into the open
- Encourage creative and divergent thinking
- Combine ideas where possible
- Summarize the group's progress at intervals
- Ensure everyone feels ready to make choices, decisions
- Ensure everyone feels committed to decision or solution

Promote decision making

Like problem solving the process of decision making is a fundamental feature of group life. In order to achieve anything every group needs a method of determining and setting about its objectives. This is the function of decision making which in its simplest sense means initiating proposals and securing agreement to do something.

It almost always involves a choice between several different possibilities and this immediately creates a power dimension because frequently there can develop a spread of competing desire and interest among members. When we remember that each member at the control stage of group development is concerned with his position and influence it becomes apparent how bound up decision making is with the core issues of power, influence, and authority.

Decision making can come to be viewed by members as a way of engaging in the ongoing power struggles, acting aggressively, gaining in personal significance and esteem. The way in which the group resolves its control issues through the decision-making process in this phase will determine whether or not the group will be able to survive and work in any meaningful fashion and so facilitating and teaching effective decision making is a primary concern of the worker at this time.

There are a number of ways in which a group can reach a decision and each is appropriate in certain situations:

- Agreement (consensus) of the whole group
- Majority vote
- Decision of the member with most expertise
- Decision of the member with most authority

Of these, I believe the most effective method of group decision making is by consensus. It also takes the most time. Consensus means that everyone agrees what the decision should be and feels that they have been involved. Consensus is reached when each member understands and is prepared to support the decision. Even those members who may have had differing views will be prepared to give the decision support for an experimental period of time.

To achieve consensus takes time because all members must be encouraged to state their views and, in particular, their opposition to other people's views. This can be a lengthy and at times conflictive process but is essential if each member is to feel he has been listened to with respect and has had a fair opportunity to influence the outcome. Here are some guidelines for developing consensual decision making in your group.

- Try to involve everyone in the discussion and decision making.
- Look for and bring into the open disagreements and differences of opinion. They are natural and to be expected. If properly used they are very helpful in widening the range of information and opinions, developing creativity and inventiveness.
  Do not avoid conflict and settle for easy options like majority vote or tossing a coin! Encourage people to see conflict as *part* of what goes on in groups and as healthy when dealt with in the open.

- Insist that people listen carefully to each other, accord each other basic respect and courtesy, particularly where they disagree or clash. Avoid blaming, scapegoating, unpleasant personalizing of discussion.
- Discourage rigid and fundamental position taking. Encourage members to explore underlying assumptions and to examine issues and facts.
- Because decisions are best based on facts, ideas, and values ensure that the relevant information is available and people know what values are at stake. In this way members can become aware of the reasons for their choices.
- Do not accept a stalemate position. Look for the next most acceptable alternative which will engage all members. This might mean working through various preferences until the dissenting or disputing factions can find one that offers the possibility of resolving the position with honour and without losing face. At times this may involve an element of *compromise* where each side may give a little in order to progress.

    At other times it is possible to create or invent a new possibility into which both sides can fit and be respected. When this happens the resulting integration can be very exciting and may open up new horizons for the group.
- At all times provide support for any member who wishes to make a contribution.

Decision making is a very dynamic process and one which will involve you closely with group members in sorting out possible alternatives and anticipating consequences. Try, where possible, to avoid making decisions for the group but rather give members as much practice and experience as they can tolerate in handling their own affairs. Members need to know that they have a right to make decisions and that you accept and safeguard their right to autonomy. As you encourage this, decision making will become more rational, less impulsive and egocentric, and more group-oriented.

If you wish to structure part of the group programme to provide opportunities to practise decision-making skills turn to Chapter 10 for some simple exercises and suggestions.

Review

- Control stage of group process is like the period of adolescence
- Behaviour at this stage reflects each member's attempt to establish an optimum degree of influence and autonomy
- Members need clear direction and control and yet must be allowed an appropriate degree of rebellion
- The worker needs to adopt a style of leading which facilitates these issues
- The metaphor of the group father is a way of engaging and activating the qualities and attributes of the will principle
- The worker engages in a series of tasks with the group designed to identify, acknowledge, and resolve the power control issues of members

Chapter 6

Work at the later stages of the group
Affection issues

Following some resolution of the various control issues the group is now usually ready to settle down to work on its tasks and goals, whether this be dealing with the personal problems and anxieties of members in the therapeutic setting or defining a job and making plans to achieve it in the work group.

This impulse towards a more mature use of the group energy and resource comes about because of the emergence of an interpersonal structure which is supportive of group activity and concerned to further the best interests of members. What has happened is that individuals have come together to form a group; they have organized themselves in terms of responsibility and power and now they are ready to explore what it means to be emotionally involved with each other.

We can view the transition from the turbulence of the control stage to the relatively more cohesive and mature experience of this latest phase of group life as yet another manifestation of the dynamic tension between the ever-present love and will energies in the group. Under the aegis of the will principle the important structural issues of power, leadership, status, and position have been confronted and resolved to an appropriate degree. Now the love principle comes to predominate and relationships and alignments between members become based more on personal affection, mutual interest, or other attractions and less on consideration of strength, power, and influence.

There is a developing sense of 'we' or 'us' and members are more concerned to seek agreement or approval from each other than from the worker as previously. You can see this quite clearly in those instances where one member brings along a friend to a session and suggests he is eligible to join the group. The antagonisms and jealousies expressed towards the new person and his sponsor in such statements as, 'He won't know how we do things in this group,' 'I can trust everybody here but I don't know him,' 'Why do you want him here?' 'What's wrong with us?' and the threats to leave the group or be less active if the new person gets in all show the emergence of a new degree of in-group feeling, cohesion, and personal involvement. In other instances the appearance of imitative or idiosyncratic behaviour in dress, language, seating arrangements, and so on reveals more explicit agreement, identification, and group harmony.

As the group assumes more importance for members they work together often and more effectively and in turn this clarifies and stabilizes relationship patterns. With the passage of time there is more open acknowledgement of personal needs and prerogatives, mutual acceptance, and support. Because the group environment is becoming more permissive and caring there is more tolerance of individual differences and a heightened sense of personal identity; members increasingly come to differentiate between each other as unique persons. This can prove to be both an exciting and painful experience because members may be more explicit about their positive and negative feelings for each other and this can generate jealousy and hostility. However, the process of clarifying and coming to terms with intimacy gradually creates the freedom and ability to be different and acceptable if not always likeable.

As roles become more flexible and group energy is increasingly channelled into task activities, you may observe among members a growing ability to plan and carry out projects relevant to the purpose of the group. While there is a high degree of integration, consensus over tasks, and a thrust towards goal satisfaction, there may occur episodic conflicts and dissatisfactions as a result of particular crises faced by individuals. Generally, however, members are more aware of the relationship between group experience and personal growth and are usually well able to work through any crisis.

It is important that you look for interaction which revolves around these three clear issues:

- Being liked and being close
- The quality and satisfaction of work
- Individuality

These issues will generate questions and concerns for members such as the following.

Being liked and being close

Do the others like me? How much do they like me? Are the people I like interested in me? Do I have rivals for one person's affections? How close do I want to be to specific others in the group? How close will they permit me to come?

The quality and satisfaction of work

Do we work well together? Am I satisfied with the way we work and the results we achieve? Can the work be improved? What are the best means of achieving my/our goals? Is the work exciting, stimulating, demanding enough for me?

Individuality

Can I be different from the others and still be liked/accepted? Can I be more myself and still be liked/accepted? Will the group constrain me in any way? What opportunities does the group offer me to explore and discover new experiences, resources, abilities, and skills?

These underlying concerns will manifest in certain typical behaviours at this stage. (See page 116)

Guiding the group at the affection stage

If the inclusion stage of the group is analogous to infancy and the control stage to adolescence, then the affection stage can be said to resemble early adulthood and subsequent maturity in that members are less self-absorbed and more other-centred.

They are willing to give more of themselves, get on with each other, and work co-operatively on the goals of the group. Quite clearly an ethical system, social etiquette, and culture unique to the group can be seen to be emerging which suggests a developing maturity and self-confidence. This has obvious implications for the worker's relationship with members and the scale of his activity in the group.

Moving towards other group members (Love principle)	Underlying needs and motives
• Imitative behaviour, dress, language • Appearance of we/us/our words • Less leader-centred, more group-centred • Emergence of more stable relationships – pairings, triads, and subgroups • Cohesiveness and identity • Humour, joking, teasing • Sharing of opinions • More immediate expression of personal feelings • Confrontation, jealousy • Increasing self-revelation • Increasing self-awareness • Dismantling of facades and images • More tolerant, caring atmosphere • Emergence of other-centred values and ethics: compassion, altruism, idealism, love, service, desire to care/support, religious sentiment, etc. • Emergence of a worldview, growing awareness of social, political, and international issues as they affect group life	• To connect and belong • To be liked and sought out by other members • To be regarded as significant, valuable, worthwhile • To give affection to others • To be of service to others • To be authentic and genuine • To share, support

Moving with or for other group members (Will principle)	Underlying needs and motives
• Increased generativity, ideas, suggestions, proposals • Increased productivity – projects, tasks • Interdependence, teamwork, sharing, co-operative ventures • Emergence of task-centred roles, a division of labour • Flexibility and creativity • Individualism in behaviour, values • Ability to differentiate between members, acceptance of the individual	• To be generative • To be productive • To contribute • To be regarded as • significant and valuable • To co-operate • To individuate

You may recall that at the inclusion stage, members needed help to deal with issues of attachment and *dependency*, and the 'mothering' or nurturing stance of the worker was designed to facilitate this. As the group moved into its control stage the major issues for members centred upon power and *independence* and the worker responded by adopting the role of 'group father' which permitted a degree of rebellion while maintaining boundary and purpose.

Now the members are beginning to explore the opportunities and potential for involvement and *interdependence* and require from the worker an approach which permits and enhances group functioning on its own behalf. In practice, this means the worker begins to move into a less central role and encourages the group to do more of its own work. This does not mean that the worker abandons the group to its own devices or retires, comfortable in the expectation that members should now be entirely self-sufficient. The group members still need the worker although in a much more subtle and sophisticated way than previously.

At this stage of its life the group is increasingly in tune with its purpose and senses clearly the steps to be taken which will fulfil this purpose. Difficulties and crises still arise of course and the group requires from the worker a style and quality of intervention which will direct its awareness and mobilize its energy towards resolution of its problems.

An image which I find useful to employ in sustaining my intervention and activity at this stage is that of the 'guide'. A distinct impression of 'journey' can often spontaneously emerge in the group at this time and may be revealed in behaviour and language such as 'We've come a long way together,' 'Who would have thought we could get this far,' 'We've come this far together, we might as well stick it out.' The idea of the guide as someone who journeys with, and facilitates the process of journeying can be very appealing and helpful.

Assuming the perspective and stance of the guide enables me to create a context in which I can consistently be available to members without interfering or over-involving myself in the very necessary process of the group finding its way. It evokes for me ideas of gentleness and compassion and suggests a style of intervening which aims to stimulate and develop a sense of knowing, of inner authority, or rightness at the personal and collective levels. And in times of crisis the stance of guide reminds me to actively encourage members to open up to a deeper awareness of self and find resolution and meaning by sharing and using individual and group resource.

The central aspect of the guide stance is perhaps the idea of 'service' implicit in the worker's actions at this stage of group life. For me the image of the guide speaks very directly to a quality of 'presence' manifested by the worker with the intention of unselfishly helping the group achieve increasing integration and become more functional. It provides a practical and conceptual framework which permits me to engage and influence the potential of the group for intimate, productive, and compassionate activity in the best interests of everyone.

We have seen that members are less self-absorbed and more other-centred, more generative and productive at this time and it is also my experience that group members actively seek out experiences which bring with them an awareness of human interdependence and the value of loving and serving one's fellow man. Members will look for opportunities and ways of making compassionate responses to each other and clearly demonstrate a need to support and be of service. It is in this area that the 'service' aspect of the guide's role is most important.

Where possible I endeavour to mobilize and channel the group energy and potential for caring and connecting, and model for members a way of being which seeks to serve the best interests of all. In practice, this means that I look for those incidents or episodes which permit me to advance the value of sharing or working together to build a context in which meaning or resolution can emerge, and which demonstrates the lack of creativity and goodwill involved in manipulating or overwhelming each other.

Typically, I engage in behaviour which appears to be:

- Encouraging, stimulating, inspiring
- Nurturing, supportive, allowing

Often these behaviours are less discreet than they appear here and the more common occurrence is a continuum of worker activity that can be said to be distinctly guiding in style and effect. The guide then is a worker who is not caught up in the struggles and striving of the group but one who unselfishly offers a practical vision of how the group can interact and allows members to internalize it at their own pace, build on, and develop it in their own fashion.

I want now to explore in more detail how the worker manifests this 'practical vision' at the affection stage.

Guiding at the physical level of group affection

Intimacy and high group cohesion at this stage can develop out of members working together in a manner which is both satisfying and productive. It is important therefore that you pay attention to group activity and procedures at the physical or structural level in order to ensure that there is a unity between people's desires and how they go about achieving them. Look carefully at your group and ask yourself:

1	Are there clear goals?	Page 17
2	Are members committed to these clear goals?	Page 93
3	Do these clear goals allow for co-operation?	Page 97
4	Is there an appropriate level of trust, cohesion, and support?	Page 92
5	Are there effective decision-making procedures?	Page 112
6	Are there effective problem-solving procedures?	Page 109
7	Is there distributed participation and leadership?	Page 121
8	Is there constructive management of power and conflict?	Page 103
9	Is there effective communication of ideas and feelings?	Page 119
10	Is there a culture which fosters collaboration and teamwork?	Page 109

If you were able to answer yes to each question posed in the box above then you have a successful group and a very effective team of people. If you were unable to answer yes to each question then you need to think about ways of promoting teamwork and the next section will be of interest to you. You might also need to review earlier chapters which cover these various features.

Promoting teamwork

Promoting teamwork in this context means that the group must learn to see itself as a team rather than as a set of individuals. In a team people are aware of each other's strengths and weaknesses and will seek to act in a way which uses their diversity to serve the collective as well as the individual. In a team set-up, problems which arise are seen as confronting the group as a whole and not just separate individuals. Team thinking results in the group seeing itself as a pool of communal resource to be deployed whenever new forms of involvement are required or situational needs demand.

To assess the quality of teamwork at this stage I ask myself two basic questions:

- Does the group have the necessary skills and structures to work together co-operatively and effectively?
- Does the group have the relevant attitudes, values, and norms which encourage and support the use of these skills and structures?

The answers I obtain based on my observations and experience of the group help me to decide how much time and energy I need to invest in teaching collaborative skills or developing a teamwork ethic or both.

Let us look now at some of the skills and values needed to work as a team that we have not encountered before.

Fostering communication

Effective communication is a fundamental prerequisite for every aspect of group functioning. In particular, the co-operative activity so characteristic of this stage demands that people are able and willing to exchange information competently, co-ordinate their actions, and reach some understanding of each other. Usually communication is adequate because the worker has endeavoured to create good communication habits and procedures from the start of the group, but it can frequently happen that methods of communication which were acceptable at earlier stages of development need reworking now. This is because the emergence of more sophisticated collaborative activity requires a corresponding evolution in group and personal communication techniques.

If this is apparent my habit is to wait for an incident or crisis which reveals or results in a fracture of communication. I then frame the problem as one which has implications for us all and as a communal affair therefore requires members to teamwork to find the factors which contributed to or were involved in the breakdown. Usually the group is able to identify one or more of the following.

Factors interfering with communication process

- Prejudices ⎫
- Attitudes ⎬ on part of receiver or sender
- Clarity of message

- Appropriateness of message
- Ability to understand message
- Ability to respond to message
- Defensive behaviour
- Environmental distractions

Having identified the relevant factors the next step in the process is to develop a short programme using exercises and experiential activities to correct any skill deficiencies. Depending on the need this programme can run over part of the session, one or two sessions, or even longer.

I tend to focus on three distinct skills of communication at this stage:

1   Sending messages effectively
2   Receiving messages effectively
3   Giving feedback

In Chapter 10 there are examples of exercises which will help develop these skills but for now I want to present the basic teaching points that need to be conveyed to members.

Sending messages effectively

- Take responsibility for messages by clearly owning them
- Make messages clear, simple, and specific
- Make verbal and non-verbal messages agree with each other
- Look for feedback about the meanings being attached to your message
- Repeat messages until understood
- Make the message and its medium appropriate
- Try to avoid judging or interpreting

Receiving messages effectively

- Indicate your desire to understand the message
- Avoid judging, interrupting, imposing solutions, or finishing the message for sender
- Restate the message in your own words and to the sender's satisfaction
- Check your perception of sender's message
- Negotiate an agreement about the real meaning of the message if necessary

Giving feedback

- Give feedback as soon as you can after a particular behaviour or incident
- Make your feedback concrete and specific
- Describe your own feelings about the event but avoid judging or moralizing
- Look for and allow other perceptions and reactions
- Do not give a superficial answer or statement. If you have nothing to say – say so

While teaching members these skills will undoubtedly facilitate communication within the group it is important to be alert for other factors that can block effective communication:

- Acoustic/sonic levels in room
- Seating arrangements (aim for circle or horseshoe; avoid rows/lines; consider effect of type of seating – hard, soft)
- Ventilation and temperature
- Quality of lighting and mood induced
- Time of day (after lunch/before breaks/morning/evening)
- Proximity of other groups, activities

Once you are aware of these physical factors you can alter them or in some way compensate for them.

Exchanging information

An important part of communicating effectively and functioning smoothly as a team is people's ability to exchange information relevant to the task or issue under consideration. Failure to do so can cause anger, resentment, and separation among members and impair the work of the group.

Very often a group has the information it needs to solve a problem or make a plan of action, but is unable or unaware of how to retrieve the data and put it together in such a way that an accurate or creative solution emerges. I find it valuable with most groups at this stage to spend time looking at ways of encouraging members to be assertive and energetic in eliciting and contributing information and knowledge about given problems and situations.

Exercises can again be helpful in creating positive experiences of information exchange and Chapter 10 gives examples of exercises that I have found particularly useful.

Promote collaborative norms and values

I said earlier that the group should have appropriate norms and values which encourage and support the use of the various skills involved in working together. You can do this by reinforcing such norms and values as they appear through praise, acknowledgement, and approval. Alternatively, you can actively intervene in particular ways to promote certain values and attitudes.

Encourage mutual relationships

If someone reveals a problem or difficulty, ask other people if they share some aspect of this problem. Do not jump in immediately to resolve the problem. Let the problem become a group theme for a while and encourage people to talk about it from different personal angles.

Make confrontation a communal affair

Occasionally you may have to challenge or confront someone in the group. On another occasion it may well be that you draw attention to some of the unspoken or silent rules that operate in groups and make them less than they could be. Try to avoid this appearing as a personal attack on your part:

- I'd like to tell you about something I've noticed.

Point out the implications of the incident for everyone in the group:

- Because I believe it has a great deal to say to each of us about the way we work together.

Present it as an opportunity to develop more awareness or try out new behaviours:

- Perhaps there is something that we have been missing or need to change.

Invite members to explore it collectively:

- Could we take a look at it?

In this way challenge and confrontation become a productive and normal part of group life and something that every member has an investment in.

Promote dialogue instead of monologue

Try to prevent yourself or group members making speeches and sermons. Encourage the art of short delivery. Get into the way of asking for feedback: 'What do you think?', 'Would anyone like to comment on this?', 'How do other people feel about this?' If people do go on, do not be afraid to interrupt and point out what is happening in the group or what it is like for you to experience this monologue.

Look for any opportunity which will allow you to initiate conversation and draw in as many people and viewpoints as possible.

Insist on acceptance and respect between members

Frequently members disregard, dismiss, or undervalue each other's contributions and communications and this can cause bitterness, feelings of inferiority, and resentment. Make it a rule that people are heard out, that a contribution is considered and even if not used, that the member is appreciated. It often happens that in a project, members with a strong interest in the task can be dismissive of others who are not as proficient but may be able to make a contribution at the emotional level to the maintenance and well-being of the group. In these instances it is important to point out the value of maintenance behaviours and demonstrate how complementary the members and their talents are. Maintenance functions are frequently ignored when a group gets absorbed in a project so it is essential to teach the group to respect its need to work on this level and value its experts in this field.

By paying attention to these necessary skills and values you can help the group get a real sense of itself as able to collaborate, exchange information, and co-ordinate its activities. In turn this improves the quality of group experience and deepens the degree of closeness with fellow members.

Guiding at the emotional level of group affection

At this stage of its development the emotional life of the group is very rich, intense, and powerful and manifests in every aspect of activity. The basic theme for the individual concerns his efforts to determine the degree of closeness he wants to give and wishes to receive from other group members. In some situations this is not always going to be what the member desires and feelings of jealousy, antagonism, resentment, and frustration are common. In other instances two or more members may form deep and intimate attachments which, while satisfying for them, can enrage the rest of the group who may feel excluded and devalued.

Throughout, the group has to face up to the rights, expectations, obligations, responsibilities, and consequences of intimacy and the deepening of feelings. Helping individuals and the group negotiate the complexities and demands of interdependence requires sensitivity, tolerance, and compassion from the worker which I believe is in keeping with the notion of guide as it has been outlined earlier.

Legitimizing feelings

People are continually encountered in group settings who are uncomfortable with certain or all of their feelings, and their attempts to deny or block the expression of these feelings not only makes life very difficult for them but deprives the group of power, colour, and depth. These people often feel guilty or ashamed of their emotional needs and experiences and may require some extra help during this stage to open up a little more or manage feelings which are rising up within them.

It is valuable to spend some time exploring the range of emotions available to the individual and encourage people to talk openly about their experiences of anger, jealousy, attraction, and joy with each other. Frequently members will say that certain feelings are positive and others negative or to be avoided. What I often find is that feelings which one might expect to be positive – tenderness, sympathy, affection, respect, and expressions of need and attraction to one another – are difficult for people to allow or express publicly.

It is important to remove any accompanying guilt or shame about these feelings and encourage members to express themselves more openly. Exercises will help but what I find most influential in legitimizing the expression of feeling in the group is my willingness to reveal my own feelings about members and events. I have often noticed that after

I disclose feelings in the group, people seem less awkward and more spontaneous with their feelings.

So do not be afraid to lead with your own feelings in situations. Tell people about the effect the group is having on you. Discuss with members any difficulties you have in relating to them and how you feel about it. Your own relationship with the feeling function, attitudes, and behaviours concerning emotions does determine what is implicitly or explicitly communicated in the group. Members pick up quickly from you what is acceptable or not, so do try to develop both in yourself and in the group an ethic which encourages expression rather than repression of feelings.

Chapter 9 contains a section on working with feelings which contains more suggestions and practical advice. The important point to remember here is that at the affection stage, emotional issues abound for people and you must help the group become more comfortable with its feelings since it is through the expression and acceptance of emotion that members will begin to reach out and come into contact with each other.

Sexual and romantic relationships in the group

Because of the dominance of affection and intimacy issues at this stage you may not be surprised in some groups to discover that two members have become sexually involved with each other. This can be an extremely sensitive area for all concerned and one that can appear to present worrying ethical and technical problems for you:

> - Is this a matter for the couple themselves?
> - Does the group have any rights or interests?
> - What is private and what is communal in a group setting?
> - Should you raise the issue or wait for it to emerge (if at all)?
> - How do you handle such a sensitive matter?

These and a dozen other questions raise issues about privacy, responsibility, the personal, and the political, and tend to centre upon the relationship of the individual to the group. They can impose severe strain on you as a worker because you need to find some way of balancing group needs and individual desires if they are not to destroy one another. Let us look at some issues which from my own experience in this area may help if you have to deal with the emergence of sexual relationships at this stage in the group.

How it is raised

I have experienced four main ways in which members' intimate relationships have come to be on the agenda of the group:

- The couple involved raised it; felt it was important to inform colleagues of their relationship because it affected their perception of and relationship with other members. They believed, rightly as it turned out, that it could affect how other members related to them.
- The relationship emerged as the causal factor when exploring presenting problems of conflict, jealousy, or resentment between some group members.

- I have on occasion challenged when a couple's relationship was interfering with the work of the group through them splitting off in sessions.
- The group would refer to a relationship indirectly through jokes, hints, or comments but were unwilling to look at it directly. I addressed the group's difficulty in finding a way of dealing with their concerns about the relationship.

It is important to remember that the collective reality of the group is such that at some level everyone knows sooner or later what is happening between two fellow members. Unless this is acknowledged and varying viewpoints aired and explored the relationship can become a problem for the group and obliged to remain out of awareness. In some situations the cost of keeping this knowledge hidden or out of the public consciousness of the group is the diverting of a good deal of energy away from purpose and task and this can often result in suspicion, conflict, resentment, and a sense of phoniness.

Carefully watch for those openings that will permit the group to approach and explore a difficulty that everyone knows is around. My experience is that there is usually a pronounced sense of relief when we finally join forces on an issue that has not been openly faced before.

The issues involved

- *The head–heart split*: Group members may be understanding and even accepting at an intellectual level of a couple's right to pair. However, they can often experience great tension and conflict because they also have an opposite emotional reaction of resentment, jealousy, or anger. The psychic dissonance caused by contradictory feelings may be projected with great vehemence onto the couple who are blamed for being selfish and for disrupting the group.
- *Exclusivity*: The emergence of a sexual or romantic relationship creates the perception of a boundary and some degree of exclusivity around the couple whether it is wished for or not. This can generate feelings of anger and jealousy. There may be a sense that the original group has been diminished in some way; that the couple now form a separate subgroup or are no longer as available or accessible as they have been. One or more members may feel rejected and feelings of inferiority and worthlessness may be the motivating energy behind expressions of anger or jealousy.
- *Confidentiality and trust*: Particularly where relationships have a strong sexual dimension, issues of confidentiality and trust become important. There may be consequences for the couple and other members if their relationship became known outside the group and this can affect how open or defensive people are in their sharing and exploration. Similarly, the presence in the group of particular moral or religious viewpoints plays a significant role in whether and how the relationship is acknowledged and in what manner it is received.

The worker's role

The complexities of human relationships are too intricate to be dealt with as if they are simple problems with simple solutions, particularly in the area of sexuality. What you can be sure of is that you will be faced with apparently contradictory and irreconcilable demands from all sides. However, a workable approach to this kind of person versus group situation can be developed by thinking out the needs and values you are trying to meet and preserve. Some of them might be:

> • The need to provide good leadership
> • The group's need to be productive
> • The needs for personal affirmation felt by each member of the group

Extending this thinking to the couple and the group it is apparent that they also have needs and values which they are trying to meet:

> • The need for affirmation of personal worth
> • The need for personal acceptance
> • The need for influence

It is clear then that there are certain values and needs which you and each group member have a common investment in meeting and maintaining. What you set about doing now is converting these values into procedures for action and resolution.

In some situations it may be appropriate to talk to the couple first and obtain their permission to bring up their relationship and the relevant issues in the group since it does involve everybody. Talk about the values you hold for the group and about the values that are important for them. Try to create some sense of the relationship between the couple and the group and their reciprocal responsibilities. Note any conflicts or differences between you that could be amplified negatively in the group. If the couple are unwilling to bring it up do not insist. A situation will invariably arise which involves members' emotional reactions to the pair and this may offer a more appropriate opportunity to look at what is involved.

When and if the matter is brought to the group try to work on the assumption that there are shared concerns and mutual needs which if explored sensitively and thoroughly can benefit everyone. Help and allow members to express their thoughts and feelings and look for opportunities to bring out the underlying issues. Challenge attempts by the group to avoid or deal covertly with issues as this will only increase suspicion and distrust. Above all, do not look for or accept instant resolution. The struggles with intimacy and sexuality may bring to the surface very real and painful conflicts for the men and women in your group which in the end may have to be lived with rather than resolved.

In Chapter 13 (page 257) I mention a group phenomenon called 'pairing' which might be helpful for you when working with a sexual or romantic relationship in the group. Pairing occurs in situations of real or imagined stress such as a change in group membership or a trauma to its functioning and so the group acts as if certain behaviours are vital to the group's survival. These behaviours are like some unconscious and emotional basic assumption that group members hold in common but never speak about. In the basic assumption activity of pairing

> • The group behaves as if salvation will come through the sexual or romantic pairing of two members within the group
> • The group may become inactive as it depends on the pair to do the group's work
> • The focus may be on the future as a defence against dealing with the difficulties of the present. Hope for the future (messiah) replaces actual work or facing the group's difficulties in the present

The concept of pairing is helpful in that the sexual or romantic relationship can now be seen as some sort of communication about the group and you can present it therefore as something that needs to be examined and thought about by the group. The group is using two members to literally join together to solve a problem or create a new possibility or imaginary future for the group. Your job as facilitator is not to attempt to control members' behaviours but rather to focus on them as communications that can be thought about by the worker and members in order to make more meaningful and exchangeable interactions about what is going on in the group. It is important to relate to the group as a natural partner or co-worker when exploring the mutual needs and shared concerns and see it as having an investment in taking responsibility for its own behaviour and success. This difficult and challenging pairing behaviour can be brought to the group's attention and the group is expected and encouraged to manage its own response and think about what the intimacy might mean as a communication within the group. The behaviour has now been delivered from an unhelpful moral perspective and reframed as a psychological issue for the group to reflect on. The following sections will also prove helpful in working with these issues of intimacy in groups.

Foster goodwill

It is my experience that there exists in the group, and particularly at this stage, an impulse to manifest goodwill. By this I mean that members exhibit spontaneous altruistic and self-less tendencies (see also page 232). Members will show compassion for each other, behave generously, and act in a way which demonstrates awareness of their interconnectedness. They may also show awareness of and concern about social, political, and international issues and connect them with events in their own group life. A discussion about the need to keep the group room tidy can lead to indignation being expressed at environmental pollution; consideration of alternatives to exploitive behaviour in the group can give way to revulsion with wars, racism, sexism, and prejudice in society.

If this impulse is not tapped or is in some way repressed, group members can experience feelings of impotence, powerlessness, and shame: 'We should be doing more,' 'It's too far gone,' 'What's the point?' 'I can't do anything about it.' Cynicism and frustration can become a way of life in the group. The impulse towards goodwill is a very clear demonstration of the workings of the love principle and it is important to find ways of expressing this in action.

It can be helpful to encourage your group to meet with other groups through sports competition (although be careful the competitive element doesn't take over), hosting visits, sharing residential experiences, or joint work on a project. Your group might also be interested in working with handicapped or underprivileged groups in the community – children, elderly, prisoners' wives, and the like. Projects to clean up the neighbourhood, collect money for famine victims, or assist in funding a kidney dialysis machine at the local hospital may provide other ways in which the group can express its goodwill, develop a healthy idealism, and engage in compassionate service.

When these impulses towards goodwill emerge, do not receive or dismiss them immediately as avoidance techniques. You must not ignore the necessity of working with group members on legitimate concerns. It is quite natural that as the group becomes more caring and compassionate of itself members become more aware of the pain and crisis around them and move to do something about it. You have a responsibility to guide the group to express their concern in a realistic and enthusiastic manner.

Guiding at the intellectual level of group affection

At this stage of group development you can see the emergence of a clearer direction and firm plans to carry out group goals. It is important that you guide the group by:

> * Praising members' ability to think creatively
> * Reinforcing their ideas
> * Encouraging members to apply their ideas
> * Creating opportunities for members to take responsibility for their plans and ideas

Encourage choice

Members will experience the group as satisfying and assume a greater degree of responsibility for tasks and projects if they feel that they can exercise real choice about the options available. Making any choice is a risky business for many people and it is sometimes easier to go along with the ideas of others. One of my tasks at this stage is to develop in the individual and the group the ability to be responsible and to freely choose a particular course of action. This means that I continually look for opportunities in which members can experience themselves initiating action rather than reacting or submitting to an event. At the simplest level encouraging someone to express his thoughts and feelings about an incident provides him with the opportunity to assert himself in relation to the situation. Even if this does not automatically result in the situation changing it can create awareness for the person that he has his own ideas and has the power to affirm and assert them.

I encourage members to see themselves as involved in an ongoing process of making choices and discerning between options about themselves and each other.

Let me give an example of a favourite method of exploring and developing the idea of choice and self-responsibility in the group. At a suitable time I select an incident or event which is emotionally alive for group members. I then ask the members to form themselves into a living sculpture or a still photograph, in a way which symbolizes the conflicts and issues involved. In turn I ask each group member such questions as:

- What are you feeling/thinking now?
- What do you want to do?
- What do you need in this situation?
- What do you see happening now?
- What would you like to happen?
- What do you think would happen if . . . ?
- What are the possibilities in this situation for you?
- What are you afraid of/avoiding?
- Is there anything else you could do?
- What choice could you make if this should occur again?

These questions reveal the underlying feelings and themes in the critical incident and give a fuller picture of what is going on. They also open up the possibility that the situation can be changed and that people can choose alternative behaviours. It can be interesting to repeat the sculpture or photograph to show the transformation brought about by aware-ness of choice potentials.

As far as possible I try to make my interventions capitalize upon, and enhance whatever choosing capacity exists in the person or situation. This can lead to more mature self-assertion, willingness to risk, and an openness in acknowledging mistakes or the need for help. Invariably this results in more honest and smoother relationships. So do try where possible to devolve as many choice-making opportunities onto individuals and the group as you can. By increasing the number of choices which the group and its members have to make, you encourage cohesion, collaboration, maturity, and self-esteem.

Foster creativity

There are many occasions when a group considering a problem or an aspect of a project reaches an impasse and is unable to go any further. This can cause frustration, tension, or discomfort due to the failure to produce an adequate solution and members may become disheartened and even give up. It is important that there is a tradition within the group which supports the view that the problem is a challenge and invitation to be creative and that with time and effort a constructive solution can be found.

You can promote such a tradition by inculcating values and norms which encourage criti-cal thinking and questioning, reformulation, originality, and innovation. The development of this type of value can be facilitated by practice and training in creative thinking, so do consider devoting a portion of time in some of your sessions to training members to seek out alternative perspectives, reformulate problems, and develop their imagination and intui-tive ability. Brainstorming, for example, is one short but powerful procedure for encourag-ing divergent or creative thinking while involving every member. The next three chapters contain ideas and exercises which I have found valuable in my own practice and which I am sure will help you improve the creative quality and productivity of your own group.

Review

- The affection stage of the group is analogous to maturity
- Members explore opportunities for intimacy and interdependence
- The worker plays a less central role. The metaphor of the guide is useful as a way of encouraging the group to do more of its own work
- The worker engages in a series of tasks with the group in order to develop teamwork and foster intimacy, goodwill, creativity, and choice

Chapter 7

Work at the ending stage of the group
Separation issues

The date of ending for some groups is determined at the outset. The number of sessions or the length of time that the group will run for is established before the group begins. In other groups termination is expected to occur upon completion of a particular task or whenever it is decided that members have achieved their goals and objectives.

However, there are other situations where a group does not coalesce; there is a heavy loss or turnover of members; workers may leave the group and termination can occur. I am not referring to these instances when I discuss ending of the group in this section. I want to look at the natural and planned termination of the group and the separation issues that are part of this stage.

The approach of termination is a psychic shock which group members react to according to their preferred method of coping with anxiety. The group is finishing and the basic issue for members is how to handle separation with the least personal discomfort. Members look for ways of avoiding or denying the reality that their group is to end and when this fails to work may regress to previous states of group disorganization.

At the same time that members are trying to avoid the ending of the group there is a growing acknowledgement of the finality of termination and a willingness to face and accomplish it. However, right up until the final moment there may well be a strong tension between these two desires that can manifest in a wide variety of confused and contradictory behaviour.

There are a number of themes to look out for in the final stages:

- *Denial*: Members may express surprise or claim to have forgotten that the group would end. Members may plan to continue on their own after the formal ending or look towards reunions.
- *Regression*: This involves a sliding back into earlier group experiences and relationship patterns accompanied by increased dependence on the worker. Attempts may be made to reactivate the problems or needs that led to the group being set up originally.
- *Flight*: Destructive and aggressive behaviour may be directed towards each other, the worker, equipment, and activity. People may drop out early or join other groups.
- *Reviewing*: This involves going over group experiences and reminiscing about past events and memories. It can be integrative in that it is an attempt to evaluate the meeting of the group experience and prepare members for letting go of each other.

These themes generate ambivalent behaviours and feelings which are confusions and distortions of the love and will energies (see page 132).

In general, I find that the longer members have been together the more visible and pronounced is their anger and mourning of the passing of the group. A group which has been meeting weekly for nine months will experience themselves as losing more than a group which has met for six sessions. The shorter group, however, will still experience a scaled-down version of what occurs in its older relative if it has at all bonded. So whether your group lasts for a day, six sessions, or nine months you can expect to find some of these manifestations of grief and anger at separation.

Let us look at the role of the worker in this final stage.

Working with the group at termination

As groups move towards their conclusion the worker again becomes a central figure and his major task is to help the members let go of the group and move away. As we have seen, this is an emotionally distressing time for members and can make huge demands on the worker who in all probability is trying to deal with his own separation issues.

I find that members look to me to be group mother, father, and guide all at the same time: because of their anxiety and distress they need nurturing but they also need reminding that there are clear boundaries and limits. At other times, members are well able to contain their feelings and review their work with little need of my intervention.

Manifestations of ending and separation	*Underlying needs and motives*
• Denial that the group is ending	• To avoid separation
• Delaying or prolonging work	• To maintain group experience
• Frenzied work activity	• To begin again
• Rejection of work	• To deal with painful feelings
• Sabotage and destruction of programme and materials	• To punish worker and 'bad' members
• Clinging together for comfort	• To destroy group
• Reduced interaction and involvement	
• Absenteeism	
• Lateness	
• Premature endings	
• Abdication of responsibility	
• Overdependence on worker	
• Rejection, provoking, challenging of worker	
• Rejection, anger, challenging of other members	
• Blaming, scapegoating, finding fault	
• Irruption of unresolved incidents	
• Feelings of guilt, shame about levels of contribution	
• Depression, despair, anxiety, grief	
• Feelings of loss and abandonment	
• Planned reunions	

Here are some suggestions that might help you work with your group at this stage.

Working with the group at the physical level of separation

Members' interest and investment in the group is beginning to wane and your main job now is to emphasize movement away from the group and towards other groups, members' own community, or workplace.

Complete group tasks

Aim to complete and resolve any remaining tasks left to the group and draw attention to any delaying or prolonging activity. Be alert for any overenthusiastic approach to work which might suggest a desire to deny or preclude the group ending. I find it important to be visible with my expectation that members will complete individual tasks and join with me in concluding group projects. This seems to make ending less threatening and more in the nature of a normal passage or development.

Permit activity to become less rewarding

There is a thin line between allowing activity to become less attractive and rewarding and letting your programme collapse into boredom and monotony, which increases the risk of precipitating early withdrawal by members. What you should aim at is a gradual reduction in attraction and interest in activity, as a way of increasing members' motivation to conclude the business of separation and look outside the group for new and more stimulating relationships and experiences.

To encourage this, avoid any activity which challenges the group to further accomplishments such as competition or new projects. Activity which is stimulating, exciting, gives high rewards, or encourages a lot of group interaction should also be avoided. If you find that members are complaining of boredom you may have made activity too bland and it would be important to reintroduce some favoured activity if you are not to force members to leave prematurely. However, complaints about boredom may also reflect resistance and anger about the impending termination. In other instances I have found that the group has naturally come to an end and attempting to continue until the official end is uncreative and tedious.

In some groups you can facilitate the idea of moving out by arranging visits outside the group which prepare members for transition into workplace, community, school, or college. Visitors or guest speakers may be invited into the group to help members with enquiries about welfare rights, accommodation needs, and other points relating to life apart from the group.

Encourage ritual and celebration

I am always surprised at the attitude of those groupwork teachers and practitioners who view the farewell party as contrived, false, and beneath the dignity of the worker. By encouraging group workers to see the farewell party as an immature attempt to deny or sublimate the end of the group I believe we miss something important and deep in human experience.

The ending of the group is a kind of death and will be experienced by many members as the passing of a particular time in their lives. They need to mark this passing in a way which celebrates the importance of the experience in their lives and gives a sense of completion. At the same time they are aware that with the ending of the group there comes opportunity for new relationships and experiences and the invitation to transfer the growth and learning that took place in the group.

All cultures have recognized the pain and celebration, the death and transformation inherent in times of transition and have marked these occasions with a rite of passage – birth, death, initiation and marriage ceremonies and rituals. Similarly the ending of the group is an experience of separation and initiation, finishing and beginning which can speak to something real and deep in us. I believe it demands and warrants its own rite of passage. Obviously this will vary according to the purpose for which the group met, the time spent together, intimacy generated, and so on. It can vary from a party for members in the last session to a drink in the pub or a meal together after the last session. The important point is that you should create an end for the group which celebrates, synthesizes, and symbolizes for members what the group was all about.

If you want to be more prosaic about the ending of the group you can see the ending ritual as a way of helping the group to relax and wind down. Many groups are very task-oriented and minimize or forget the need to slow down, rest, and take pleasure in their labour. Marking the end of the group in the ways I have suggested brings home to members the necessity of maintenance activities and provides an opportunity for informality, fun, and saying goodbye.

Working with the group at the emotional level of separation

As soon as people know that the ending of the group is really going to come they deal with this knowledge by using strategies that often come from earlier in their lives. This can cause a great deal of emotional disruption among members depending on the purpose and intimacy of the group. Here are some ideas to help you to work with the feelings and emotions that are prevalent at this time.

Sort out your own feelings

The first thing to be aware of is that you have been very closely involved in the life of the group. You have been a part of the conflict, the resolutions, and the decisions that were made. The group has been a satisfying, frustrating, exciting, boring, painful, and happy experience for you. You have nurtured members through the difficult and awkward stages of their life, provided them with stability and boundary when they were in open revolt against your leadership, and you have had to sit back and let them learn through their own efforts when you could have done it faster! The point is this – the group is also ending for you and you have your own feelings and thoughts about this.

You may be glad, sad, or a mixture of both and so it is important to spend time preferably with a supervisor or colleague, looking at your own feelings about the group ending. Being clear about how the ending affects you ensures that you do not get swamped or overwhelmed by members' feelings and are free to support the group at this difficult time. Acknowledging feelings of sadness or loss, to yourself first of all, enables you subsequently to be visible with them in the group and model for members a more appropriate way of being in relationship with their own feelings. It also helps you identify the emotional themes that are likely to be around in the group and develop strategies for highlighting and facilitating them.

Deal with separation anxieties

Give members permission to have feelings about the end of the group and encourage them to share these collectively. I try to give some structure to this by building in small sessions where members can talk about what they appreciated in the group and what they resented. This has the effect of bringing feelings to the surface, balancing them, and channelling them effectively.

View expressions of guilt, failure, and incompetence as signs of sadness or repressed anger and do not allow them to be put forward as reasons for the group ending. Allow appropriate levels of grief and anger to be expressed while maintaining boundary and avoid being hooked into punitive behaviour or made to reject members. I find the simplest way of working with such behaviour is to describe what is happening and wonder aloud what is behind it. Members are usually able to verbalize and reflect on their motives quite quickly.

Members may need help to complete unfinished business with each other or find it difficult to say goodbye to each other. It can be useful to spend time in pairs doing this or you may prefer to use exercises in which everybody can participate.

What can often make ending more difficult for members is their association of group termination with other unresolved or painful life experiences of separation, loss, abandonment, and bereavement. It is not uncommon for some members to talk openly about the death of parents or relatives and bring into the group emotional material from these events. Although the ending of a group can activate very deep feelings of pain and shock you should not allow yourself to be frightened or put off by this. You can create a positive experience of termination for your group which can go a long way towards healing and redeeming past endings, and showing people that not all separations have to be brutal and bloody.

As you help people deal with their good and bad feelings you will find that they are better able to accept separation and dissolve the group. Allow this to be a difficult time for members and respond to them with compassion, understanding, and acceptance.

Working with the group at the intellectual level of separation

It is important to help members conceptualize what the group experience has meant to them and be clear about what they are taking away from the group. A major activity at this stage is to create time and space where members can evaluate their involvement and progress. This is a different procedure from the reminiscing type of review that members typically engage in. Evaluation is a structured part of the group's work and has clear objectives:

* To determine the value of the group to the individual
* To gauge progress in achieving individual goals
* To assess whether group objectives were achieved
* To determine what aspects of the group require modification

The particular purpose of your group will determine what you evaluate for and how you conduct this. I have a particular format that I use in most groups because I find it a simple but powerful way of generating meaning, making connections, and focusing members on their future outside the group. Depending on the type of group I am working with I will ask members to write or draw in response to my questions. I preface the evaluation by repeating familiar themes to my group members – the idea of journey, of unfolding, and of process.

- Where have you come from?

  o   What were your goals/objectives at the start of the group?
  o   What were your hopes/ambitions/fears/anxieties?
  o   What was the group like for you?
  o   What were the times of joy/pain/highs/lows?
  o   What did you enjoy/regret, appreciate/resent?

- Where are you at now?

  o   What have you achieved/changed/learned?
  o   Are you satisfied/frustrated with what you have accomplished?
  o   What comments can you make about yourself now?
  o   What would you change/modify about the group/programme/sessions?

- Where are you going to in your life?

  o   What is the direction you wish to go in?
  o   What do you need to do in your life?
  o   What is your next step/goal/possibility?
  o   What do you still need to change/achieve/learn?

- What is in your way?

  o   What prevents you from changing/achieving/learning?
  o   What blocks you from going in this direction?
  o   What are you avoiding/overlooking/refusing?

- What will help you?

  o   What do you need to help you change/learn?
  o   What do you need to develop in yourself?
  o   What skills/qualities/knowledge do you need?
  o   Where will you get them from?

These five headings provide a framework for members which begins to help them understand their experience in the group and creates context, orientation, and perspective so that the group is not perceived as an isolated event but is woven into their lives.

Encourage people to reflect and abstract what learning and growth took place; what personal and interpersonal skills they acquired. This will help individuals view their membership in a more objective light and lessen feelings of grief or sadness by showing how personally beneficial involvement in the group was.

You may wish to spend time helping the group plan more specific follow-up needs. This may require you to be available to offer help after the group terminates or may take the form of a 'reunion' to gauge 'success' on a longer timescale. Be careful that follow-up is seen for what it is and not used as an attempt to continue or prolong the group.

The experience of leaving the group is not an easy one for either the members or the leader so make plenty of time available for the group to work through the separation. Don't avoid or skimp on this stage of the group's life, because if handled well the experience of ending, despite feelings of sadness and grief, can foster personal satisfaction and self-reliance, with members leaving the group feeling that they can make it on their own.

Review

- The separation stage of the group is analogous to death and brings up issues to do with ending, termination
- Members can experience this as a time of great anxiety
- The worker is more dominant in this stage and may intervene as group mother, father, and guide, as appropriate
- The worker helps members to deal with feelings about ending, to review involvement, and to separate

Chapter 8

The foundations of creative groupwork

The practice of groupwork involves a dialectical and syncretizing process and the group worker, if he is to be in any way creative, is required to embrace and reconcile a number of contradictions and opposing truths. Indeed the power and efficacy of the medium is a function of the degree to which a worker can creatively transcend two apparent paradoxes. These paradoxes can be stated in the form of assertions which I believe represent four cornerstones of groupwork practice.

- Groupwork is a rational activity
- Groupwork is an intuitive and spontaneous activity
- The group worker is separate, non-directive, value-free
- The group worker is involved, sympathetic, and committed

Any one of these statements can be acknowledged as 'true' by a group worker who may then proceed to construct a philosophy and operate on the basis of his truth. I have done it myself with each of these statements, at different stages in my career. Increasingly, however, I have found that my practice is enhanced by affirming the presence and validity of all four statements on all occasions.

The process of moving to this position has been somewhat like allowing oneself to be, first, influenced by one ideology and then to allow experience to challenge and shatter it, and finally to transcend the contradictions in a synthesis which unfolds through a new commitment to more comprehensive goals. The experience is confusing and painful and there is a tendency to avoid or minimize frustration and stop the process by adopting one particular party line: groupwork is either rational or it is not; the worker is either non-directive or he influences the group explicitly.

I believe the truth is nearer to a position which is inclusive of the potentials and properties of each of these perspectives. Creative groupwork is able to reconcile apparent opposites and see the complementarity in contradiction. Unfortunately there is a tendency on the part of many beginning group workers to slip into a rational, technical style of intervention which can limit the worker's capacity for relevant response and dialogue and confuses means with ends. In order to redress the balance and show the importance of a supra-rational approach to working with people, the remainder of this chapter is devoted to considering and rehabilitating the more experiential aspects of the foundational groupwork paradoxes.

Groupwork as art, faith, and science

I am convinced that working with a group is more of a synthesis between art and faith than the logically evolved and dispassionate procedure that some applied social scientists would have us believe. While it is clearly essential to have a body of theoretical concepts and technique, I would suggest that groupwork is more than the 'appliance of science', and needs to include and express those other dimensions of human experience.

If it is to be a powerful and humane medium, groupwork requires:

> - That the worker intervene at least as stylistically as the artist who bases his work on intuitive, affective, and aesthetic judgements
> - That the worker function out of a deep conviction and vision of the wholeness, creativity, and possibility inherent in the group, which matches the faith of the believer who knows what is and what can be

I am encouraged in these views by recent research from the field of group therapy which explores the various factors and processes contributing to improvement in the patient's condition.[1] Probably the most famous work was carried out by Irvin Yalom who in 1970 identified 12 'curative factors'.[2] Some of the more important of these curative or therapeutic factors are:

> - *Self-understanding*
> - *Interaction*
> - *Universality*: member's realization that his problems are not unique
> - *Instillation of hope*: belief that participation in the group will be beneficial
> - *Altruism*: benefit derived from recognition that group members can help each other
> - *Guidance* ⎫
> - *Identification* ⎭ worker's influence
> - *Cohesiveness*: the degree to which each member feels accepted and valued
> - An *'existential' factor*: being authentic, taking responsibility for self

I have worked in a wide variety of group settings and it is my experience that these curative factors apply not only in therapy groups but contribute greatly to the well-being and productivity of most, if not all, group situations. I believe they reveal the existence in groupwork of deep taproots into the realms of art and faith and clearly make the point that working with a group is about the creation of a fellowship bond in which the worker cannot avoid being other than an active and influential moral agent.

The discovery of these therapeutic factors seems to me to devolve a special responsibility onto the worker to create just those conditions in the group which will foster awareness, perception, and belief among members and help them achieve their goals. To do this the worker must not only intervene in an aesthetic way but he must also have clear beliefs about the value and importance of what he is doing.

If he is to work imaginatively and sympathetically with people and bring a quality of presence to the group which is spontaneous, genuine, and enabling, the worker must aim to synthesize in his practice many different aspects of the human experience. This is very much a personal and ongoing part of being a group worker and not one that can be taught. However, it can be encouraged and developed and we will now consider some of the basic values, resources, and attitudes that will help you become a more effective and creative influence in the group.

The importance of values and vision in groupwork

These therapeutic factors that we have been looking at really seem to revolve around possibilities in the group setting which are considered desirable. However, while one might desire to include in one's group design variables such as the existential factor or altruism, their inclusion is not something which can be very easily planned or replicated in any setting. If we are to have any regular access to these processes, a shift in perception is required from a mechanistic view to one which allows that groupwork is more than a rational activity and that in its 'irrationality' is revealed a deep affinity with the spontaneity and sympathy encountered in painting, poetry, or music. And at the heart of groupwork, as at the core of these supra-rational activities, is a concern with the transmission of values and the incarnation of a vision.

Values are really what are most important to people and will exert influence on group members to act in their direction.

Values motivate behaviour and give us a general direction to move in. They provide a vision of what is possible; of what we may be. If you have what appears to be an intractable problem, participation in a carefully constructed group experience with its promise of support, care, and opportunities to learn, can provide you with the hope that things may be different and stimulate more creative coping and management behaviours. Frequently the major inducement which a group can offer its members is the opportunity to select and engage with values which will assist and motivate them to change.

This is important news for the group worker. Values create vision and vision creates goals. Our work can only be as effective as the vision and range of possibilities that we hold out to group members. Without a sense of what we may be – a goal to aim towards – members can have no hope; they experience no enthusiasm. So it is incumbent upon the group worker to be clear and thoughtful about the values the group strives to generate and the vision of possibility he wishes to manifest for members, until such time as they can see clearly for themselves.

For some of you this may appear patronizing and even interfering. Frequently I come across an attitude among group workers which asserts that it is essential to be value-free or at the least neutral. The group worker is one who believes in the client's right to self-determination; does not make value judgements and would never seek to impose upon group members. That such an attitude is in itself a value judgement seems to escape its adherents.

With a little thought it is evident that this particular attitude is neither realistic nor desirable. While in no way wishing to compromise the integrity of another person it should be obvious that it is not possible for a worker to eliminate the impact of his own values.

There is simply no situation in a group which does not imply choice at some level of consciousness or suggest that one action has been selected or preferred as more desirable than another. Intervening to protect, support, or challenge a group member, for example, all indicate that a worker regards this activity as having some advantage or value. Another problem I find with the value-free perspective is that it fails to understand that values are essentially self-determined. It is extremely difficult to change another person's value system. Value change will only truly come about when it makes sense to the person concerned. Victor Frankl writing about his experiences in a Nazi concentration camp clearly makes the point that a person's values and the internal choices that related to them could still flourish amid the most savage oppression and duress.[3]

By now it should be clear that I see the group worker as a 'carrier of values', to quote Alan Klein, and like him I see the most important aspect of the worker's method as the effort to help group members 'find their own values'.[4] But if you are really going to help members find their own values, it is necessary that you think long and carefully about your own, since your relationship with group members will quickly and clearly demonstrate what is actually important to you and how you see people relating to each other as human beings. Neither can you expect members to create a personal vision of what is most expressive of them until you have offered them your vision of what it could be like in this group. You cannot even really expect members to use the service offered if you are unable or unwilling to advance your vision of the possibilities and choices inherent in attending the group.

Identification with the worker is one of the primary dynamics for change and it is inevitable that as members come to trust and like you, they will internalize aspects of your behaviour, values, and vision. You cannot avoid being a model for the people you work with nor should you try to avoid this. The most appropriate course of action is to accept with grace and thoughtfully work out a vision for the group which has as its core a desire to help people find their own way. Your values create your vision and your vision can create choices. The more choice you can create for members the more likely you are to be an effective and creative influence in the group and the more likely they are to achieve their goals.

The group worker's deadly sins

From personal experience I have discovered that certain themes recur in groupwork practice. With tongue in cheek I call these themes 'the group worker's deadly sins' as they seem to represent practice 'weaknesses' which can only be overcome by diligence, hard work, and lots of self-forgiveness! In fact these themes represent deep fears and worries which motivate workers to operate in unhelpful and on occasion quite unhealthy ways in their groups. In Chapter 2 we looked at how the promise of engagement in a group could excite fears and anxieties in prospective members. It follows that running a group will excite in workers similar and more fears and anxieties. The very nature of group experience is volatile and challenging and places responsibility on the worker to maintain, facilitate, and contain the group. These demands on the group worker can appear overwhelming, exposing workers to the public scrutiny of members and threatening self-esteem and professional authority by posing confusing and paradoxical questions to do with responsibility and control, attachment and separation, progression and regression.

Because of the complexity and unpredictability of group processes and interactions, permeated as they are by unconscious forces, it is just not possible to run a group without making mistakes and gaffes, leading to feelings of embarrassment and impotence in the best of workers. Many workers can be traumatized by these experiences and since everyone has had some sort of past encounters in family, school, work and peer group which were diminishing and wounding to self-esteem you can see how workers may approach groups defensively and suspiciously as potentially frightening and unfriendly if not actually unsafe places. I have supervised so many group workers who do literally approach their groups like the cartoon lion tamer approaching the roaring lions with a chair in one hand and a whip in the other!

Some characteristics of groups have been identified by Nitsun as creating unease and anxiety in group workers.[5]

- The group is a public arena
- The group is a plural entity
- The group is a complex experience
- The group creates interpersonal tensions
- The group is unpredictable
- The group fluctuates in its progress
- The group is an incomplete experience

In essence what Nitsun is saying is that the group is a public space with multiple opportunities for blaming and shaming to take place and that this can agitate and trigger anxieties and concerns to do with loss of face, criticism, rejection, scapegoating, competition, rivalry, envy and a plethora of social tensions and emotions. The prospect of unwelcome surprises, unforeseen events, and irregularities in attendance can make the group at times a volatile and unpredictable place. The lack of constant and linear progress can give the group an oscillatory or see-saw feel and make members disillusioned and disappointed. Since the group can only deal with a limited amount of material at any time this can leave members feeling dissatisfied and critical of their group experience.

Small wonder then that group workers can take their members' criticism and hostility personally and feel impotent, threatened, and exposed. From such traumatizing feelings it is only a small step for workers to constrain their spontaneity and take up cautious, overly controlling, and correct positions in the group. This desire for worker potency and efficacy can lead the worker to withdraw from a more collaborative relationship with the group and damage group cohesion by making the group's usefulness as a therapeutic or educative instrument much reduced and on occasion void.

Many of the these defensively harsh, unrealistic, even grandiose worker activities are underpinned by what Brightman calls a 'grandiose professional ego ideal'.[6] What he means by this is that many group workers have an inflated professional self-image of how they should operate and what they can do. Brightman identifies three characteristics of this over-blown professional self-image which as we shall see fuel the group worker's 'deadly sins':

- The wish to be all powerful – omnipotence
- The wish to be all knowing – omniscience
- The wish to be all loving – benevolence

This is obviously one dimension of things and is manifest in those groups wholly dependent on a wise, heroic, overly caring leader to guide or curb them. Like a solar system these groups revolve in fixed positions around the central sun.

From what was said earlier we might identify the other dimension of the worker self as a devalued and reduced professional self-image characterized by:

- The dread of helplessness – impotence
- The dread of confusion and not knowing – incompetence
- The dread of anger and hatred – malevolence

Continuing with our astronomical imagery we could say that for the worker, leading such groups is like struggling with a cosmic black hole that sucks in and extinguishes light and life and energy.

Perhaps the most common position for workers involves a continual oscillation between the two poles of inflation and deflation. We shall see the interplay of these polarities constantly at work in what I have called the group worker's deadly sins:

- Power
- Ignorance
- Pride
- Envy
- Nostalgia
- Indifference

Let us consider how these dynamics actually operate in group leaders' actions and orientations.

The need to control the group or the sin of power

The most common practice weakness is the worker's attempt to overly control the group. This is based on two main fantasies:

- The controller is afraid of the group. If asked to reveal his worst fear, it is that the group will suddenly fly out of his control. His unconscious fantasy is that the darker side of human nature will escape in the group, overwhelm him, and cause others to act in a destructive way. He dreads being flooded with unbearable feelings. He is frightened by the number of people in the group, feels alone, and threatened by the spontaneity and unpredictability of group members. So he tries to programme people and events in order to avoid the imminent chaos and searches out routines and formulas which will provide him with security and predictability. Needless to say, those stages of the group's life that are naturally more provocative are a nightmare for him.
- Another type of controller appears to believe that she is responsible for the group and so must do whatever is necessary to ensure that the group is successful, well-attended, and orderly. Frequently this worker is afraid of being blamed if the group does not work out in some way and so she must exercise constant vigilance in order to avert failure. In other cases the worker reveals an unconscious contempt for group members since she is unable to allow them to be autonomous and self-determining but must continually

chivvy them in the desired direction like some 19th-century missionary or imperialist among the colonial natives. Some workers are insensitive to group process and promote individual relationships with themselves and do not stimulate or allow enough interaction between group members. This frustrates and blocks group development and movement and generates a much diluted experience for all.

The controlling worker is usually not very experienced with groups or may have been a participant in a destructive and unhealthy group and their inappropriate parental and controlling behaviour is a way of maintaining order in the face of potential chaos. Unfortunately, this rigid stance often energizes the rebellious adolescent in group members. Most people resent inappropriate control and will react to it in various ways. If this expression is not permitted or its form is unhealthy and immature, a negative spiral of repression and revolt, oppression and sabotage, can ensue with disastrous consequences for worker and members.

It is essential that you work out carefully your attitudes to control, discipline, and authority, preferably in the planning stage of the group – and with a colleague or supervisor – if you are going to be able to 'let go' in the group. You will need to think very seriously about the nature of responsibility. Obviously you have a responsibility to guide, protect, and facilitate the group members but equally they have responsibilities to you and to each other. Members must be expected, and allowed, to be responsible!

The particular purpose for which your group was set up and the nature of membership should largely determine the control levels in the group. If you become aware that you are having to discipline, organize, or control more than before, ask yourself:

- What is going on in this group?
- What does the individual/group need?
- What are they trying to say to me?
- Are the group goals clear, agreed, realistic?
- Are members fearful, unwilling to focus on goals?
- Are members inviting direction for some other reason?
- How do I feel about group members now?
- What am I avoiding?
- What do I need now?
- What is the best way of getting the group to work with me on this control issue?

As far as possible try to:

- Create a situation where people are not afraid to express themselves
- Expect members to be responsible
- Listen carefully in order to find out what people need
- Find and use a common language
- Find any common ground/values between you
- Do something together about the control problem rather than you acting alone

---

The sin of ignorance

This is a weakness for many facilitators and one that is really brought about by a lack of knowledge and understanding of the properties and qualities of the medium of group-work. I find that many novice workers are blissfully unaware of:

- The organic and energetic nature of the group
- The dynamic tension of the love and will energies (members' urge to attach and the urge to separate)
- The relationships between content and process interaction, task and mainte-nance behaviours
- The need to include and work at the process and maintenance levels in a group
- The typical stages of development that a group goes through
- How to match their style of leading to the group's needs at different stages of development

Typically this results in:

- Behaviour being seen at an individual level rather than in terms of group process
- Failure to recognize the need motivating the behaviour
- Failure to intervene appropriately
- Loss of creativity, productivity; anger, resentment, frustration, withdrawal
- The other deadly sins

This is an example of the importance of the rational side of working with groups. With-out access to the theoretical and intellectual knowledge many group workers stumble around not knowing what to look for, influence, or co-operate with. Once they become conscious of the nature, properties, and characteristics of groups most workers find that they are more spontaneous, perceptive, and skilful in their practice. Theory is as essential to working with groups as any skill set. After all good theory is distilled practice wisdom, gathered from close observation and thoughtful work with many groups over time. The earlier chapters in this book provide helpful summaries of the main points you need to be aware of when working with a group and also contain practical suggestions.

Addiction to perfection or the sin of pride

When I first started working with groups I had a strong desire to be a good group worker. I wanted very much to be successful. Success to me meant sessions in which I intervened with perceptive and sparkling interpretations, members resolved their problems, got a lot from the group, and wanted to come back. To ensure such success, I meticulously planned each session. I worked out my objectives, selected the best exercises with care, and consid-ered in great detail the most suitable interventions to make if this happened or that hap-pened. Looking back I see now that my over-planning resulted in a rigid, staccato, formal style that could not cope with spontaneous or unpredictable events.

And sure enough one day in a session a young girl disclosed some detail about herself that I just could not relate to. I did not know what to say or do. The copious session notes on my knee offered no appropriate intervention. After what seemed an eternity, I blurted out that I just did not know what to do. To my amazement the other girls in the group came in immediately and affirmed and supported the girl in a very caring and down-to-earth way. I realized that my compulsive attention to detail and preoccupation with getting it right was creating in me a very arid, unimaginative, and unfeeling way of working. I was fast becoming a technician, a mechano-therapist.

The drive to be a successful group worker and my need to get things right were really a manifestation of that grandiose professional ego ideal that we looked at earlier based on unrealistic and unrealizable fantasies and expectations. I was afraid of being a failure as a worker, looking as if I did not know what I was doing; making mistakes. I wanted to impress, to be liked, to achieve, and above all to avoid the shame of falling below impossible standards. This had resulted in over-planning and a loss of creativity and empathy. It was a revelation to me that my fear of failure and pursuit of perfection was actually slowing up progress in the group, lessening cohesion, and undermining any attempts to co-operate or collaborate. From then on I began to teach myself different attitudes and develop other ways of being in a group.

Much later as a trainer, I found that fear or shame about failure and the compensatory addiction to perfection lay at the root of a lot of the novice group worker's activity:

- Over-planning, perfectionism, fussiness
- Working at a content level
- Avoidance of process work on feelings, atmosphere, etc.
- Self-defeating behaviour – not beginning or completing projects, delays, cancellations
- Excessive intervention
- Preoccupation with technology – video, two-way mirrors, etc.
- Desire for co-workers
- Anxiety reflected in constant course attendance, acquisition of ideas, techniques, 'skills'

On page 151 you will find some suggestions which can be useful in lessening the fear of failure in the group setting and helpful in replacing a shame and pride based professional self-image with a more realistic worker self.

Comparison or the sin of envy

I remember working with a group of teachers on ways in which they could be more creative and informal in the classroom setting. After a time I became aware of a sullenness and lack of response from them. When I challenged this and asked them to look at what was happening, it soon became clear that the teachers were comparing their own work situation, where they had 30 'unwilling' students in classroom conditions, with the current setting where I was working with a polite, 'willing' group of adults. They were contrasting their own fears, anxieties, and clumsy efforts in the class with my apparently confident and proficient approach to them. These comparisons resulted in feelings of inadequacy, lack of competence, powerlessness, and helplessness that were then projected onto me in the form of envious anger and resentment.

Since then I have observed on many occasions how a group worker may enviously compare herself to her co-worker or another colleague. Sometimes the comparison is with a mental picture of how the 'ideal group worker' – a composite of experience, reading, fantasy, and wish – would behave in a certain situation. Sometimes the comparison is triggered by a co-worker's more insightful comment or the group's explicit appreciation of that worker. The consequence of such comparisons is usually the same as it was for those teachers. Workers find themselves resentful and jealous of a co-worker or team member. They feel inadequate, deficient, and may begin to compete, try to impress or dominate. In some instances workers may render themselves impotent or powerless in the group because they cannot see how they could work like 'Dr Jack' or Carl Rogers.

One of the disturbing things about these negative comparisons is that the group worker is often unable to become involved with members because he is convinced that another person would be more effective in his group. The negative comparison activates deep-seated feelings of unworthiness and inadequacy and can create self-fulfilling patterns in the group, resulting in unhappy and frustrating experiences for everyone. If you observe in yourself or in your co-worker:

- Sudden criticism and signs of intolerance
- Rivalry, competition, need to win, achieve, impress
- Withdrawal, depression, loss of interest
- Evidence of feelings of inadequacy, incompetence, worthlessness, inferiority, jealousy
- Panic, helplessness, impotence, powerlessness
- Obsessive behaviour
- Anger, resentment, hostility
- Sudden interest in acquiring skills, attending courses

It could be that this type of comparison and self-depreciation is happening. It is vital between co-workers that this is acknowledged openly and dealt with. This may mean having to involve a third and neutral party. Similarly if you find that some of your behaviour in the group is motivated by jealousy of 'what the previous worker did', or other comparisons, it is important that you pay close attention to this if you are not to be overwhelmed and de-skilled. Talking with your supervisor or another worker can help a great deal. Disclosing some of your feelings in the group can also yield surprising insights and discoveries. As soon as you recognize the presence of a tendency to compare yourself or your group with another setting, act quickly to deal with it because these comparisons can distort reality very easily and release negative energies in the group.

Attachment to the past or the sin of nostalgia

A variation of the last two practice 'sins', attachment to the past, manifests in workers and members, as a nostalgic yearning back to an enjoyable session, activity, or group.

Statements or thoughts like, 'This group isn't the same any more,' 'I wish the group were more like it was when . . . ' indicate a turning away from what is happening here and now and an avoidance of possibly painful but necessary growth. At other times it may be evident that a worker is unable or unwilling to move forward, is stuck at a particular period of a group's growth or endeavour, and is repeating this in subsequent groups. Usually there is some feeling of helplessness or disillusionment operating to deflate the worker and only when this is brought into the open and can be processed can you and the group move on.

As soon as you become aware of this tendency in yourself or your co-worker, acknowledge it and look for someone to help you deal with it. Bring it up in supervision sessions or failing that, try as honestly as you can to identify your fears and anxieties in the situation. See the pattern as indicating the need for your practice to develop and grow. Try to get a sense of what you need to help you move on or face up to a particular issue, activity, or stage of growth in the group, and work out specific ways of changing your behaviour. It can be valuable to share your insight with the group if you feel capable of converting the issue into a group theme.

The truth about neutrality or the sin of indifference

Many group workers like to believe that they are neutral, non-directive, and value-free about the people they work with. I have already said that this latter belief is untenable without its opposite and on its own is in my experience very often the major source of difficulty in establishing effective interpersonal relations in the group and promoting healthy task and maintenance behaviour.

We have here in a very stark form one of the fundamental paradoxes of groupwork and indeed of the helping professions. In offering help to others the group worker must respect the personal integrity of members and must not impose his own personal preferences. And yet we have seen that the very effort to initiate the work with a group is laden with beliefs about its value, power, and efficacy, otherwise it could not be offered or accepted. The worker's relationship with members is a major instrument for promoting change and it is clear that absolute neutrality would manifest as indifference that could only alienate members and at best make the experience a bland and superficial one.

The way in which I try to resolve this paradox is to make it a central feature of what the group has to offer members. I am clear and explicit about my vision of the range of possibilities inherent in the group experience and of the value of this, but I will not impose this vision on people for at its core is a belief that individuals can make choices for themselves, can determine their own reality, and must be expected to assume responsibility for this. In other words I will be involved and will actively engage with members but I will not do for them what they must do for themselves. The group represents a set of beliefs about how people can coexist together but each group and every member has to work out whether this is relevant for them and if necessary create alternatives and other ways of working. I advocate the value of mutuality and reciprocity while maintaining the individual's right to choose differently. I involve myself fully in the process while endeavouring to remain outside it. In the next section we will explore a practice that I find crucial in helping me resolve the paradox of neutrality which exists side by side with passionate involvement.

The importance of right relations in the group

If members are to achieve personal goals and help accomplish the group task they require a healthy environment which encourages them to have intimate relationships with each other and fosters interdependence. Assagioli, who developed psychosynthesis underlines this point. He believes that 'each man may be considered as an element or a cell of a human group' and that the problems which inevitably arise can be solved by creating circumstances in which the different group members learn to work together as one.[7] From this perspective we could see the group as a constellation with all the members interacting and supporting their own particular configuration rather than as the solar system we discussed earlier in which the members revolved around a central leader. In Assagioli's view these circumstances come about whenever people begin to practise 'right relations' with themselves, each other, and their environment.

Right relations is a practice which I find has exciting and powerful implications for work with groups. It includes some of the therapeutic or curative factors that we looked at earlier.

- Friendship
- Co-operation, teamwork, sharing
- Empathy
- Goodwill
- Altruism
- Sense of responsibility
- Service
- Understanding

I use right relations as a way of helping members recognize and affirm the value and uniqueness of each individual in the group; as a method of creating space in which members can learn, give, and receive, without trying to convert, convince, or impose on each other. I introduce the idea of right relations at the beginning of the group and depending on the type of membership, I may use standard trust exercises, or individuals' personal experiences to make a few simple points:

- Relationships are necessary for survival, growth, and development
- Relationship means being a part of something rather than being isolated. (However, being a part of something does not mean being inappropriately dependent on it.)
- Right relationship is about creating interaction and balance between people, and helping members experience the benefits of sharing and working together
- Right relations means being with other people in the way that you would wish them to be with you

In a discussion or review, conversation usually focuses around:

- What right relations means personally for members
- What would block/prevent right relations in this group
- What would facilitate right relations
- The importance of trust
- What values, norms, rules are appropriate in this group

Introducing the notion of right relations at the start of the group is more than a way of dealing with members' inclusion issues. It is the start of a practice that will influence every aspect of group functioning. The motivation which underlies the practice of right relations is one of goodwill and a desire to be in relationship with other people in a way which creates awareness, respect, and acceptance of the needs of both parties. If the group is to be a satisfying and productive experience, right relations must become the ongoing interest and concern. Certain fundamental personal and group interactive skills and values need to be encouraged.

In a group setting expression of a member's experience determines and contributes to the overall flow or process of the group. Withholding self-expression limits and starves the potential in a situation and can activate and amplify negative feelings which will disrupt right relations within the group. I try to inculcate in members an awareness of their responsibility for the quality of group experience and of their obligations to each other. I encourage members to be more visible and express what is happening for them in appropriate ways. Initially this raises issues for members about risk-taking, self-revelation, and the consequences for them and for other people. These issues have to be addressed and I find that being able to present members with a concern for right relations in the group is a useful way of providing a context or framework in which these issues can be worked through.

Frequently communications in a group are diluted or withheld because one person is unwilling to be seen to be angry or hurtful towards another, or because he is afraid of being rejected for his remarks. In these instances I encourage people to connect to their goodwill when they send and receive messages. This can often transform situations and people can give and accept feedback which they would previously have perceived as hostile or wounding. Thoughts and feelings can now be expressed as friendly information with the aim of exploring the dynamics of a situation or looking for resolution rather than seeking to obliterate the other person.

Some members can find it difficult to allow or accept the pain and distress of a colleague and will rush in to rescue the person or fix things up. In these situations I encourage the rescuer to express his own discomfort and become more aware of how efforts to help the other person are largely designed to relieve his own distress. By locating the exchange within the context of right relations it becomes possible for both the rescuing member and the distressed member to have their own reality and uniqueness without one needing to change or disallow the other. Another way in which I use and create right relations in the group is to urge members to check out their assumptions and perceptions of each other. Frequently you will see members assuming knowledge, or attributing ideas and feelings to each other which are not based on reality and which can have explosive repercussions. By checking out what they perceive or understand with the other person's experience, members can remain in some degree of harmony and balance with each other.

Beyond these specific examples, the chief value of right relations is that it provides me with a context or holding frame within which the great paradoxes of groupwork can be contained and lived with:

- Each member is, and is not, his brother's keeper
- Members are interdependent and yet autonomous
- The worker is separate and he is involved
- The worker is neutral and he is committed
- Groupwork is a rational activity and it is spontaneous

Right relations recognizes, affirms, and grows out of the essential contradiction and complementarity inherent in these antinomies. The work, values, and concerns of members, group, and worker emerge out of the tension generated by seeming opposites and the practice of right relations offers a context in which the necessity of each can be permitted and explored without one having to dismiss or obviate the other.

With practice, and continual reminder and encouragement from you, right relations can become a reality in the group, as well as a goal to aspire towards. Gradually members become more active and assertive in the group and the collective experience is healthier, deeper, and more genuine. Members come to see that there is an assured mutuality between self and other which means that the individual member benefits as the group experience is enhanced. Have a look at Chapter 12 for more examples of how to implement right relations in the group.

Creating a realistic group worker self-image

Modifying a grandiose professional self-image and replacing it with a realistic worker self is an ongoing and essential task requiring a willingness to engage in self-examination and a desire to cultivate in oneself qualities and attributes that will serve the group and not just one's own need. What can contribute greatly to a humble but dignified worker self is a correct understanding of two important activities on the part of the worker. Group leaders need to provide opportunities for members to value them without becoming inflated and grandiose and they also need to reflect and mirror back members' own capacities and individuality with compassion and understanding.

The work of Heinz Kohut and his circle musters compelling theoretical and clinical evidence to demonstrate that personal well-being is the result of an empathic environment in early childhood that has the two principal and crucial functions of providing the developing self with appropriate mirroring and opportunities for idealization.[8]

Kohut asserts that empathic maternal attention and caring provide the infant with a mirror in which she gradually comes to recognize and experience herself as a total entity – as a self. This mirroring is crucial for the gradual emergence and development of an enduring sense of identity and a self, which may eventually mature into adequate ambitions and competence and realistic self-esteem. Because of failures or inconsistencies in empathic mirroring, the individual's self may become unstable or disturbed, and there can be a tendency to narcissistic vulnerability and disorder.

In a second line of maturation during the formation of the self, not only does the infant want to be admired by her caregiver, she wants to psychically fuse with the caregiver whom she experiences as omnipotent and perfect and therefore soothing because of the parent's ability to regulate the infant's troubled emotions. In other words, the parent is idealized, and the infant wishes to merge with this powerful and perfect other to preserve her own cohesion and security.

Kohut and his colleagues believe that we continue to need throughout life and search for empathic mirroring and idealized objects and situations to maintain healthy psychological well-being. So this is an entirely natural process in which suitable experiences provide a platform for more mature choices. From this perspective, we can see how many people would be attracted to various group opportunities and political movements or spiritual traditions to create a context for living. Groups mirror important self-images that are essential for a meaningful sense of self, identity, belonging, and acceptance and also importantly provide opportunities for self-identification with and idealization of revered secular, political, and saintly figures. Individuals and groups need and seek out people and experiences which will mirror and reflect their self-esteem and ambitions, and secondly individuals and groups need and seek out people and experiences which will inspire and motivate them.

The group worker as an exemplar

Is important for you as a group leader to be aware of the absolute necessity of your role as a suitable and temporary exemplar that the group members individually and collectively can esteem and value. Some workers may inappropriately seek out idealization and exploit members' adulation as a means of avoiding or compensating for their own inadequacies and limitations. Others may fear being revered and push away or puncture members' valuing of them. Both behaviours are wrong and damaging to the group. You do the group no favours seeking out esteem or prematurely diminishing it. Accept the temporary nature and need for the group to idealize you because you will find quickly enough that the group will move to the next stage of its life cycle and bring you down to earth.

Example of a group needing to idealize its leader

A psychotherapy group was left traumatized by the tragic and unexpected death of its longtime leader. The group did not meet for some six weeks until a replacement leader could be found. As one might expect, when the group did resume the predominant feature of the subsequent sessions was the ongoing narrative of members' responses to the shocking loss of its leader and the ambivalent feelings of affection, gratitude for what the deceased worker had done for them, and anger and hatred at having been abandoned and left to fend for themselves. The new leader was much admired for having stepped into such a difficult situation and for a long time was regarded as a sort of superhero who was really superior and preferable to the disappointing past leader. The new leader was content to let the group idealize him as a way of regaining its shaken confidence and find a way of dealing with the unbearable possibility that he too might let them down. He knew that to refuse the adulation of the group would only plunge them into a hopeless state which would add to their existing trauma. The group needed to depend on a reliable authority which for now would not let them down and could help them hope for a better time.

After some seven months the new leader noticed the members beginning to express the slightest grievances against him and was able to tolerate the lessening of the group idealization as they began to relate more realistically and authentically with him. The leader did not try to defend himself or seek to regain the previous esteem he had been held in. He was able to recognize that the group felt more stable and confident about their viability and that they were moving on to form a more real relationship with him and each other. They no longer needed to persuade themselves and each other of their luck in acquiring such a talismanic leader. In due course the group were able to resume a robust relationship with the leader knowing that they could be angry with him and knock him and he would not collapse.

The group worker as a mirror

It is essential to provide an appropriate mirroring response to individuals and groups in which they can feel validated, see themselves as competent and valuable, and build up a positive and dynamic self-image. Mirroring by the group worker involves an empathic monitoring of the condition and quality of individual and group feelings and self-images. It requires an understanding of the stage of development in the group's life cycle and a suitable and sensitive response. It is important for the worker to avoid excessive mirroring responses when there is little or no appropriate effort or success or merit on the group's part and equally to avoid withholding praise or attention for fear of inflating the group.

Example of how a leader provided mirroring for the group

In the group just described the new leader decided after nine months to introduce two new members to the group. He took this decision because in his careful assessment the group had adequately grieved the loss of their previous worker and were successfully engaged in therapeutic work again. Understandably the group was anxious about the newcomers for all the usual reasons that groups find expansion difficult. But they were also worried about what newcomers might think about them when they heard about their recent history and they expressed anxiety about how they might cope if the newcomers decided that such a group was not suitable for them. It took some time to work through the feelings about stigma and rejection that were stirred up.

The group worker pointed out to the group members that he felt sure that the group was strong enough and healthy enough to be able to include the prospective members, and because of what they themselves had come through and survived he was clear that they could offer the newcomers a helpful experience and opportunity. This was a very powerful validating and affirming mirroring response by the worker and greatly encouraged the group, confirming to them that they could live creatively after suffering a great trauma.

The group as a mirror

Foulkes who developed the therapy model of group analysis likened the group to a 'hall of mirrors'.[9] What he meant was that it was easier to see in others what one could not see in oneself and that over time this mirror-like attribute of the group could result in expanding awareness as members came to recognize unwanted aspects of themselves and accept this without shame or reproach.

Seven centuries ago Dante Alighieri in his great work the *Divine Comedy* describes the ideal group made up of 'each soul a mirror mutually mirroring'.[10] This is a beautiful image to bring to groupwork practice: the idea that the group members can offer mutual authentic and affirming responses to each other and that this can be powerfully transforming and enlivening.

One of the easiest ways to promote the idea of the group as a mutual mirror to its members is to continually engage the group as your co-worker. Make the group your partner in investigation and consideration of its own responses and experience. In this manner you catalyze the rich collective resources and memories of the group and emphasize the practice of reflection and self-reflection and giving considered and empathically attuned feedback to each other.

A realistic group worker self-image

Conducting a group places huge demands on a worker as we have seen and it takes a long time to learn to steer a path between the Scylla of inflation and the Charybdis of deflation and arrive at a place where one can be realistic in recognizing that one necessarily has authority and influence in the group but that there are limits to one's power and knowledge and compassion. Eventually one realizes that group members do not learn from the leader only but receive emotional support, understanding, and education from each other. Groupwork is revealed as a powerful method of intervention and change when the group worker understands that the job is really to build and serve the group.

- You are not responsible for providing right answers or even any answers to problems
- Do not refuse the role of expert: members need to esteem and believe in you
- Avoid being cast in the role of permanent expert
- Explore members' experiences of failure and identify favourite ways of avoiding, coping, hiding. Identify idealized self-images, parental and self-expectations that contribute to a fear of failure or preoccupation with success
- See more in the group and its members than they can see in themselves
- Believe in and cultivate a collective or group wisdom which can be called on
- Insist on a communal approach to work, teambuilding, problem solving
- Develop and encourage values and norms which emphasize and allow the creative and positive aspects of failure, risk-taking, decision making, spontaneity and intuition, compassion, forgiveness
- See the work of the individual or group as an ongoing process rather than a static project. Work more with process levels of experience
- Do not hide your mistakes in the group. Use them as an opportunity to model new behaviours and develop suitable norms

Review

- Groupwork is an activity which arises out of the acknowledgement and synthesis of contradictions and opposing truths
- Groupwork is a supra-rational activity which involves intuitive, subjective judgements as well as rational, technical prescriptions
- There are a number of curative factors or values which must be present if the group is to be effective
- Values create vision and vision creates goals
- The group worker must be a carrier of values while aiming to help members find their own values
- The group worker is an exemplar, model, visionary
- There are common practice weaknesses to be recognized and overcome
- It is important to establish right relations in the group as a practical reality, a goal/vision to aspire towards, and a context in which the paradoxes of groupwork can be reconciled
- Be alert to the presence of grandiose or inflated views about groups or your role as leader
- Be alert to the presence of deflated and diminishing views about groups and your role as leader
- Accept the importance of providing a suitable and temporary exemplar who can be esteemed and valued
- Look for appropriate opportunities to mirror individual and group strengths and capacities

References

1   Butler, T. and Fuhriman, A. (1983) 'Curative factors in group therapy: a review of the recent literature', *Small Group Behaviour*, 14, 2: 131–42.
2   Yalom, I.D. (1970) *The Theory and Practice of Group Psychotherapy*, New York: Basic Books.
3   Frankl, V. (1963) *Man's Search for Meaning*, New York: Pocket Books.
4   Klein, A.T. (1972) *Effective Groupwork*, New York: Association Press.
5   Nitsun, M. (1996) *The Anti-Group: Destructive Forces in the Group and Their Creative Potential*, London: Routledge, pp. 48–54.
6   Brightman, B. (1984) 'Narcissistic issues in the training experience of the psychotherapist', *International Journal of Group Psychotherapy*, 10: 293–317.
7   Assagioli, R. (1980) *Psychosynthesis: A Collection of Basic Writings*: 131, Wellingborough: Turnstone Books.
8   Kohut, H. (1977) *The Restoration of the Self*, Chicago, IL: University of Chicago Press.
9   Foulkes, S.H. (1964) *Therapeutic Group Analysis*. London: Maresfield.
10 Alighieri. D. (1320) The *Divine Comedy*, Purgatorio Canto XV, Line 78, in *The Portable Dante* (ed M. Musa), New York: Penguin, 1995.

Chapter 9

The skills of creative groupwork

Creative groupwork is a phrase that I use to describe the means by which a worker creates the psychological space necessary for the range of possibilities inherent in his vision of the group to emerge, and intervenes in a way which affirms members and facilitates the achievement of the group purpose. Here are some examples of what might be termed creative groupwork:

- Being able to work intuitively and imaginatively when familiar or traditional approaches do not seem appropriate in a situation
- Feeling comfortable working at different levels of the group experience at the same time
- Being able to work with process to help individuals or the group when stuck, flat, or tense
- Working effectively with feelings
- Using a variety of techniques to work through difficult situations in the group
- Developing the practice of right relations
- Knowing when to leave a task or programme to deal with process or maintenance issues
- Helping members articulate and work at their own operating principles rather than imposing a structure or vision upon them
- Helping members see the consequences of their behaviour, developing options, creating choice
- Encouraging the resolution of interpersonal conflict in a way which does not negate either party

If you consider this list it is clear that there are three major skills which the group worker uses to engage the group with imagination and sympathy:

- Use of self as a model or exemplar
- Perceiving what is happening in the group and aligning with, or encouraging certain values, norms, behaviours
- Providing structure and experiential work which will foster and train desirable behaviour and attitudes

These skills are not new to us. In the last few chapters we have looked in detail at how you may use these practice behaviours or some combination of them in different situations. Now I want to consider them in relation to four activities that you are most likely to need to develop in your work with groups.

> - Working with feelings
> - Teaching members how to maintain themselves
> - Teaching members how to analyze group process
> - Working with difficult situations

Working with feelings

In some ways feelings are the common denominator between people in a group setting. Unconsciously each member is preoccupied with feeling states: wanting to feel happy, good, approved of, and well-regarded; feeling bad or rejected and wanting to change that. Much of the colour, diversity, and richness of group life is provided by the feeling tone of members' interactions. This is because feelings and emotions are multidimensional, containing instinctual elements, intuition, physical and sensational experience, as well as an evaluative aspect.

Frequently members of a group may have difficulty expressing their feelings about events or situations. You can observe two main patterns.

> - Members keep a tight rein on their feelings because they are afraid things will get out of control or because they see expression of feelings as weak and immature. These members do not trust feelings and try to avoid them either by consciously suppressing or unconsciously repressing them. However, unwanted feelings do not just disappear. They continue to try to enter awareness and behaviour directly or covertly and they often encounter more opposition. The result may be an unhealthy group with a flat, dead feel, or a tense, anxious group where things seem to be constantly simmering but never actually coming to the boil.
> - When feelings are revealed they may be poorly or inappropriately expressed. Some members can express lots of feelings but in ways which alienate other people or disrupt group activity. One person may flare up at the least imagined slight, while another may sulk or cry at the drop of a hat.

The unhealthy thing about both of these patterns is that through a process of amplification, members can be invaded by other people's unexpressed or inappropriate feelings. This can result in a distorted perception of reality, intolerance, confusion, and hysteria. Feelings can enrich and enhance interpersonal life but all too often they disrupt it with conflict and grief. It is essential that you help members be more straightforward with their feelings if emotions are not to stand in the way of better relationships in the group. You need to teach members how to ask directly for what they want and to express appropriately what they like and dislike. Here are certain guidelines that I find useful for helping people work with feelings in the group.

Feelings are OK

In Chapter 5 I talked about legitimizing feelings and there is not much more to add. The important thing is that you help people recognize that experiencing feelings and emotions is an integral part of being human. No one has to apologize for having feelings. It is really how we act and behave around our feelings that makes them negative or positive.

Become aware of feelings

Often a group member may be unaware of what feelings he is experiencing and in some cases how to define them. It is important to draw attention to this because recognizing that he has thoughts and feelings about a situation can help an individual be less passive and more active in the group. Sometimes a simple question, 'How are you feeling right now?' is enough to evoke awareness. At other times drawing attention to visible cues and body language is valuable.

> - What are you doing with your fists?
> - You seem to be holding your breath
> - I notice that you are drumming your fingers
> - I see you're looking worried

Once a feeling has been recognized I often ask a few more questions as a way of evoking greater understanding and experience of the feeling and helping to release some of its energy.

> - Where in your body do you experience this feeling?
> - What does that suggest to you?
> - If your feeling had a voice what would it say?
> - What image does this feeling suggest?
> - Can you become this image in your imagination, speak, act, behave as this image?

Accept responsibility for your own feelings

Difficult or irrational feelings do not go away by being censored or denied. They go away by being recognized, accepted, and worked through. In groups people have many different ways of not taking responsibility for their own feelings. Three of the most common are:

> - Blaming others
> - Projecting onto others
> - Distancing feelings

Frequently you will observe one member blame you or other colleagues for how they are feeling:

> 'If you hadn't insisted on talking about this, I wouldn't feel depressed now.'
> 'All this group does is talk about unhappy things. It makes me really angry.'

Usually what is happening here is that the person has been bottling up a particular feeling and the discussion has brought up emotions that he would prefer not to be aware of. It is important that you point out to the individual that such contact with someone who makes him angry or depressed is often because he is feeling this way already. Invite the person to explore what he is feeling and help him get it out of his system.

Watch out for people blaming others for what they are feeling. This often indicates a personal difficulty with a particular feeling and a need to reject or avoid it.

Try to use blaming situations to help people identify feelings that they find difficulty in expressing, as a way of improving and developing interaction in the group. Some of the more difficult feelings for people in groups are:

- Feelings of being no good/inferior/not able to do things
- Not being able to handle affection/interest from others
- Feelings of being dependent on a person/attracted/interested in someone
- Feelings of being hurt/rejected/vulnerable/visible
- Guilt/shame
- Helplessness/powerlessness
- Being angry/wanting to punish/hurt

Another way that people in groups avoid taking responsibility for their feelings is to attribute or project onto other people qualities or emotions which in fact belong to them (see page 201). Whenever I hear people making critical comments towards others I generally ask them if they can own some of the statement for themselves. In other words I ask them to consider if there is anything in their statement which could possibly apply to themselves. Very often the initial remarks can change drastically when the person takes responsibility for what he really feels instead of projecting it onto other people.

Statements like:	*Can be more honestly expressed:*
- You're always angry with me	- I'm angry with you
- You're always showing off	- I want some attention too
- You confuse things in the group	- I'm jealous of the way you get what you want in the group

People may distance their feelings by disguising them in question form: 'Does anyone feel angry about this?' usually means 'I feel angry about this.' 'I wonder if you're annoyed with me?' really means 'I feel upset/anxious/angry that you are upset/anxious/angry with me.' I strongly discourage people asking this sort of question in the group because members are seldom requesting information but really masking their own experience.

Many questions start from a hidden agenda and can be put in the form of a statement which is more explicit and less open to game playing. Another form of distancing feelings is to use 'it' or 'we' instead of 'I'. 'The group feels tense' decodes as 'I feel tense.' 'We don't seem to be in great form today' translates as 'I feel down today.'

It is important to challenge any attempt to avoid or disown feelings in the group. First, because helping members own their feelings is to encourage them to be more powerful and responsible in the group. People can quickly learn to stick up for their emotional rights in the group and to be assertive without invading others or being deprived themselves. Second, accepting responsibility for our feelings allows the feeling to exist and therefore to change. Feelings are not static or permanent unless they are disallowed in which case they become chronic. Feelings are naturally transient, and if allowed and accepted will change appropriately. This is a prominent feature of the therapy group, where unacceptable or frightening feelings are often seen to dissipate when encountered and accepted, and a feature that I try to build in to all the groups that I work with. Irrespective of task or purpose, people need to recognize and take responsibility for their feelings if they are to relate to each other honestly and create opportunities for growth and transformation.

Exploring feelings

There is always some risk for members expressing feelings in the group because they can never be sure how others will react. Nor can you be sure that you will be able to facilitate the situation and prevent it getting out of control or frightening the group. However, if you have encouraged people to be more aware and accepting of their feelings you have reduced much of the risk and unpredictability and members will be more likely to express their feelings in an appropriate fashion.

One way that I encourage people to become more comfortable with feelings is to demonstrate the importance of expressivity in determining the quality of group experience. This fits in easily with the ideas about right relations that we looked at earlier. I teach members that behind every feeling, conflict, and disturbance is an unfulfilled need that the person is trying to meet through his emotional responses and behaviour. This is not only important for the individual but has major consequences for the group. So it is in the group's interest to allow and respond to the feelings of its members. If the group and the person can become conscious of what is really needed when angry, depressed, or tearful then they can consider options and make choices to meet the need, which will be more constructive and will enhance group and personal experience.

I ask questions which open up these deeper needs and give me the flexibility that is necessary to deal with feeling problems:

* What do you need right now?
* What would help you cope with this?
* Is there anything that you need from the group?
* How could things be different for you?
* What are your feelings telling you about yourself/the group?
* What are you avoiding/preventing yourself from doing?
* What are you being deprived of?
* Is there someone in the group who could help you now?

Often these sort of questions reveal the underlying need in the situation and can serve to refine and reframe the problem. It is usually not difficult to enlist the support and resource of the group to help create meaning and resolution:

- Does anyone know how John is feeling?
- Has anyone ever felt like this before?
- What was it like for you?
- What did you need?
- What were you avoiding; deprived of; being prevented from doing?
- What did you do/want to do?
- What do you think John could do?
- What would you advise John not to do?
- How do you feel about John's emotional reaction?
- What do John's feelings tell us about the group communication/trust/decision making/task/process, etc?

Sometimes penetrating to the deeper levels of a feeling reveals an emotional block which requires some release or discharge of energy. Depending on the purpose of the group, time available, and temperament of the person or couple involved you may wish to provide ways and means of expressing strong feelings. Here are some ideas taken from my work in a therapy context which I have found useful in a variety of group settings.

Stay in the here and now

If you watch people in a group you will see that they often distract themselves from uncomfortable feelings by talking about or discussing their feelings rather than experiencing them. It is important to draw attention to this and encourage members to be concrete and specific about their feeling experiences in the present tense. This simple but powerful technique creates the potential to go deeper into a feeling and co-operate with the natural impulse to discharge and complete the experience. Often this involves encouraging the person to stay with distracting feelings of frustration, being blocked, or confusion in order for the real feeling to emerge and be dissolved.

Repeat and exaggerate

Another simple technique for helping a person contact and discharge feelings is to use repetition. Sometimes a person may disclose that he is angry or sad, in a way which shows that he is inhibiting or checking the energetic aspect of the feeling. I try to identify a key phrase in the person's disclosure and ask him to repeat it several times. Usually the person is helped to contact the basic feeling and discharge it quickly. A helpful variation is to ask the person to exaggerate the phrase in some way – say it loudly, softly, shout it. Repetition and exaggeration can also be used on non-verbal language very effectively. I might ask someone to exaggerate drumming his fingers on the table to help him get in touch with some frustration or anger he is feeling. You can request a member to repeat and exaggerate any gesture, posture, behaviour, statement, or attitude.

Dialogue

Another way in which members can explore strong feelings and conflicts is to encourage them to converse with an absent person or a part of themselves which is causing distress. In the famous Gestalt empty chair technique the member imagines that the absent person or contrary part is sitting in a chair opposite and he expresses fully his feelings and all the things he is prevented from saying. This is a simple method of resolving intrapersonal and interpersonal conflicts. It can seem artificial at first but artificial does not mean false and your respect and compassion for the person will usually encourage them to get involved. A way of involving the group is to do a psychodrama where other members play different parts or people in the individual's conflict (see Chapter 10, page 180).

Physical release

Since feelings always have a physical expression, it is valuable to give practical ways of discharging feelings. Again, depending on your group, members can, among other things, do the following:

- Use a cushion to kick, punch, jump on
- Stamp on the floor
- Push against the wall
- Tear up paper
- Wring a towel (neck substitute!)
- Shout, scream
- Squeeze a tennis ball

This sort of expression of feeling need not be confined simply to therapy groups. Strong feelings arise in the work group or the classroom and being able to acknowledge them and offer an appropriate discharge is a valuable and creative service to give any group of people. These few techniques do not require a lot of knowledge or expertise and will carry you through most situations which involve feelings. All they require on your part is sensitivity and a willingness to be attentive and imaginative.

Some things to be aware of when working with feelings

- *Deal with emotions as they arise rather than storing them up.* Try to keep conflicts or disagreements current if you are to avoid major confrontations. Explosive situations arise because group members are unable or unwilling to handle emotional crises as they encounter them.
- *Challenge any attempts to rescue a member from a painful but perhaps necessary experience*: Some members consistently try to:
  o Console/be kind
  o Plaster over the cracks
  o Sweep under the carpet
  o Make everything better

If this is not explored, energy in the group can be dissipated and unhealthy behaviours can be institutionalized.

- *Do not allow gossip.* People in groups often talk about another (present) member as if he were not there. They talk to me or to someone else about the third person. I challenge this every time because it weakens and erodes many of the values and norms that we have been looking at. I encourage members to look at and address each other directly and use first names.
- *Avoid overexposure.* Most people in groups will share and reveal themselves at their own pace. Sometimes, however, in the early stages of the group when people are unsure of the boundaries, an individual may reveal too much about himself or go too far. This can frighten other members who may feel they have to perform similarly. It can also be difficult for the individual who afterwards may feel embarrassed or regretful and can find it difficult to return to the group. To avoid this, work gradually and sensitively with people's feelings at the start. Check out constantly if it is alright for the person to continue. Are they making a choice to talk or feeling compelled to talk? How are other people feeling? Be aware of your own reactions to the person and trust your judgement.
- *Avoid 'why' questions.* Questions which start with 'why' are 'closed' in that they demand an explanation or a specific answer. They are rarely helpful and are best avoided. Questions which start with 'how' or 'what' are more valuable because they allow a person to be more 'open' about their experience or feelings. Use and encourage questions like:

  o How is this for you?
  o What is happening for you?
  o How do you see/feel/experience things?
  o What is it like for you?

These are present-tense questions. They open up the process and involve the person in their own experience.

Working with members' feelings in these ways will deepen and enhance the learning which takes place in the group. It will also be evident over time that members are developing healthier and more creative ways of relating to each other based on acknowledgement and acceptance of feeling and emotion. Feelings will come to be regarded as significant, desirable, and productive and will add to relationships instead of disrupting or detracting from them.

Teaching members how to maintain themselves

Every group is set up to achieve some tasks or goals which its members believe are worth striving for and yet it cannot devote all its energy and resource to doing this. If the group is to achieve its goals and not fall apart on the way some of the collective resource must be invested in ensuring that members feel included and able to participate, are respected and valued. So from the start each group has to find a way of balancing and apportioning energy, resource, and time to its goal-oriented activity and to looking after its members.

Unfortunately few groups are able to create a healthy balance between their task and maintenance concerns. They frequently act as if these two needs are in opposition or competing for limited resources, instead of seeing them as essential and complementary. In this, most groups tend to reflect the larger societal preoccupation with striving, achievement, and success which is inculcated in the family and institutionalized in school and workplace. As a result many people will arrive in your group intent on getting on with the job and quite unskilled and uncreative in their ability to look after relationships. If this situation is allowed to develop the group can rapidly become a very unhealthy experience characterized by competition, apathy, or burn-out.

If you can identify some or all of the following behaviours and attitudes in your group and they do not seem to be obviously related to its stage of development then it is probable that your group is mishandling its task – maintenance needs and requires assistance:

> - Tiredness, exhaustion, flatness, sense of being stuck
> - Frustration, burn-out
> - Conflict, bickering, arguing over goals, programme, resources
> - Apathy, boredom, indifference, reluctance
> - Absenteeism, lateness, drop-outs, turnover of members
> - Poor concentration, decision making, problem solving, creativity
> - Slow starts, never having enough time
> - Excitability, tension, emotionality, irritability

Prevention is better than cure

I was once called in to work with a team of workers who were very exhausted and suffering from stress and burn-out. I found them to be very depressed and quite self-destructive and at a point where it was not possible to help them move on. After six months the team had to be broken up! I learned two important lessons in this group:

> - Help a group see the necessity of maintenance activity while it has a choice to take care of itself. When it reaches breakdown it has no choice at all!
> - A group which can play together is more likely to be a group which can stay together!

Now when I work with a group I emphasize from the outset the importance of paying attention to maintaining and looking after relationships in the group if the job is to get done successfully. I introduce a more organic rhythm to the programme and to each session which balances and reconciles the task and maintenance needs in the group. This rhythm starts from the simple fact that every session has a beginning, a middle, and an end and draws attention to the needs of members at each of these phases.

Try to get into the way of viewing your sessions more organically. Do not simply pitch into work after an initial greeting or suddenly stop when you become aware that you have run over time. These are patterns of activity and relating that many people have picked up in school and the workplace and if allowed to develop unchecked in your group will create a very stressful and unhealthy atmosphere. Aim to start slowly giving people time to gather and settle down. Move gradually into the main work for the session and leave time to wind down and separate. Here are some things to consider.

Beginning: a stitch in time

A 'nurturing' beginning is best, so arrange seats if necessary (in a circle), check warmth of room, greet people as they come in, offer refreshments if this is appropriate. In every group I use the check-in procedure outlined on page 92. I ask people to say how they are feeling, what they have been doing since last session, what they are looking forward to in this session, and anything else which might be appropriate. This helps members:

- Include themselves
- Connect with each other
- Settle down
- Helps the leader assess the mood and feel of the group
- Gets everyone talking at the start
- Affirms each member as important and unique

If people come in late I will briefly review what has been happening or invite members to do so. It is usually worthwhile clearing up any unfinished or leftover business from the previous session which might get in the way, and going on to outline the activity for the day or provide a context for the session. If you find that:

- The check-in is shallow or empty
- The check-in goes on too long
- People are not really interested in each other
- People are waiting or stalling
- Some people want to get straight to work
- Some people are tired, flat, depressed

Point this out to the group straight away and get them to consider possible consequences and coping strategies. Often I have found that I spend the rest of a session dealing with what was not discussed in the first five minutes.

Show people that they are important and that their anxieties and questions are worth group time. If people feel valued and accepted here they will carry these positive feelings into the next phase. Do not smother or patronize people or let this beginning stage drag on. Watch out for signs or comments that tell you people are ready and willing to move on.

The middle or formal work phase: a bad penny will always turn up

Ensure that members know what the activity and its purpose is. Check that tools, materials, resources are available if required, people understand their role and feel able to contribute. If you have adequately prepared the group for its work at this stage it is probable that difficulties which occur have got more to do with members' personal needs and relationships.

Watch out for:

- Members who are tired and need a break
- Members who are hungry or unwell
- People who may be overly enthusiastic or dominating and alienating others
- Members who are quiet or who may feel ignored, deprived, rejected
- Activity that is getting too complex, intellectual, or becoming bogged down in details, is becoming boring or unsatisfying
- The group working to unrealistic deadlines or with anxieties about time
- Only a few people contributing
- Asking too much of group members

Should any of these or other themes become apparent, the best thing to do is disregard the agenda for a while and draw attention to what is happening. Many group workers are very nervous about leaving the task to focus on the process or maintenance issues and prefer to ignore them, hoping it will all come right. This is usually a mistake. What is ignored will always come back to haunt the group so deal with issues as they arise.

Encourage members to acknowledge and respond to the needs behind a behaviour or incident which are being ignored or dismissed. Do not allow conversation to range widely or evoke fruitless resentments. Keep discussion focused on the particular incident and make sure that it is seen and dealt with as a group problem. Give yourself a time limit – 15 minutes perhaps – to open up the important issues and make space for people to share their feelings and declare their interests. Do not look for instant resolution; very little can be immediately resolved in a group. It is more of a cumulative process. Be confident that you have acknowledged the difficulty, discussed it, and involved group members. This is usually enough to take the steam out of a situation and let you all get back to work.

The end of the session: don't pour gallons into pint pots . . .

It is surprising how many groups end suddenly, with little preparation for a return to the domestic environment and a sense of being cut off or left hanging in the air. This can have a counterproductive effect in the group and will often create fear, resentment, and stress. Make sure to leave some time at the end of the session:

- To wind down and relax
- To summarize, draw conclusions, complete, contextualize the session, tie up loose ends
- To plan the next session, unfinished business
- To appreciate and celebrate
- To prepare for re-entry into domestic environment

This seems fairly obvious and yet many workers forget to help the group wind down or simply run out of time. Another type of worker fails to see the importance of giving precious time to this and demands work right up until the bell.

The ending phase need not take up a lot of time and yet it can have far-reaching effects.

- It can minimize emotional fall-out from the session
- It can allow business to remain unfinished and held over to the next session
- It gives a psychologically necessary sense of achievement and completion
- It can prepare members to handle eventual group termination
- It teaches members to pace themselves and inculcates an organic and rhythmic aspect to group experience

The simplest method of ending is to invite each member in turn to check-out. This involves members reporting what they have remembered, learned, appreciated, or resented in the session. Often issues will come up at the last, or people will report feelings or experiences that could have been looked at earlier. It is important to acknowledge this but not to go into detail or allow yourself to be manipulated into running over the allotted time. Agree with people that this issue can go on the agenda for the next meeting. You might decide to go first or last and give your own summary of what was happening in the session. You can use other ways of ending the session – a game, exercise, piece of music, or some quiet contemplative time together.

By paying attention to the way in which members come together, settle down to work, and then end their session you will gradually inculcate in the group a feeling for a more balanced, compassionate, and graceful way of being together. Members' ability and willingness to work on their maintenance issues, and develop their team spirit and camaraderie all flow from your initial efforts to create a pattern and a context in which relationships are as important as the task.

Pleasure versus striving feelings

I said earlier that a group which plays together is more likely to stay together. What I am pointing to here is the importance of a group being able to celebrate its activity and achievement, do things, and take time out to enjoy and appreciate each other.

One way in which I help a group develop a sense of play and well-being is to introduce and help members distinguish between times when their pleasure or striving feelings are in the ascendant. Striving is about attachment to a goal and the need to achieve. It can bring pleasure but often it may become an end in itself and distorts and subjugates satisfaction so that a person may come to feel driven or compelled. Pleasure, on the other hand, is about the ways a person nourishes and nurtures himself and involves choice and self-affirmation.

Early in a group's life or when it seems appropriate, I will devote part of a session to exploring these two ideas. Members easily understand their essence and relevance and are quite able to identify their typical strategies around striving and gaining pleasure. I then help people look at how their striving patterns could lead to competition, dominance, and selfishness in the group and encourage them to think about the need to develop ways of managing anti-group behaviours as they arise. I also ensure to brainstorm or compile a list of things which would bring members pleasure, as from this the group can internalize the importance of maintenance and plan an appropriate programme of activity. Familiarity with the language and practice of pleasure and striving gives a valuable context within which to explore an issue, and means that afterwards members will naturally look for something that they can do which will be healing and affirming. It also legitimizes the creation and use of particular rituals or activities which give pleasure and satisfaction and provides a simple way of presenting the need to balance task and maintenance issues in the group.

As the group develops you will find that your early efforts to teach and instil the importance of maintenance bear fruit. Increasingly, members will be able to deal with disruptions or interference to the task, attend to relationships, and work together more creatively and harmoniously. The group will develop a tolerance for the pace of its different members and will come to relate and work together in a more organic and whole manner.

Teaching members how to analyse group process

Every group faces certain common problems – identifying goals, creating a comfortable climate, developing procedures, making decisions, and the like. It is valuable if members are able to recognize and discuss the processes which occur as they are happening because it makes for greater and more intelligent involvement and agreement. However, being able to recognize group process, quite apart from commenting on it, does not take place by itself and methods of analysis have to be built in if members are to become able and willing to turn from *what* they are discussing to explore *how* it is being discussed. I use a number of methods to help members become more self-analytical.

Worker process comments

Initially the impetus for highlighting process or maintenance issues comes from you. By indicating your awareness and interest in what is going on you will:

- Illustrate how the sessions influence behaviour
- Indicate the immediate problems confronting the group
- Legitimize discussion of process
- Build in the process-analysis function as a feature of the group's activity

The important thing is to choose a suitable place to intervene and comment. Try to deal with the behaviour or activity of the group as a whole and avoid drawing attention to particular members. This makes it less threatening and easier to engage people. You are trying to encourage the group to examine what is happening, so make a short statement about what you see in front of you and then ask a question:

- 'We've spent longer on this decision than we agreed to. I wonder what's happening?'
- 'Everyone has been silent for so long now. How are people feeling right now?'
- 'No one is really saying anything new here. What's blocking us?'

At first members may ignore your comments or not speak because they are unsure how to respond or what to say. Permit this and help members look at their embarrassment or discomfort. As the group develops, your process comments will become more normal for members and will increasingly activate analysis of what is really happening in the sessions.

Member process comments

When I begin to remark on, and draw attention to group process, I introduce a basic ground rule:

> Each member has the right and responsibility to comment on what is happening at any time in the group.

As members begin to intervene at the process level you may notice that some comments are ignored, while others evoke anger or conflict. This can often arise because comments are too superficial or too threatening. In either case it can be valuable to spend time teaching the group how to give feedback (see page 121) and introduce some of the ideas about creating right relations (see page 149). The process interventions of members are not only important for their value in exploring what is happening in the group but for the opportunity they present to introduce ideas about, and practise the skills of communicating, working, and living together.

The process period

This is a period of time which is set aside or given over to assessing what has happened in the group or what is taking place in the present. In some groups I have found it useful to structure this into the session, for example, a training group, but in most groups I will suggest a process period in response to a difficulty or an incident. It is important to give a set time – between ten and 40 minutes is best – so that members can see their explorations in the context of the session.

You can decide to encourage the whole group to work together or may opt for smaller subgroups. The subgroups encourage greater participation and can be given one aspect of the problem to consider and report back to the larger group. You can help the large group focus on process by using brainstorming techniques or exploring the critical incidents and sequence of events that led up to the conflict or impasse.

The process observer

Sometimes group members can get so caught up in their experience that it is difficult to help them step back and see the process at work. I find it valuable to use a 'process observer' at these very emotive times who can then 'officially' sit outside the events and report on what is occurring. It is important to thoroughly and specifically brief this member on his role and what he is to watch out for.

Ask the process observer to focus on the way the group makes decisions, communicates, or distributes power and consider giving a checklist, like the one overleaf, to assist him.

After a set time, say, ten or 20 minutes, the process observer can report back to the group what he has seen happening and this initiates a discussion about causes, strategies, and resolutions. It is important that the process observer is able to give feedback and not threaten particular members. This is usually a very popular activity and is worth considering as a way of introducing the idea of process analysis because of its value in engaging group members.

- Is everybody included/listened to/consulted?
- How does the group handle dissent/conflict?
- Are decisions consensual, majority vote, or individual?
- What was the group atmosphere like? (Note *when* it changes and *why.*)
- Who makes suggestions, suggests procedures, compromises, rejects, asks for votes, disrupts, makes proposals, asks the others?
- How does each member hinder or help goal achievement?
- How far did the group get in achieving its goal?
- How could decision making/communication be improved?

These simple methods if used singly or in combination can provide substantial insight for members about how they influence and are influenced by the group. They also encourage members to take responsibility for what happens between themselves and begin to identify the options, consequences, and choices for change. I believe this is one of the more exciting fruits of encouraging process analysis and members increasingly move from a passive to a proactive stance in the group as they come to realize that they are in charge of their experience and perception.

Working with difficult situations

There are a number of difficult situations which crop up sooner or later in most groups and will require you to intervene at some stage.

Dominating member

The dominating member behaves in a way which will give him, or enable him to exercise, more power in the group.

Manifestations

- Constantly talking
- Having the 'worst' problems and therefore 'needing' attention
- Being the 'nicest' or 'kindest' person
- Knowing what is best – adviser, critic, 'leader', moralist
- Acting aggressively, attention-seeking

Some of the causes which contribute to one member taking over or dominating may include:

- Lack of trust
- Poor cohesion
- Feelings of inferiority or inadequacy
- Fear, anxiety, embarrassment about speaking out
- Unequal relationships, problems with distribution of power, knowledge, skill
- The dominator may feel superior, more able, needier, more distressed
- The dominator may feel afraid of silences

You may decide to wait until a crisis develops around the role of the dominant member or you can intervene at a suitable point before breakdown occurs. In either event:

- Acknowledge what is happening and make it a communal problem with consequences for the group. Do not allow one individual to be seen as the problem.
- Bring out whatever feelings are involved on all sides.
- Highlight the process by which the situation came about. Explore people's needs and motivations and look at what is missing, being avoided or made covert.
- Management structures may need to be introduced or overhauled – speaking in turn, rotating leadership of sessions, time-sharing, setting an agenda. It might be important to set up skill-training sessions to look at aspects of communication, trust, decision making, and the power structure in the group. Think about ways of reinforcing sharing behaviour and introduce values, norms which emphasize mutuality and reciprocity.

Getting stuck

Frequently one member or even the whole group can become stuck or locked in a particular feeling or behaviour.

Manifestations

- Long or recurring silences
- Resistance to advice or suggestion
- Atmosphere which feels cold, frozen, flat, wooden, dead, tense, or unreal
- Repetition of a particular feeling or behaviour
- Taboo areas and subjects: sex, race, religion, politics, anger, competition, individualism
- Difficulties in sharing, trusting, deciding, planning, working
- Loss of creativity, productivity

Some of the causes of getting stuck include:

> - Unresolved feelings or issues
> - Member or group feeling in deep water, out of their depth, in unknown territory
> - Unexpressed feelings of anger, resentment, sadness, inadequacy
> - Collusive agreements to avoid dealing with problematic or painful material, issues, dynamics
> - Difficulty in trusting, joining in, sharing
> - Opposing or entrenched viewpoints, subgroups, inequalities in relationships, power, knowledge, skill

As soon as you become aware that a member or the group is stuck draw attention to what is happening. By now the procedure should be familiar – make being stuck a communal problem, bring out the different feelings involved, and through working on the process issues help people understand why they are stuck and what choices they have about it.

If members find it difficult to talk in the group consider dividing into pairs or threes for ten minutes to talk about the problem from a more individual perspective before coming back to report in the large group. Brainstorming singly, in pairs, or in the group is also valuable as is the 'sculpting' technique explored on page 191. This is a powerful way of exploring why a group is stuck and you can ask members to sculpt themselves in terms of themes like intimacy, power, competence, and the like. Do not forget to discuss this thoroughly afterwards. Anything which involves physical activity can be a very good way of breaking open a pattern of stuck-ness and releasing people to examine what is going on, and should be considered.

The cynic or sceptic

The cynical member sets himself apart from the other members by his disbelief and constant sneering at the possibilities in the group.

Manifestations

> - Condescending or patronizing attitude towards worker/members/group goals
> - Scoffs or sneers at mutuality; professes to believe people are only motivated by self-interest
> - Nit-picks, points out flaws, weaknesses of plans or interactions, constantly deflates and disparages
> - Mocking, sarcastic, contemptuous behaviour

Some of the causes of cynical behaviour in the group result from:

> - Bad or painful experiences in the past
> - Fear of failure – the cynic doesn't try!
> - Fear of intimacy and tenderness – cynicism is used as a defence against getting close

The cynic is quite touchy and easily alienated so I usually try to deal with him indirectly at first. When a member is cynical about a situation, interaction, or planned event, I invite him to explain his doubts to the other members. Indicate to the cynic and the group that the individual may be doing some important work for the group. By making him responsible for his cynicism and reframing the behaviour as a communication to the group it is possible to eliminate much of the sarcasm and scoffing which goes with this attitude while at the same time creating a situation where a member's cynicism serves the group. Groups can get unrealistic and inflated about their intentions and exchanges so having a cynic around can ground people and draw attention to unconsidered deficiencies and shortcomings.

If there is a chronic or very severe problem with cynicism in the group it should be confronted with particular reference to its separative and distancing functions. In extreme cases you may have to weigh the degree of cynicism against the group purpose and contract and ask a member to review or consider his involvement in the group. Generally, however, I find that if I maintain an open and friendly attitude to this member and convert his contributions, in time the cynic lets go of some defences against getting close and will allow himself to join in more of the group's activity.

What to do if someone breaks down

On occasions you may find that a group member undergoes an emotional crisis or becomes very distressed. Here are some guidelines that you might find helpful in such a situation.

- The first thing to do is stay calm. Do not allow yourself to panic, blame yourself, or feel guilty. Most people experiencing distress are terrified of losing control and need to feel protected and contained. They will want to have confidence in you so decide that you are going to help and put everything else to one side.
- Listen to the person. Try to understand what is happening, what has triggered off this crisis. Do not rush in to make things better or rescue! Give yourself time and let the person tell you in their own way what is wrong. Do not try to deepen the experience by getting him to act out his feelings or try to do therapy with him. All you have to do is let him talk – you listen! When you know what is happening you can develop options and find a way out.
- Do not allow yourself to feel afraid of being useless or inadequate. No matter how distressed a person is there is always one part of him that is in touch with reality. Speak to that part and he will respond. If you find yourself getting stuck, get in touch with what you feel and think about it for a moment. Your feelings will probably mirror those of the distressed member and you can use them to get on his wavelength, create boundary, ask questions, and generate options. Follow your hunches and feelings and do not be afraid to use your feelings of confusion or helplessness to open up the situation:

'I'm confused about what you mean. Can you say that again?'

or

'I'm not sure what is the best way to help you with this. Tell me why this is happening for you now.'

Ask other members for their views and comments but do not let them analyse or make intellectual points about what is occurring.

- You may need to give the distressed member time after the session or get more expert help. Do not feel guilty if you have to refer the person on. You cannot be all things to all people.
- Help the other group members express their feelings about the situation at an appropriate time. They may be shocked or feel frightened and it is important to work through this if you are to avoid people dropping out or the group getting stuck. The distressed member may be embarrassed about returning to the group or members may be afraid to refer to the incident. It is important to talk about this. The more honest you are about what has occurred the less frightening it will be for all and the more quickly everyone can integrate and learn from the experience.

Review

- Creative groupwork is about making space for options and possibilities to emerge in the group
- There are three basic skills involved:
  1   Knowing how to use yourself as a model
  2   Knowing how to influence and co-operate with what is emerging
  3   Being able to provide structure and foster desirable behaviour
- You will need to learn how to work with feelings
- Teach members how to maintain themselves
- Involve members in exploring their own process
- Give yourself time with difficult situations and make them communal problems
- Use every opportunity to make the group your co-worker

Chapter 10

The techniques of creative groupwork

The experiential nature of group behaviour and learning requires the worker and members to engage in an interaction which, by its nature, touches on all aspects of the human experience. The quality and richness of this interaction is in part a product of the processes that the worker knowingly or unknowingly helps to initiate and the relevance of the methods or 'technology' used to assist the group achieve its ends and resolve its problems.

In the last few chapters I have talked about what I consider to be the essential processes and skills to introduce and co-operate with in your group. I now want to discuss some of the methods that make up a basic repertoire and form the 'toolkit' that you use to work experientially in most group settings.

The toolkit

I developed my own toolkit empirically and out of my urgent need to help group members find a way around the frequent and inevitable ruptures in communication. These breakdowns usually seemed to occur because members had some problem conceptualizing an event or because there was a language barrier or an emotional difficulty that got in people's way. Often there was a great deal happening in the group, but somehow it did not seem to come out appropriately or it was hard to identify a coherent pattern. The constant struggle to come to terms with language and reason seemed to constrain and confuse situations and produce only exasperation and frustration. I began to raid any other field or discipline which offered me ideas or practical advice that could be modified to create a richer and more complete experience in my groups. Through trial and error I began to evolve methods and techniques which in time I found transposed to most group settings.

These methods include and are derived from:

- Role-play and simulation
- Art techniques
- Imaginative techniques
- Games and exercises
- Bodywork
- Expressive writing and journaling techniques
- Myth, story and Archetype

Gradually I developed a structure and terms of reference within which I and group members could tackle any situation that emerged. There are four basic principles underpinning this structure and they give context and rationale to the notion of a toolkit which can be used with groups.

- Technique as metaphor
- Technique as experiential learning
- Technique as a way of involving the whole person in group experience
- Technique as a way of motivating people

Let us examine these four principles before we turn to explore the methods in detail.

Technique as metaphor

I once worked with a group of adolescent boys and girls who appeared to have mixed thoughts and feelings about each other which they were holding back and not expressing. Several attempts on my part to discuss the effect this behaviour was having on communication and trust levels in the group met with no success – members denied that there were hidden agendas in the group and would insist on moving on to other topics.

I decided to tackle this problem more indirectly and so in one session I invited the members to participate in an exercise designed to involve each of them. I divided the group and asked one half to role-play the members of a youth club committee whose responsibility was to administer the allocation and spending of a grant of £1,000. I gave each role-player a set of instructions which involved them in grossly caricatured alliances, collusions, and attempts to attract or dismiss each other but allowed them complete freedom as to how they did this. I asked the other half of the group to identify the secret motivations and agendas of the various role-players.

After a hilarious role-play we debriefed and discussed what had been occurring in the scene. Members talked about the obvious secrets of the role-players and explored some of the reasons why people might be fearful or unwilling to reveal their motives and agendas. Soon one member remarked that the role-play struck him as an exaggerated version of what took place in our own group. Other members agreed and quite quickly it was possible to bring into the open some of the feelings and sentiments which had previously been suppressed and begin to look at the factors involved in their suppression.

A number of points emerge from this example:

- Drawing attention to the facts does not always meet with members' agreement, elicit co-operation, or change attitudes.
- If you are dogmatic you can actually evoke in members a stubborn resistance or insistence on the false or unhealthy beliefs that you wish to change. This is why Paracelsus,

that Renaissance magus, warns us against simply telling 'the naked truth'. The clever group worker should use 'images, allegories, figures, wondrous speech or other hidden, roundabout ways', to convey meaning and resolve difficult situations.[1]

- It is very possible to encourage people to explore their predicament by using a technique or exercise which is metaphorical, which simulates reality, and reveals the bones of a situation. Instruction by metaphor does not depend on an objective checking of the facts or on rational thinking. Instead, working metaphorically implies coming upon an actual situation from outside, intuitively and spontaneously, rather than from within the event through more usual processes of deliberation and logic, which can lead to protectionism and defence.

- Every method, exercise, or technique then, as I use it, is a metaphor: a way of shifting perception and creating meaning. I am not interested in any medium or technique as an end in itself but as a means of engaging people and providing a context for work, which is directly related to the members' level of ability and willingness to act. From this perspective the value of any technique lies not in its skill or knowledge base but in what it points to, its ability to act symbolically, open up dialogue, and encapsulate meaning.

- This leads on to an important point – an exercise or technique which does not work is just as valuable as one which does. Let me explain. If I want to explore the need for trust in a group I can sit down and discuss the issue with members. Now this can become quite abstract since you cannot actually see or touch trust and in some groups this discussion may seem laboured. A much easier and more relevant method is to do an exercise with the group which, even if it breaks down, provides you with tangible material and rationale coming out of members' own direct experience and learning. In this way even a technique which does not work becomes an opportunity to explore the group process and develop new and agreed ways of working and behaving.

Technique as experiential learning

This last point is highlighting how you can use methods and exercises as a way of creating experiential learning in the group. Experiential learning simply means generating from personal experience, ideas, rules, and procedures which can guide behaviour, and then modifying these concepts and practices to make them more effective in the light of new experience. So in the example given above, the importance of being able to trust each other derives for members from their experience of what it is like to be together when there is suspicion or anxiety about personal safety in the group.

Experiential learning can be seen as involving four phases:

- Concrete personal experiences, are followed by
- Observation, reaction, consideration, which leads to
- Abstraction and conceptualizing of theory, principles, rules, and procedures, and
- Application

Experiential learning is based on three assumptions:

- That group members learn best when they are personally involved in the learning experience
- That members must discover knowledge for themselves if it is to really mean anything to them
- That members will be committed to learning and working if they can set their own goals within a given framework

You can see how each method, exercise, or technique that you use in the group becomes an opportunity for members to experiment with new behaviour, try things out, develop, and practise new skills. Each exercise or technique carries with it the promise of learning when it is accompanied by consideration of the experience and analysis of its process. In this way your use of techniques and exercises becomes an organic and integral part of how group members learn and work and not some alien or gimmicky rite enacted at the start of a group or when you are at a loss as to what to do.

Technique as a way of involving the whole person

A basic premise throughout this work has been that every group is a multidimensional experience which must engage the individual at the physical, emotional, intuitive, and intellectual levels of his being. A moment's reflection reveals that not all individuals operate equally on all these levels in groups – some people may be comfortable or productive on one level rather than another. However, we do need access to all these faculties and if learning and behaviour in the group is to be relevant and mature it is essential that you include and work with as many of these levels as possible.

Unfortunately many groups and workers often exhibit a style in which one mode of exercise comes to be overdeveloped at the expense of the others.

Thus:

- Some therapy groups consider the expression of feelings as the only valid form of work
- In some discussion groups verbal ability, conceptual skill, and high concentration spans are valued above anything else
- Some activity groups can become overly engrossed in the physical skills and dexterity required

The consequences of overdeveloping one level of experience in the group and neglecting the others can be far-reaching:

- Loss of creativity, depth, richness
- Getting stuck easily
- Boredom, repetition, superficiality

- Conflict, intolerance, tension
- Loss of productivity
- Reduced ability to learn
- Problems in expression and communication
- Development of elites and hierarchies based on skill, knowledge, or proficiency

If it is to be effective and creative each group must offer its members clear opportunities for direct personal participation and observation which will engage and evoke the whole person.

This means that the group leader:

- Must be comfortable and able to work with each of the major modes of experience
- Must be able to help members cross from one mode to another as appropriate
- Must be able to integrate the modes and involve the whole person

The more imaginative and expressive techniques – drama, art, fantasy are powerful and effective methods of evoking and utilizing maximum personal resource. They seem to build a bridge between the conscious self and unconscious elements and mediate between the rational mind and its more irrational, affective, and intuitive parts. They offer you very valuable methods of working through conflicts and balancing experience at the physical, emotional, and mental levels. In situations where it is often difficult for members to comprehend what is happening or verbalize about it, the judicious and discriminating use of these techniques can release energy, create awareness, and provide structure and context.

Technique as a way of motivating people

The truth of the matter is that you cannot motivate another person. Motivation is something that lies inside a person and not outside. It can be reached but not controlled. When you appear to motivate other people you are in fact tapping and aligning with motivations that already exist inside them. Motivation is about discovering and activating the highly personal desires of group members rather than producing them.

A motive is really a desire – a response to a felt need. It is desire that motivates and when you appear to motivate other people you are actually responding to their feelings in a way which enables them to gratify their desires while at the same time helping you to gratify some of yours. Real motivation is about the mutual satisfaction of desires.

You can use various techniques to boost the appeal of a subject or task and increase the motivational attraction for group members. Take, for example, work with a group of children where it might be important to talk about the principles involved in asserting oneself, saying no to a drink or cigarette or withstanding peer pressure to break into a shop. You are more likely to generate interest and enthusiasm for this project if it can be presented in a way which offers fun, activity, and opportunities for demonstration and exploration, as well as making the point. Members will be more involved and the experience will be more complete if you can create opportunities for them to tell a story, draw, or enact a role-play which will bring out the essential principles.

So when considering a session or a theme in your programme have clear what you want to come out of it and then think for a moment about the range of desires that might be around for members. Refer back to Chapter 3 where Maslow's hierarchy of needs is discussed. When you have some idea of what people want, think about using an exercise or technique as a way of engaging members' interest and augmenting their reason for investing in the project. You might want to have another look at the subject of programming discussed in Chapter 2. The remainder of this chapter is given over to looking at some techniques that I have found very effective in group settings and that might be helpful to you. Also, refer to the extensive bibliography at the end of the book which lists useful books and anthologies of exercises.

Technique number 1

Using role-play in the group

Role-play is a technique that is increasingly used in the group setting to:

> - Explore the role behaviour of an individual in a domestic, leisure, or work situation
> - Practise new skills
> - Explore and resolve a current problem
> - Replay a childhood scene or fantasy situation

Role-play is a very flexible technique which can be adapted for work in any group setting.[2] In its simplest form, role-play involves setting up a scene which represents for an individual or the group, some conflict, anxiety, or need to practise new roles, behaviours, or skills. For example, a group member may be applying for a job and will want to rehearse the personal and social skills required to perform well at interview. Other group members will role-play people on the interviewing panel, boss, secretary, and the like and help the individual identify and become familiar with what he needs to do in this situation.

Here are some of the situations in which I have used role-play techniques in groups:

> - An adolescent is anxious about an impending court appearance
> - A child is confronted by a bully and does not know what to do
> - An individual wishes to make friends with a particular male or female
> - Resolving problems with parents/teachers/employers
> - Helping individuals learn how to assert themselves/handle certain emotions
> - Helping individuals learn and practise new social and professional roles/skills/behaviours
> - Drawing attention to interpersonal behaviours and group processes – working with conflict, decision making, communication, trust, authority and control, sexuality
> - Helping group members explore social, economic, and political problems

Why role-play is useful in a group

A working knowledge of role-play techniques is an invaluable aid to work in groups because:

- *Role-play increases involvement*: Role-play introduces and legitimizes a fun and alternative way of exploring difficulties or issues in the group. It encourages participation by group members and is an effective method of reducing tension and creating space to look at a problem. Often quiet or silent members will find it easier to join in and contribute to the work of a group when they can engage in a role-play which requires them to play a part rather than themselves. You can increase the likelihood of participation by allowing people time to prepare beforehand or giving them a script which they can refer to during the drama.
- *Role-play increases spontaneity*: Even in those situations where members prepare or start formally, the actors usually identify quite quickly with their parts and start to ad lib and improvise freely. This brings a creative and spontaneous dimension to the subject of the drama which frees people to respond to each other in a more relevant and often intuitive way. There is often more immediate expression of feelings and a willingness to take risks which I find shifts interaction from a contrived or an intellectual level to one characterized by personal investment and authenticity. I have frequently heard members remark on the freshness, genuineness, and relevance of a particular role-play.
- *Role-play enhances awareness and understanding*: Frequently group members report an increase in understanding and empathy after they play the role of a significant other or observe a colleague play them in a scene. Exchanging roles increases a member's feeling for another person and encourages acceptance of him. Often if there is interpersonal difficulty in the group I will encourage members to exchange roles in a representation of the incident. In the actual drama and in the review afterwards, members tend to be more accurate in their perception and portrayal of what is happening, more sensitive to each other, and less anxious to prolong the conflict.
- *Role-play facilitates problem solving*: You can take any problem, relationship, or situation and create a role-play from the central elements involved. The flexibility of the technique means that you can stop scenes and discuss options, rework, alter scenes, try out different strategies and endings; all of which enhances creativity, risk taking, and problem solving.
- *Role-play deepens group cohesion and mutuality*: Because members can see everyone working together to solve individual and collective problems, role-play is a valuable way of emphasizing and developing mutuality, interdependence, and goodwill. You can use it to nurture reciprocal helping relationships and foster intimacy and acceptance of members' problems.

Guidelines for using role-play in the group

WHEN TO USE IT

Role-play may be used to explore any difficult or complex situation but it is most suitable when:

- A member is having trouble trying to describe a problem and the people involved
- A member is trying to clarify his relationship with a significant other
- There is an internal or interpersonal problem in the group
- Members need to practise or rehearse a skill or particular situation

INTRODUCING THE ROLE-PLAY

Role-play can be presented as an impromptu opportunity to rehearse or try out new behaviours. In order to ground the role-play in people's experience, I relate it to a particular problem:

> 'Mary, it must be discouraging when your mother doesn't appear to believe that you can make your own decisions. If you like, we could help you practise talking to her. This might show you better ways of handling the situation and help you convince your mother that you are serious. Would you be interested in this?'

It is important not to make a fuss over role-play or to force members to participate. Present it as something which is interesting and useful and explain its potential in the situation.

HELP MEMBERS EXPRESS THEMSELVES

Help the member whose problem suggested role-playing to describe the situation and the primary characters involved:

> 'First we must know who was involved in the situation and what they said and did so that you can select group members to play their roles.'

I encourage other members to ask questions and comment, in order to involve them and obtain the best possible picture of the situation. This also helps the initiating member increase his understanding of the event.

INVITE MEMBERS TO VOLUNTEER FOR ROLES

- *Brief role-players*: I encourage role-players to make up whatever speech and action they believe best conveys how their character feels and behaves. When people are new to role-play I permit them to spend some time preparing their part or considering a script. However, once the drama starts members are instructed to express their character as best they can, using their own words and feelings, instead of sticking rigidly to a format.

  Just before the scene starts, check that everyone understands their roles. Answer any questions and provide help where necessary. Agree a time limit for the action and then start.

DURING THE DRAMA

- You can stop the role-play at any stage to assess what is happening or what options are available.
- In some situations you may ask particular members to reverse roles in order to help someone express what he senses the other to be feeling. This is a very valuable little technique and can open up dialogue, create empathy, and awareness.
- Sometimes an actor feels unable to proceed or runs out of material. You can examine this in terms of what it says about the problem or you can enlist another actor or

change to another scene. This sort of freedom helps people feel more secure and willing to join in.

- If you become aware that something is not being expressed between role-players it can be useful to ask other non-playing members to double for the particular people and say what they think is going on or not being expressed. I use this technique a lot and find it essential in opening up the fantasies and covert communication which role-play can draw attention to. It is also a lovely way of including every member of the group since you can put doubles on the role-players and even in some situations post doubles on the doubles.

AFTER THE DRAMA – DEBRIEF

The first thing you must do is de-role each player. Get them to say their proper name as this helps them step out of the part they have been playing. Frequently members can become very identified with their part and this may spill over into the session. I then go around each player and ask them to speak about:

- How they felt, behaved in role
- What they thought, felt about other roles
- What they thought about their character
- What they understand now about the situation

After this I invite non-playing members to comment. From the discussion that ensues, it is possible to highlight particular points, develop coping or skill strategies, and learn from the experience.

Do consider using role-play in your group. It need not take long – sometimes only a few minutes – and can be very valuable because of its potential for mobilizing group energy and resource.

Technique number 2

Using art and drawing in the group

Artwork is a term which I use to describe a series of collage, pictorial, graphic, or other media which enable group members to communicate symbolically. These techniques emphasize the feeling and intuitive aspects of personality and offer a valuable way of exploring events in the group life which are not always logical or are hard to talk about in a coherent way.[3]

On occasions a group may not have the linguistic or conceptual ability to deal with an issue and if members are not to act inappropriately out of frustration or helplessness it is important to provide them with a means of developing awareness about what is blocking them, strengthen their ability to cope with events, and facilitate the release of feelings. Various artistic and expressive techniques like painting, collage, and modelling lend themselves admirably to these objectives and it is important to be familiar with their use.

While at times I may use a wide range of media and artistic techniques to help members express themselves, I find that drawing is usually the quickest and easiest medium to introduce and use in sessions. Drawing is a particularly good technique because:

- Every aspect of group life can be portrayed and communicated visually even if it is only an angry slash on a page or the depiction of members as matchstick men
- Materials are basic and clean – pencils, crayons, felt-tips or ballpoint pens. Unlike paints they require no preparation or cleaning afterwards
- Drawing requires minimal skill or expertise and can penetrate to the heart of a situation immediately and spontaneously
- Drawing channels the emotional energy in a situation. It gives substance to what may otherwise be vague and uncomfortable and makes it possible to be more conscious and to talk about one's experience
- It builds a bridge between the verbal and the visual spheres, the rational and the intuitive mind, and the inner and outer worlds of experience
- Drawing is more evocative and revealing of members' experience than words There is often less defensiveness and more depth in a drawing than in the words a person may use to describe an event

Here are some examples of how drawing can be used in group situations:

- To help people introduce themselves in a new group – self-portraits, self-advertisement, badge, motto, symbol for self
- To explore members' self perceptions – private and public self, masks, strengths and weaknesses, aspects of self, good and bad self
- To help members become familiar with emotions and feelings – quick line drawings of love, hate, anger, fear, etc., drawing opposites, brave/afraid, happy/unhappy, theme drawing on fear, etc., emotional masks, drawing feeling memories
- To explore family or interpersonal relationships – family portraits, sociograms, family trees, particular events or incidents
- To develop cohesion, co-operation, and working together – group drawings, team, and pairs drawing. Themes can include communication, group symbol or badge, sociograms, any aspect of life in the group
- To solve a problem, develop creativity or explore group process – drawing a particular theme, for example, how the group handles conflict, makes decisions, etc.; fantasy themes – life in outer space, draw a novel animal; make different drawings which represent a problematic situation, pictorial brainstorming, draw feelings generated by the incident

Guidelines for using drawing in the group

WHEN TO USE IT

Drawing can be used to facilitate or open up any aspect of group life or process but it is particularly useful when:

- A member is having trouble describing a problem
- Feelings and emotional material are getting in the way of expression
- Problem solving is blocked and members need access to intuition, imagination, and creative parts of themselves
- Members find it difficult to talk about or explore interpersonal relationships or group processes

---

INTRODUCING DRAWING

I usually introduce the practice of drawing early in the group's life when members are more open to new ideas. I follow a particular sequence which starts at the individual level and ends with members working together to produce something of relevance to the group. Initially I ask people to draw doodles, lines, squares, etc. and I counter assertions by members that they are not able to draw by asking them to use the hand they are most unfamiliar with. Abstract drawings in an awkward hand are usually enough to get everyone joining in since it now becomes permissible not to be artistic and makes it safe to put pen to paper.

From this I go on to asking people to draw more everyday objects and experiences, still in the unusual hand – telephone, flower, feelings, and the like. At a later stage I suggest that members pair up and I set them tasks which they must draw on a shared sheet – member A can draw circles and member B can draw squares, for example. These more abstract sketches involve people drawing in a non-threatening way and this helps them become used to working together. After a time it is quite easy to introduce themes such as 'time I stuck up for myself' or 'a situation which made me feel sad', which members can draw on the same sheet and talk about afterwards. I use a lot of these themes and tend to keep people in the same pairs in a session to deepen the experience and build intimacy, although over a number of sessions I rotate the pairings.

You can give more intimate and personal themes as members show themselves responsible and capable of working with them. From pairs I then move to subgroups which can tackle various aspects of a theme such as communication. Each subgroup takes a topic such as non-verbal language, methods of communicating, or problems in communication and draws on a shared sheet whatever comes to mind on the subject. After ten minutes each subgroup presents its work verbally and visually to the others. When all the subgroups are finished it is quite easy to have a group discussion about the particular theme because members have been stimulated, involved, and made more aware of their feelings and opinions.

The same process occurs in doing a group drawing on a theme. This time everyone joins in on a large shared sheet to visually brainstorm their thoughts and feelings about a subject. I start with innocent themes like shopping at the supermarkets or going to a party, before tackling more complex aspects of relationship or group process. By following a sequence like this over a few sessions it is easy to develop attitudes and approaches to drawing which are not based on needs to compete or be skilful but which see drawing as a valuable way of generating more information and involvement of members.

SHARING AND DISCUSSING THE DRAWINGS

It is very worthwhile to spend time after a drawing session in sharing and discussing. This is particularly important where you are using drawing to highlight process or open up a problem. Invite people to share their drawings – as much or as little as they wish. Do not insist on sharing! You can work in pairs or subgroups initially, but do spend some time in the large group sharing and discussing. The questions in Chapters 8 and 9 will help you structure feedback and discussion. Avoid interpreting or imposing your beliefs about people's drawings and always try to evoke what the drawing means to its creator. You can usefully ask other people what it means for them, but the emphasis must be on their experience and associations to the picture rather than on its technical or artistic merits.

Think about using drawing in your group. You will find it an easy, valuable, and practical technique which transforms inner forces into visible shapes and creates conditions in which these visible shapes can then be transformed into ordinary words and understanding.

Technique number 3

Using imaginative techniques in the group

Imaginative techniques are ways of evoking and creating symbols and mental images to deal resourcefully with the problems and circumstances of group life. Often a group and its members may find the everyday mode of rational thinking more of an obstacle than an aid to understanding what is happening between them. In these situations it is fruitful to ask questions like:

> - What colour is the group atmosphere right now?
> - What image/picture/symbol comes to mind about what is happening now?
> - If you were a fly on the wall how would you describe what is going on here?
> - If you had a bird's eye view of this group/interaction/problem what would you see happening?
> - If you were the ship's captain what would your first order to the crew be now?
> - Imagine a wise person were available and willing to help you with this problem – what advice do you think he would give you?

On first sight these questions seem strange and you might imagine that it would be an awkward experience asking these of a group. And yet they are a powerful and natural means of evoking or drawing out feelings and experiences which already exist – though they may be hard to describe – and providing a structure and vehicle for their expression.

These questions employ the language of mental imagery and symbolism in order to help members connect to and communicate with areas of the self which can supplement and enhance the analytic mind. They consciously call up, or build an image to represent some aspect of individual or group experience and aim at focusing attention on the problem and increasing awareness and expression of personal experience.

Imaginative techniques include:

- Visualization – seeing pictures, images in the mind's eye
- Guided fantasy – offering the individual or group a series of images which they can visualize and explore in imagination (see page 28)
- Symbolic imagery – images with deep symbolic meaning and regenerative properties such as the wise person, the path of life, water, sun, etc.
- Meditation – body relaxation, generating new ideas, insights, contemplative meditation

---

These techniques are based on two simple assumptions

- *Psychological energy and feeling can be channelled by a symbol or image, transformed by it, or integrated by it*: Roberto Assagioli, who developed psychosynthesis which uses imaginative techniques a great deal, believed that when someone was offered a symbol or situation to imagine, they projected thoughts, emotions, and qualities onto it which came from their own experience.[4] This has obvious implications for work with groups, particularly in situations where members have difficulty expressing themselves or working out a problem.
- *Energy and behaviour follow thought*:[5] Visualizing a symbol, or any thought indeed, can lead to an identification with it and this can be used to establish new and more desirable attitudes and behaviours in the group. When we create something we always create it first in a thought form. A thought always precedes its manifestation. An artist first has an idea and then creates a picture. 'I think I'll make dinner' is the idea that precedes creating a meal. The idea is like a blueprint; it creates the image of the end product and then magnetizes or attracts physical energy to make the idea occur in reality, as the media advertising companies are very well aware.

So by visualizing or thinking about an idea or symbol, group members can create, vitalize, identify with, and evoke its potential and qualities in their interactions with each other. As you encourage them to observe the possibilities, the idea becomes more clearly defined. Feelings are attracted to it and the idea becomes a desire seeping into members' everyday experience. Thus by inculcating and developing thinking about teamwork, co-operation, sharing, goodwill, and the like you can help members gradually to create these very conditions in the group.

Here are some of the situations in which I have used imaginative techniques:

- Using symbols to explore group process – resistance, conflict, quality of communication/ trust
- Using symbols to explore individual experience – body, personality, sexuality, relationships

- To help members identify changes which they would like to make in their lives, to make a decision or choice – useful exercises might be:

  1   Fantasy journey to the Temple of Silence[6]
  2   Encounter with the wise person/advice-giver[7]
  3   'Ideal model', life/career/relationships, etc.[8]

- To evoke a desired situation and mentally rehearse skills and behaviours:

  a   Mixing socially with other people, making friends
  b   Asserting oneself
  c   Job interview, sports performance
  d   Training groups – professional performance and presentation of skills and behaviours

- To visualize and work through a difficult, frightening, or embarrassing situation in the future:

  1   Making a speech, presentation, job interview
  2   Making friends, self-introduction
  3   Asserting oneself, ending a relationship, saying no
  4   Worst fears, phobias, and compulsions, shyness, stammering, blushing, drying up, getting stuck

- For healing and regeneration:

  a   Developing positive self-image
  b   Developing particular aspects of personality
  c   Relaxation and body awareness
  d   Overcoming illness or emotional disability
  e   Strengthening and developing the will

- To end a session and help members wind down and relax
- To develop creativity, problem solving, intuition, and imagination
- To promote norms and values in the group – sharing, mutuality, reciprocity, goodwill, etc.
- To help members evoke and connect to meaning, purpose, essence in their lives, work, relationships

Guidelines for using imaginative techniques in the group

WHEN TO USE

You can use imaginative techniques at any stage to explore individual or group experience but I find it best to use them:

- To help a member who is having difficulty describing a problem
- To channel feeling or emotional material which is obstructing expression
- To develop or augment problem solving, creative imagination, intuition
- To teach members how to relax
- To help members mediate and confront reality
- To promote particular values, norms, and behaviours

INTRODUCING IMAGINATIVE TECHNIQUES

Familiarize your group with this way of working as early as you can and introduce the technique as an alternative way of understanding and thinking about situations. Ferrucci,[6] Whitmore,[9] Fugitt,[10] and De Mille[11] contain numerous exercises and imaginative activities that can be used in any group and will give you tips on how to introduce and modify this medium to your own particular setting. Do try to read these books if you can.

Some people like to participate in imaginative games with their eyes closed. Others prefer to keep their eyes open. Either is permissible but you may have to check that an eyes-open attitude does not indicate fear, suspicion, or distrust of the group or the medium.[12] Encourage people to be appropriately silent and not to talk or distract others. Initially a certain amount of talking and even giggling may be inevitable but if you persist with the approach, members will become accustomed to the need for silence and goodwill and respond accordingly.

AFTERWARDS

I often accompany imaginative work with drawing or writing. This serves to ground the experience and begin the process of manifestation and expression. Drawing or writing frequently unfolds other insights or ideas and is a valuable way of consolidating and making more complete the process of understanding. Sharing and discussion can then take place in twos, threes, or in the large group. You should try to relate the imaginative experiences to the here and now reality of the group. Ask members how and in what way the experience is reminiscent of or arises out of their everyday or group interaction. Do not force or insist on this because sometimes a person's imagery does not immediately speak to a situation and it may be that it only fits into place later. Usually, however, the experiences do contain simple answers and insights and will illuminate personal and group process with humour and grace.

Do consider using imaginative techniques in your group. You will find them not only a playful and creative way of working but a powerful medium for channelling psychological energy and generating new alternatives and solutions.[13]

Technique number 4

Using games and exercises in the group

I was working in the first session of a group recently with professionals who wished to explore their practice with ex-psychiatric patients. People had introduced themselves but still the atmosphere was tense. I invited people to join me in some games and exercises as a way of breaking the ice. Group members proceeded to have a sword fight using their index fingers only, make statues out of each other, and have a conversation without words, amongst other games. This activity only took 15 minutes and yet it was successful in reducing the tension and inhibition in the group and generating fun, excitement, and shared experience.

These and other games offer a valuable source of activities, exercises, and strategies for working with groups. They can be used and enjoyed by everyone as they usually involve simple and easily understood procedures. Here are some of the reasons for using games in groups:

- At the beginning of a group games can help people introduce themselves and become better acquainted
- Team games encourage members to do something successfully with others, promote trust, co-operation, teamwork, cohesion
- Communication games help members become aware of the importance of listening to each other, non-verbal language, and the various skills involved in self-expression
- Games can stimulate imagination, develop resourcefulness, and teach problem-solving and decision-making skills
- Games can help members develop awareness, sensitivity, and control – when to be quiet, noisy, still, active, responsive to others, dependent, independent, interdependent
- Games teach the necessity of rules, procedure, and framework. They promote discipline, control, self-responsibility, teamwork, and the exercise of personal will and choice
- Games provide opportunity for fun, adventure, excitement, risk taking
- They generate interest and enthusiasm and can stimulate a group which is tired, bored, or just after lunch! Games help a boisterous or excited group channel and expend surplus energy
- Games involve physical contact, can enhance motor co-ordination, and develop poise, confidence, and self-esteem
- Games can simulate reality, aspects of group process, problems with relationships, and can be used to explore dynamics and create resolution and meaning

You can see that while the objective may vary, I am interested in the purposeful and constructive use of games. Without a context or rationale, games are just a way of filling time or can be a frivolous, empty activity. I often come across workers who use games in their sessions but are vague as to why they do so. They may have attended a conference or course which started with the obligatory games session and believe this is how groups are supposed to be run. Other workers would like to use games as an alternative to more traditional verbal and conceptual ways of working but are uncertain as to how to do this.

Remember there are only four reasons why you should use games in a group:

- As a metaphor to simulate or represent reality
- To generate experiential learning
- To motivate people
- To engage the whole person

When your use of games arises out of one or more of these contexts then you will find that the game or exercise is relevant and meaningful and it is possible to use the game as a springboard to discussion, problem solving, or exploration of group process.

Guidelines for using games in the group

- *Build up a repertoire of games*: This will help you if the group is bored, tired, rowdy, shy. At the end of this book is a list of manuals and compilations of games which make profitable reading.[14] Over time you will develop a personal library of games which you can adapt to suit any particular occasion or need. Do remember to work out and rehearse a game before you try it in a session.
- *State the purpose of the game*: It is usually best to state the purpose and objective of the game in advance so that people have some idea of what they are getting into.
- *Invite participation*: Do not force or insist on members joining in. Members who sit out of a game are still involved through their laughter, enjoyment, encouragement, and appreciation of the others. Permit this and next time you will find them joining in.
- *Be positive and encouraging*: Maintain an attitude which asserts, 'You can do it, would you like to try?'
- *Time*: Allow adequate time for a game but pay close attention to how the group responds to it. A manual may advise 20 minutes but your group may only need half this time or may require more. So do not be afraid to improvise, change the rules, stop, or introduce another game. Remember boredom means trouble!
- *Review*: Most games benefit and enhance the work of the group if you devote some time afterwards to reviewing the experience with members (see page 194). Sometimes it is not appropriate or necessary to look at how members found the activity but as a general rule you should help members see the relevance and meaning of the games session for their work in the group.
- *Invite suggestions from members*: Many members will have experience of games or activities that they have found enjoyable and which can be easily adapted for the group. Not only does this more easily involve members but it provides you with material that you know works!
- *Always be sure you know why you are using a game or exercise*: If you cannot give members an explanation that makes sense then you should not be using a games approach. Make sure the game fits with what is happening and will lead to clarification.

A miscellany

Sculpting

Sculpting is a technique that can be used to explore themes such as intimacy, power, or relationships in the group. If used in a loose, flexible way it need not take up a lot of time and can be very effective in illuminating the interpersonal dynamics in a situation. Because it involves a spatial and emotional language rather than words or concepts it is a valuable tool to use at certain times in the group life.

I sometimes use sculpting with individuals in the group who may be experiencing some difficulty in describing a problem or incident. I will ask the person to assume a physical posture or gesture which expresses their feelings in the situation or conveys the main characteristics of the event. It can be valuable to include group members' comments on the posture as a way of helping the individual begin to articulate the experience. Sculpting can generate powerful emotions but with a willing and trusting group it is possible to deepen communication between members and heighten consciousness about the dynamics and processes involved.[15]

Creative writing

Some individuals and groups find writing a useful method of reflecting upon and expressing their experience. With these groups I often encourage people to write a few notes after an exercise or jot down their thoughts about an incident in the group as an aid to discussion. Encouraging members to keep a personal journal or establishing a group diary is another valuable method of helping people think about what is happening in the group and pick out the significant factors in a situation.

Creative writing is also a way of helping members communicate emotions which are often too painful or compacted to be released verbally, and accustoming people to the expressive and cathartic value of image and metaphor. A technique that I find particularly effective in exploring a problem or some aspect of group process is to engage members in writing a group poem about the incident. The rules are simple – I write a first line pertaining to the situation and any member can then write any word, sentence, or lines which spontaneously come to mind. There is no attempt to create rhyme and the emphasis is on immediacy, intuition, and discovery. I have found this to be an excellent way of stimulating a quiet, silent, or withdrawn group.[16]

Storytelling

Many of the problematic features of a group can be dealt with through the medium of myth and storytelling. Sometimes an incident may be too painful or obscure to confront directly and inviting members to construct a story around the incident can be an effective way of expressing emotion and raising consciousness. You can ask willing members to supply one word in turn around the circle, a sentence, as much or as little as they wish to contribute. Storytelling can enhance conversation and communication skills and can be used to promote self-esteem, build confidence, and foster co-operation.

A wonderful metaphor for groupwork is to be found in the story of *The Wizard of Oz*. The story is about isolated and disconnected individuals who, feeling a lack of something essential in themselves, band together to seek out a wise person who will help them regain that which they have lost. In the coming together, the individuals learn to care for each other, protect each other, and look out for each other – the very qualities that were perceived to have been lost! The wizard turns out not to be an expert but a man of compassion and good intent who tries to help the companions as best he can. Through his efforts the travellers learn to work and live together as a group, which in effect requires them to recover their lost qualities in service of the whole. A perfect story for exploring individual and collective dynamics!

Over 700 years ago Dante Alighieri wrote his classic poem the *Divine Comedy* which describes his imaginary journey through the states of consciousness described as Hell, Purgatory, and Paradise. After finding himself depressed and in an existential midlife crisis Dante meets a guide, Vergil who conducts him skilfully through the frightening regions. Along the way Dante converses with a series of characters who instruct him on their downfall and means to avoid the same fate. You can see how such a vivid story of a lost individual and a skilled helper who have to undertake a journey of self-examination and redemption can be very helpful for those frequent times when groups get stuck or sidetracked.

You can develop story making and narration by asking members to describe what they think is happening in photographs cut out of magazines, pictures on tarot cards, and the like. It is surprising how skilfully members can use the story method to uncover the elements of a situation and communicate with each other, when in other circumstances they might prefer to remain silent.

Music

At times I use music as a way of altering the mood of a group or channelling energy. An active group can be helped to relax by playing some suitably soft music and an inert group can find reggae or pop very energizing. Many group members have particular musical favourites and will respond to an invitation to share their musical memories with the others. This can augment exploration of a theme or problem and is an effective method of stimulating and generating discussion. The use of music also leads quite naturally to drama, role-play, and movement.

Developing a suitable climate for the use of techniques

When you first propose using role-play, drawing, visualization, or any game to explore group process or help members communicate and express themselves, you may encounter objections:

> - I can't draw/act/do this
> - This is stupid
> - I don't like this
> - What is the point of this?

It is important to allow these and other protestations and quietly point out that what you intend to introduce has nothing to do with the aesthetic or skill aspects of a particular medium. Clearly state your intentions and objectives so that people understand that they are participating in an experiential exercise which is for the purposes of learning, creating resolution, and meaning.

Emphasize that:

> - This is a different way of working in the group
> - It is a way of developing more creative, imaginative responses to situations and problems
> - There is no right or wrong, best or least. The emphasis is on inquiry, discovery, expression, and change

If objections persist you may have to give some time to exploring underlying issues in the group revolving around competition, exposure, trust, and confidentiality. Do allow for a certain amount of embarrassment or awkwardness as many group members may not be familiar with work involving modes other than the rational and verbal, and it will obviously take time and practice to become accustomed to some of these ideas.

You may find members acting in a provocative or undermining manner when they first try out these techniques. People may giggle, disrupt, or misbehave. Do not be put off by this! Most of us find new and unfamiliar situations threatening and behave similarly. Acknowledge the fear, embarrassment, or anxiety generated and repeat the technique in another session. Do not abandon the technique believing it is failing or is inappropriate. In most cases you will find that persistence creates familiarity and acceptance. Having said this, however, you must always respect members' freedom of choice about involvement in an activity. Participation should be on a voluntary basis and you should never force or coerce anyone into experiential work.

It can be valuable to agree a contract with group members determining the purpose of the exercise, the length of activity, how it is to be used, confidentiality, members' rights and responsibilities, and the like. This is usually sufficient to persuade even the more timid or suspicious members to join in. It is important to spend time reviewing and grounding the experience afterwards in order to evoke and articulate consciousness. Again no one should be forced to share and I usually preface this phase of experiential work by reminding members that they can share 'as much or as little' as they wish. The way in which you handle this review stage can determine how willing members will be to do this work again so be sensitive in eliciting feelings, question judiciously, and demonstrate that you are listening and appreciative of a member's experience.

You might wish to ask:

- Does anyone wish to share what that was like?
- How do you feel about what happened?
- What did you discover about yourself?
- Have you experienced anything like this before?
- What does this remind you of/suggest/what comes to mind?
- What does this experience say to you about what happens in the group/about your life?
- How can you use this experience to move on?
- What was missing?
- What could have been improved?
- What do we need as a group?

Through your questioning and your approach to the review of experiential work you can create an atmosphere which suggests that members are free to find their own way and that what they think and feel is fundamental. The review can become an opportunity to reflect and think critically, talk through issues, and try out new ideas, guesses, and hunches. This may be very exciting for members and can come to be positively associated with the new techniques.

Do not necessarily confine yourself to reviewing in the large group. Think about using pairs or subgroups as an alternative to sharing and talking in the large group. The smaller units provide more time, opportunities for intimacy and depth, and a chance to practise conversation skills, empathy, and acceptance.

By your being clear and open with members, firm, warm, and supportive, these techniques can come to be seen as an exciting and acceptable way of working mutually on group issues and personal concerns. Initial reluctance or embarrassment will come to be replaced by enthusiasm and satisfaction and your use of techniques will become an integral part of the way the group operates and a means of engaging the member in a creative and complete manner.

A postscript

It is clear that the variety of problems and situations encountered in working with groups is great and the actual methods adopted range widely. And yet the rationale remains the same – a vision of and belief in the power and creativity of fellowship, mutuality, and reciprocity. This leads me to believe that one technique alone underlies all efforts to work creatively with a group of individuals and help them achieve their personal and collective goals. This technique is based on love and understanding. The point can hardly be overstated.

Ultimately, vision is more important than techniques and methods. The group worker who has a thorough understanding of what happens whenever people come together, and who knows how to co-operate with influence and allow these processes, will be able to adjust his activities to the problems at hand rather than follow a prescribed technical procedure. Such a worker has a flexibility and creativity which has been acquired by building his work on principles and vision and not by memorizing routines and methods. Techniques are important, but they are meaningless and mechanized unless grounded in a vision of the possibilities inherent in fellowship and shared experience.

Review

* Techniques can be used metaphorically
* Techniques are a way of generating experiential learning
* Techniques are a way of motivating people
* Techniques are a way of engaging the whole person
* Techniques should be used purposefully and with intent
* State an objective for the technique, invite participation, review the experience, contextualize the learning
* Develop and build a repertoire of techniques that can be adapted to any situation in the group
* Remember that technique follows vision and goals!

References

1 Quoted in Baynes, C.F. (1950) trans., *The I Ching or Book of Changes*, Princeton, NJ: Princeton University Press.
2
   * Badaines, J. (1977) 'Psychodrama: acting your problems away', *Psychology Today*, December: 38–40.
   * Badaines, J. (1977) 'Psychodrama: concepts, principles, and issues, *Drama Therapy*, 1, 2.

- Keysell, P. (1975) *Motives for Mime*, London: Evans.
- Pemberton-Billing, R.N. and Clegs, J.D. (1968) *Teaching Drama*, London: University of London Press.
- Rayner, P. (1976) 'Psychodrama as a medium for intermediate treatment', *British Journal of Social Work*, 7, 4: 443–53.
- Way, B. (1975) *Development through Drama*, London: Longman.

3
- Goodnow, J. (1977) *Children's Drawing*, London: Fontana.
- Liebman, M. (1982) *Art Games and Structures for Groups*, Bristol: Bristol Art Therapy Group.
- Oaklander, V. (1978) *Windows to Our Children*, esp. pp. 21–52, Moab, UT: Real People Press.
- Remocker, J. and Storch, E. (1979) *Action Speaks Louder*, Edinburgh: Churchill Livingstone.
- Storr, A. (1976) *The Dynamics of Creation*, London: Pelican.

4   Assagioli, R. (1980) *Psychosynthesis*, esp. Chapter 5, London: Wildwood House.
5   Assagioli, R. (1980) *The Act of Will*, esp. Chapter 5, London: Wildwood House.
6   Ferrucci, P. (1982) *The Visions and Techniques of Psychosynthesis*, Wellingborough: Turnstone Press.
7   op. cit., p. 144 ff.
8   op. cit., p. 167 ff.
9   Whitmore, D. (1986) *Psychosynthesis in Education*, Wellingborough: Turnstone Press.
10 Fugitt, E.D. (1983) *He Hit Me Back First: Creative Visualization Activities for Parenting and Teaching*, Fawnskin, CA: Jalmar Press.
11 De Mille, R. (1972) *Put Your Mother on the Ceiling*, New York: Viking Press.
12 Gawain, S. (1978) *Creative Visualization*, Millvalley, CA: Whatever Publishing.
13 Masters, R.E.L. and Houston, J. (1983) *Mindgames: The Guide to Inner Space*, Wellingborough: Dover Publications.
14 See:
- Brandes, D. and Phillips, H. (1979), *Gamester's Handbook*, London: Hutchinson.
- De Boro, E. (1980) *Lateral Thinking*, London: Penguin.
- Hopson, B. and Hough, P. (C.R.A.C., 1973) *Exercises in Personal and Career Development*, Cambridge: Hobsons Press.
- Jelfs, M. (1982) *Manual for Action*, London: Action Resources Group.
- Pfeiffer, J.W. and Jones, J.E. (1975) *Handbook of Structured Experiences for Human Relations Training*, 5 vols, San Francisco, CA: Jossey-Bass/Pfeiffer.
- Stevens, J.O. (1973) *Awareness*, New York: Bantam Books.
15 For an introduction to sculpting read:
    Hopkins, J. (1981) 'Seeing yourself as others see you', *Social Work Today*, 12, 25: 10–3.
16 For more on poetry and creative writing see:
    Carradice, P. (1981) 'Ode to a tiger', *Social Work Today*, 13, 7: 22–3.
    For journalling techniques, see:
- Progoff, I. (1978) *At a Journal Workshop*, New York: Dialogue House Library.
- Rainwater, J. (1979) *You're in Charge*, Chapter 4, Wellingborough: Turnstone Press.

Chapter 11

Working more intensively with groups

Focus and context

In the last few chapters I have sketched out the essential processes and skills which I believe you need to master in order to lead your group effectively. Knowledge of stages and patterns in group development has been outlined in Chapters 4–7 and process skills articulated in Chapter 9, which will enable you to be in tune with your group and intervene effectively. But I now want to draw attention to what underlies this. I want to turn now and consider the role and importance of the two practice skills which, as you become ever more familiar with them, will enable you to work more intensively and at deeper levels with your group and to include more of the members' preoccupations and concerns.

A central concern for the group worker

It is clear by now that any group is a volatile, dynamic, and rapidly shifting system of individual and collective experiences and interactions, with multiple levels of need, activity, and performance. At times the group experience both for the members and the worker can seem and feel overwhelming, even incomprehensible, impulsive, random and, at worst, chaotic. Typically, at these times and in such situations a worker may be required to intervene in order to help group members clarify what is happening and make appropriate choices or assist in managing some change or event which is impacting on them.

A key problem for the group worker is where and at what to direct his attention.

- What am I looking at?
- What does it mean?
- What is required of me/us now?

The question of what the worker pays attention to is about *focus*, and the question of making sense of the data or phenomenon observed is about how the worker creates a *context* for meaning. You may recall that I first mentioned the need for context in my introduction (page 2) when I said that context provides a frame of reference which informs and disciplines how and when you intervene. So, knowing what you are looking at and what it means provides the worker with the opportunity to intervene effectively and systematically throughout a spectrum of member preoccupations and concerns. We shall consider this spectrum of preoccupations shortly, but first I want to say some more about focus and context.

Focus is about:

- Attention   Noticing an effect, topic, feeling, behaviour, or its absence in the group or oneself.
- Observation   Studying for a time the *location* of the event; where is the centre of activity, the point of greatest energy? *Configuration*: what is the shape and size of activity? Who is involved and who is not? *Dynamics*: what are the feelings involved in the phenomenon? How does it develop or diminish?
- Definition   Is there a clear image, theme, or event which can be presented to the group for consideration?

Context is about:

- Connection   Weaving together a mass of responses connecting events and behaviours which precede and follow a particular passage in the group.
- Reflection   Thinking about what is occurring both separately and collectively, creating words, sentences for what is happening, discussion, composition of themes and motifs, creating a hypothesis.
- Interpretation   Generating meaning, giving orientation, determining what the individual or group is preoccupied with.

Example of worker's use of focus and context in a group

A therapy group for adults had been meeting for about a year with a constant set of five members, when three new members joined.

They were well received by the old members, but after about six sessions I noticed that I was feeling vaguely dissatisfied with the quality of group interaction. I could not determine what my discontent was about so I set myself simply to observe for the next session or two what was occurring in the group.

What soon became clear was that there was really little interaction. Each member seemed to take a turn in presenting their current life experience to a seemingly attentive but silent audience. This was in marked contrast to the established pattern of more spontaneous and reciprocal interaction engaged in by the senior members before the new arrivals. It was clear that in some unspoken way the whole group – but in particular the large subgroup of senior members – were relating with each other in a manner which seemed to promise attention but not mutuality or engagement. I became more aware of a sense of impatience in myself with the senior members whom I thought should know better and should be inducting the newer members into the norms and ways of the group. I knew now that I had located a disturbance in the group and I had some sense of the size and shape and who was involved in that disturbance.

On thinking about my impatience with the lack of mutuality and my irritation with the senior members for withholding real contact while seeming to give attention, I began to conjecture that the senior members were punishing me for introducing new people while at the same time withholding the benefits of group experience from the invading arrivals, and that I was reacting to this. I now felt able to draw the group's attention to a clear theme of distant and uninvolved contact and invite discussion. The senior members in particular denied that they were uninvolved and asserted that they were only sharing out the group time so that everyone had a turn and that no one felt excluded. They were oblivious to the point that the emphasis on fair shares was not only about equity but must also indicate a fear of losing out to others and a defence against the wish to exclude the newcomers from getting more.

It was not possible to get much further with things until two sessions later, when two senior members missed the group session without notice and most untypically. Members who did attend worried that the absentees might not come back, though there were no grounds to believe this; they feared that the absentees were not getting enough from the group and became anxious that the group had got too big to provide everybody with what they needed.

When the two absentees turned up the following week with weak excuses for not attending, it was now much easier to invite reflection and discussion about what was really going on in the group as it was manifested in the quality of relationship and engagement.

Gradually, senior members began to reveal their displeasure with me for suddenly introducing three new members and not staggering the entrances over time. The experience of feeling swamped and no longer the focus of my attention had rekindled old feelings of anguish and rage at the thoughtlessness of parental figures, displacement by younger siblings, and the rivalries and family allegiances that this generated. This had been re-enacted in the group rather than spoken about and worked with.

With these revelations the group now had a context in which to speak about their feelings and experiences of change, loss of the familiar, new beginnings, disruptions, newcomers, and reorientation. Early experiences of change, loss, and adaptation within the family were now seen to create a template which moulded individual response to similar experiences in later life. Only by talking about these experiences in the containing and permissive environment of the group which each member had to build and contribute to, could the individual be freed from repeating the old patterns and choose a novel response.

Investigative and facilitative attitude of the group worker

You can see from this vignette that what enables the group members to move to a more mutual interaction is the persistence and capacity of the worker to ask the group to focus on a particular problem and put it in a context which generates some meaning and opens up possibilities for development. Focus and context are the two poles of an investigative attitude which characterizes what a group experience can offer an individual.

Focus draws attention to some phenomenon in the group life, and context provides a container for holding and generating sense and meaning for that phenomenon.

The group worker is the representative of an investigative attitude which places singular importance on considering process issues. The worker is the embodiment of an ethic which is based on the idea that the essence of group membership is shared experience, and that anything which inhibits this development requires examination and discussion.

> - The essence of the human being is social, not individual
> - The essence of the group is shared experience
> - The individual is part of a network of social processes (family, occupational, political, religious, etc.)
> - Disturbance in these networks can be re-enacted in the current group
> - The current group can help individuals become aware of their unhelpful patterns of social disturbance and make new choices

Over time, this function of inquiry and curiosity becomes distributed among the membership, as the worker emphasizes the active participation of all members and their involvement with each other.

There are a number of major concepts which contribute to the investigative attitude in the group.

But here is the crucial one:

- All events and incidents in the group can be viewed as types and forms of communication, both conscious and unconscious, verbal and behavioural. These communications can be focused upon by the worker and members, and contextualized in order to make meaningful and exchangeable interaction.

We can even identify different contexts and levels of communication which can help provide the worker with an initial frame of reference and guide.

These contexts for group behaviour are characterized by decreasing awareness and ability to think and talk about what is really preoccupying members and an increased propensity to act out the core issues behaviourally.

The explicit context

The group is a public forum where everyone can see and be seen by everyone else. This generates many opportunities to be blamed and shamed in front of others. To enter a group, an individual surrenders some degree of privacy and autonomy, and that brings with it a fear of rejection and a wish to conform to hypothesized or explicit norms and values and real or imagined authority. So one often sees in the group individual members asking for permission to speak or apologizing for themselves – 'Can I just say . . . ?' 'I don't mean to upset the apple cart but . . .' These and other protective and controlling measures were first learned in the family and school as part of the process of social conditioning and soon become evident in ordinary group interaction.

It is possible for the worker to recognize and categorize these explicit and conscious communications of members as operating within a context which is to do with and influenced by members' concerns about public opinion, social standing, and self-esteem, community, authority, law, custom, and the like.

The transference context

Transference is a psychoanalytic concept which refers to the tendency of individuals in an unusual or clinical setting to relate and treat others as if they were significant figures from their personal history.[1] So group members might relate to the worker as if to a parental figure rather than as a person in their own right or to each other as if they were siblings rather than colleagues.

Since the first group is the family group, all groups thereafter resonate to some degree with the dynamics, tensions, and yearnings of the primary group experience. The individual has to manage the presence of others in the current group as the inevitable struggles for dominance and status can so easily ignite re-enactments of the sibling rivalries of the primary family group. Members will compete with each other for the worker's attention, become preoccupied with the identity of the 'favourites' in the group, and show surprising sensitivity and jealousy around the worker's interactions in ways which re-enact and are reminiscent of earlier child–parent–sibling relationships.

When such behaviours and communications surface in the group, it is invaluable for the worker to have an understanding of the inevitability and almost 'normal' nature of transference phenomena in order to provide that containing and reassuring context which relieves the pressure and encourages members to think and talk about what is happening.

The projection context

'Projection' is another psychoanalytic term which refers to an individual's unconscious tendency to disown unacceptable parts of themselves for fear of being rejected.[2] These unwanted qualities – like anger or desire – or unacceptable parts of the self – like the clingy child or flirt or bully – are then projected onto others, who are often reproached for the very things feared in oneself.

I think that much of the difficult and intensive work in groups is really about working with these projections – so pervasive, mobile, and slippery. The desire in the group is to present a good image, and since group involvement entails a loss of privacy, individuals engage in a great deal of projection in order to hide shameful or unacceptable parts of themselves. Much of the worker's intervention in these circumstances is aimed at demonstrating to individuals and the group how they create situations where expectations and predictions about the world are fulfilled.

Once the self-fulfilling prophecies can be illustrated, work can then begin to help members accept the repressed primitive and instinctual parts of themselves and abandon the self-hatred and fear which gives rise to projection in the first place.

What helps me identify the presence of projective activity is to think of the group as a hall of mirrors in which everybody sees themselves reflected by the others present. Members can see others reacting to events in the same manner in which they do, or in marked contrast to their own behaviour. Often members will comment on this: 'You remind me of how I used to be . . . ' Frequently you will hear people say, 'You know it's like looking in a mirror . . . ' Sometimes these mirror reflections are helpful and enable members to get to know themselves through seeing the effect they have on others and the pictures they form of themselves. Sometimes the mirror reflections are so distorted or alien that empathy and contact are impossible and confusion and conflict are the prevailing moods in the group.

The worker endeavours to help members realize that it is parts of the self and not the whole of oneself that are being reflected, and that the power of the group is its capacity to provide different angles, perspectives, and levels so that one cannot avoid seeing oneself through others' eyes.

It is the unique property of the group that quite quickly it can provide each individual with a multiplicity of self-reflection – a picture in the round, so to speak – a refracted picture of oneself to reflect upon and consider, in any one moment immeasurably more complex and multilayered than the simple view of one's own self up to that point. Through proximity and contact with others, the possibility emerges of correcting distorted images of oneself and discovering new dimensions and depths in one's being. But this is always a painful process and groups need a lot of training in order to understand and contextualize their behaviour at this level. The worker must always be alert and vigilant for how members are using each other and the group to deal with inner parts of themselves.

The somatic context

At times you may hear members talking about their experience of the group in somatic or bodily terms. Frequently, members will report how some emotional conflict or event in the last session made them feel sick afterwards. Another member will angrily describe how all this talking is giving her a sore head or the lack of co-operation is a real pain. Often, in a new beginning group, members will report sweaty palms, butterflies in the tummy, heart palpitations, and other physical sensations prior to talking or speaking out. It is as if the member's experience of group life is operating at a very primal and direct level and is expressed in physical terms.

People may perceive or experience group involvement as doing something to them somatically and producing painful or uncomfortable symptoms or making them worse in some physical way.

What is happening is simply that a very common experience for us all in times of crisis or emergency is being magnified in the group setting. In a highly charged or stressful situation people regress to primitive functioning in order to cope with or manage the real or perceived threat. We are all familiar with the instinctual nature of the fight–flight phenomenon. Now, in a group situation there is a loss of privacy, the experience of being in the public gaze, and the ever-present sensation of feelings swirling around and being amplified and magnified.

If something is happening in the group which is new for us or threatens our vulnerabilities, like introducing oneself to strangers or finding oneself part of a quarrel, we can respond to the heightened emotionality of the encounter with feelings of panic. It is these feelings of panic that engender the instinctual and reflexive nature of fight–flight responses, because panic undermines and attacks our capacity to think about what is happening. Not being able to think coherently about what is going on results in members feeling flooded with feelings and sensations, leading to that hypersensitive awareness in which the group is misguidedly believed to be causing the individual's pain and distress.

I will say more about this somatic context of group life and behaviour later (page 217) but for now I just want to suggest that you need to learn to recognize that individuals and groups do operate at these sorts of levels and that it is an entirely natural feature of group life which must be allowed for by the worker. I said in my introduction (page 4) that the group is organic and natural and that the group is an energetic experience. This means that there is ebb and flow in the condition and quality of the process and that the group can be emotionally and physically experienced and lived. This is why often, in interviewing individuals for prospective membership, you will come across fears of contamination and contagion and fantasies about the group swamping the individual.

Just as these fears and fantasies are dealt with in individual sessions by bringing them out into the open where they can be discussed and tested, so in the group the worker has to normalize these somatic phenomena and, by going towards them with interest and attention, recontextualize the circumstances as something to be explored and talked about rather than being overwhelmed by.

The archetypal context

The concept of the 'collective unconscious' was developed by Carl Jung and represents a landmark in the history of psychology.[3] Before Jung, psychoanalysis had concerned itself exclusively with the exploration of the personal and individual unconscious.

Jung then showed the great extent of collective psychic elements and forces which exercise a powerful effect on the human personality. According to Jung, the collective unconscious is a vast world stretching from the biological to the spiritual level, and contains latent memory traces of human ancestral development. This psychological residue of evolutionary development manifests in patterns or predispositions which can determine the individual's response to life experiences and even what sort of experiences he has.

These predispositions or blueprints are called 'archetypes', and are the crystallization of human experience over countless generations. They appear in the human psyche as a readiness to behave and experience life along broad lines, themes, or motifs.

The importance for the group worker of the collective unconscious and its archetypal energies is that the individual is now linked not just to the past of his infancy but to the past of his tribe, culture, and species. This means that both the individual and the group are resonating to cultural and tribal symbols, stories, and myths, and that these impact on group life, shape it, and can serve it if the worker is tuned in to this particular context.

One of the first archetypal manifestations of the collective unconscious in any group is the scapegoat and its close cousin the sacrificial lamb. You may know that the scapegoat as a phenomenon dates from biblical times, when the wandering Jewish tribes used the animal actually to bear the burden of the sins of the tribe.

The scapegoat was then separated and exiled from the tribal group and sent into the desert to die. By contrast, the sacrificial lamb was not banished from the group but offered up on behalf of the group to appease God. The sacrificial lamb was therefore a martyr within and for the group.

What this all means is that groups throughout history and up to the present day share certain recurring dilemmas and tend to come up with identical solutions.

Indeed, I would assert that group involvement and membership centres on a core dilemma which can be stated thus:

> Being a member of a group requires an individual to surrender part of their autonomy in service of the whole but not to surrender so much that they merge with or are overwhelmed by the group, whilst at the same time asserting their individuality but not in such a way that they are alienated from the group or narcissistically preoccupied with themselves at the expense of group involvement.

The tensions for individuals and groups which ensue from trying to solve this dilemma are such that, inevitably, conflicts around dependency, independence, desire, status, power, sex, property, and the myriad of human concerns have to be split into good and bad parts and acceptable and unacceptable qualities.

As we saw earlier, the easiest way of coping with perceived negative or shameful impulses and desires is to project them into others selected for that purpose. People look for others to blame so as to avoid the pain of responsibility or the helplessness of need. So the scapegoat is invoked in the member who embodies the negative or disowned aspects of group life.

The scapegoat is always somehow different and in some way – because of age, gender, colour, religion, or personality – goes against the implicit or explicit rules of the group and is easily selected to bear the 'sins' of the group. By attacking and exiling the scapegoat the group membership hopes to absolve itself from its own unacknowledged and often secretly longed-for desires.

In the case of the sacrificial lamb, a member offers himself as a martyr for the group. Such a member may carry the group's aggressive feelings about the leader and engage in a hostile relationship with the worker until the behaviour is understood and contextualized. All sorts of resistances and ambivalent feelings in the group can be taken up and suffered by the sacrificial lamb, resulting in much misunderstanding and lost opportunities until such time as the worker can see what is really happening.

There are all sorts of archetypal patterns and motifs which are evoked and which influence groups. For example, most people as they settle into the group have a sense of journeying towards some goal, and a means I have consistently found helpful in contextualizing and illuminating the dynamics of a group in question is, at an appropriate stage, to invite the group to examine the story of *The Wizard of Oz* and find correspondences with this story and their own experiences. We discussed this wonderful metaphor for groundwork in the previous chapter and considered how it provides a joyful context in which members can situate their woundedness and isolation and both identify with the various characters and be inspired to continue with the journey and its perils and hazards.

The myth of Narcissus and Echo has resonant power in groups. Narcissus is a beautiful and profoundly self-absorbed youth who falls fatefully in love with his own reflection in a pool. The nymph Echo seeks intimacy with him but is cruelly rebuffed and eventually herself dies. The story is about unhealthy and stagnant relational dynamics and what happens when people are unable to relate to each other meaningfully because they are too preoccupied with their own agendas.

In the same vein Milton's great poem *Paradise Lost* details the narcissistic dynamics of Lucifer and his demonic group when they are cast out of paradise because of their insurrection. Lucifer would rather 'reign in Hell than serve in heaven'. He has many modern descendants in groups. These are what I call the kings and queens of Hell. They are the members of groups who are unwilling to give up their solipsistic self-absorption and surrender a degree of autonomy in order to join in with others. They fear rejection and contempt if they let others close and so they treat intimacy with contempt and refuse to conform with the requests of peers to relate to them.

Another archetypal motif that we discussed previously was Dante Alighieri's classic poem the *Divine Comedy* which describes his imaginary journey through the states of consciousness described as Hell, Purgatory, and Paradise. This remarkably vivid story of a lost individual and a skilled helper who have to undertake a journey of self-examination and redemption can be very helpful for those frequent times when groups get stuck or sidetracked.

This is the power of the archetypal context for working with certain dynamics in groups. The archetypal dimension can be utilized to contextualize and transform behaviours and feelings which otherwise would bring chaos to the group. The aggressive member can be seen in the context of the warrior and taught to respect their capacity for aggression and use it in service of what is valuable rather than waste it in petty squabbling. The attention-seeking member may be misusing the hero archetype. The member who monopolizes and dominates the dialogue may need some help to connect to the poet/ bard or storyteller archetype.

The archetypal motif of birth–death–rebirth gives context and meaning to the experience of beginnings and endings, and members leaving and joining the group. I like to incorporate the old pagan and Christian festivals of Halloween, Christmas, and Easter as part of the sense of rhythm and development in the group year.

The important thing to be aware of when including the archetypal perspective in your work is the interactional synchrony between the collective unconscious and the individual. Individuals in the group are acting out their own personal needs as well as replicating and re-enacting great mytho-poetic dramas and stories. And at the same time, collective myths serve the evolutionary process of the group and are re-embodied through individual action.

Use of the worker's self to provide focus and context

At the beginning of a group few members have much understanding of the power and value and the opportunities offered by the group experience, nor can they be expected to have much sense of community. So they need quite a bit of help in order to come together and intermesh. Initially, the worker accepts leadership responsibility as a way of:

- Engaging, motivating, and encouraging new members
- Defining the purpose of the group
- Clarifying expectations about what is possible, what is not, what is required, what is not

in order to:

- Create commonality, collaboration, and community

Because the essential property of the group is shared experience, the worker endeavours gradually to wean the members from their early dependency on him. The power of the leader is based on projections onto him of parental and authority images and experiences in each member's personality, and their expectations that the worker will behave in the traditional hierarchical mode of authority and leadership. Rather than fight this the worker accepts it as natural and appropriate, but slowly, and at the group's pace, moves in the direction of leadership which is more collaborative and participative. In this way leadership becomes more a function of membership than the automatic preserve of one person. The group learns to replace the worker's authority with that of the group and its members, thereby subtly modifying attitudes to and the exercise of authority.

The worker modifies traditional attitudes to authority among members and helps to deepen and intensify the group experience by:

> - Modelling new positions
> - Sensitizing members psychologically
> - Acting as a catalyst to activate and mobilize what is latent in the group

The worker aims to foster the development of a shared psychic life in which everyone participates, to which everyone contributes, and for which everyone is responsible.

This means cultivating and emphasizing the investigative attitude which I referred to earlier (page 199):

> - Group relationships could not exist or be made visible without communication
> - Anything at all in a group which can be observed, perceived, or reacted to is a communication
> - The group worker is open to all and any communication which will locate and clarify what is really going on in the group

but especially:

> - Relationships formed with the worker and other members are also the object of communication and investigation

This is to focus on the worker and member relationships and to use them as a context for inquiry and understanding and working with deeper issues of group process. This is a very radical and catalytic position which the worker adopts, and one which at times proves irritating and uncomfortable for most, if not all groups. Most people enter a group of whatever kind with some conflicts and problems around managing relationships. Participation in a group over time generates the desire for intimacy with others, but as these feelings arise members can become anxious about them.

You may recall that I said on page 203 that a core dilemma in groups was how to get close but not too close, and how to be separate but not too separate.

To resolve this dilemma, members throw up their characteristic defences against the disturbing feelings and as part of the process they may stop people getting close to them. However, the commitment to the group contract requires them to attend and not to flee the threatening relationships, as previously outside the group they might have done. What now happens is that the group becomes permeated with members' typical devices for avoiding intimacy and sabotaging relationships, because whatever defences are employed outside the group become manifest and re-enacted in the group. This material is what the worker repeatedly draws attention to and what members find so difficult to engage with, because if the group is to achieve its goal, members need to assume responsibility for the difficulties and complexities of group interaction and take some time to engage with and investigate the group process.

The worker's emphasis and insistence on deeper and more intensive examination of the problems thrown up by belonging to a group can activate rebellion and exaggerated independence in some members, compliance and dependence in others, and this can stimulate the emergence of transference relationships to the leader.

Part of the worker's function is to be a transference figure, and it is the worker's understanding of his role as a transference object and his willingness to take on and focus on the transferences as a context, in order that they can be worked through and dissolved, that contributes so much to the group's capacity to transform member attitudes towards power, authority, and self-responsibility.

We will take up this theme of the transference relationships again in terms of how to work with them in the next chapter, but I want to now consider how the necessary self-examination of the worker in the group is another vital source of focus and context.

Here is an important principle:

> • What characterizes and distinguishes the group worker is his capacity to be both in the process and able to reflect upon it

The group worker is not outside the group looking in, but is a part of the group – a member with particular administrative and process responsibilities. I have continually emphasized the capacity for shared experience as the central property of the group, and such an idea is based on the belief that worker and members alike are inextricably linked with one another in a psychic system which they co-create.

This is what is meant by the very useful concept of 'matrix', which is a term derived from the discipline of group analysis and refers to the existence of a web of intrapsychic and interpersonal interrelationships which grow in the group over time and which everyone in the group shares in, contributes to, and is influenced by.[4]

The group matrix consists of interacting processes between a number of closely linked and interlocking people and inevitably gives rise to the phenomenon of 'resonance', which simply means that all group members, including the worker, intuitively and unconsciously tune into each other and to the relevant preoccupations and concerns of the group.[5]

This means that, since the worker influences and shapes the matrix and the pattern that the group takes and is also impacted on by the presence of the others, the feelings, hunches, intuitions, and fantasies of the worker can, on reflection, provide important clues about:

> • The internal life of the group
> • What is not being spoken about
> • What is not being thought about
> • What is fearsome and to be avoided
> • How members are feeling

- Why they might be feeling this
- What the anger/silence/depression might be about
- What members might be thinking about
- Why the group is stuck
- Why a behaviour/event is being repeated
- What the loss of creativity means
- Why there is difficulty sharing/trusting/deciding/working together
- What is happening between people
- What is not happening between people
- What is unfinished
- What is trying to emerge in the group

The mental, emotional, and instinctual responses of the worker in the group are profoundly important and not to be ignored or discarded. I would encourage you to cultivate your inner awareness of your impressions and reactions, and try to think about them as a way of focusing on the group. This requires time, patience, and great effort and discipline to build and maintain skills of self-examination and scrutiny so that they become second nature. This skill of self-analysis in the context of the group is akin to the use of the counter-transference as a therapeutic tool by the psychotherapist or psychoanalyst.[6]

Counter-transference originally referred to the feelings and conflicts stirred up in the therapist as a result of working with the client and was seen as an obstacle to be eliminated.

Just as transference was held to be unfinished business from the client's family history which got in the way of things and required dissolving, so counter-transference was seen to be the therapist's infantile reaction to the client, which equally needed to be dissolved. In recent years, counter-transference has come to have a broader meaning, which includes the therapist's conscious and appropriate emotional reactions to the client and has been recognized as an extremely valuable clue about how the client typically reacts with others and the sorts of responses which he generates in others.

Like any powerful tool, counter-transference is a difficult instrument to master and effectively depends on the worker's ability to be empathic and to be aware of and in contact with his emotions without defending too vigorously against whatever unpleasantness might arise.

Example 1

A woman in one of my therapy groups reported that she had recently attended a weekend personal growth group even though she knew that this was contrary to the rules of the therapy group which did not permit such extra-curricular activities. I found myself annoyed with her for this breach, and irritated with the other members who knew of the rule and did not challenge her on this. This happened on a second and a third occasion, and I found myself angry with the rebellious woman and the passive and acquiescent members. I refrained from saying anything because I wanted the members to confront her and because I did not want to appear the omnipresent authority.

When the third occasion occurred without challenge from the group I felt very angry with everyone and felt I had to say something. I did not know what to say except to be angry but I felt if I expressed my anger I would be going along with something unclear. At this point I tried to think about things and ask myself some questions:

> - What on earth is happening here?
> - Why am I so angry?
> - Because the woman is breaking the group rule and provoking me
> - Because the other members are going along with it
> - Why is she provoking me?
> - I don't know, but I feel like a father telling his adolescent daughter to be home by midnight and she keeps pushing the boundary

At this point I experienced immense relief because I had a possible context in which I could locate my anger and make some sense of what the woman and the group were doing. I told the woman that I was angry with her for the boundary breach but that I was curious as to why, knowing the rule, she would want to provoke me, and said that I felt like a father trying to curb his daughter. She replied that she too had been thinking why she had broken the rule and that I must be reading her mind because she had found herself thinking about her adolescent struggles with her father. We were now able to discuss her behaviour in this context and examine how she still reacted to authority figures today in the same inappropriate ways.

What also became apparent as the others took up this theme was how the group members were acting like younger siblings and letting this elder sister question and push the family rules and boundaries.

Example 2

This is the third session of a support group for staff in a young persons' residential home, and two female members of staff are talking about the strain of caring for their own children at home and looking after the disturbed adolescents in the unit.

They describe their guilt and the stress at leaving their own children at home and their sense of failing the young people in the unit.

The worker's internal response was as follows: 'I feel depressed and quite overwhelmed and find myself thinking about these staff as burdened and drained mothers who cannot get it right with their children.'

Two of the male staff join in and talk about how badly treated they feel by the young people in the unit and how they want to master the violent behaviour of the kids. One man produces the image of Ranulph Fiennes, the Arctic explorer, trekking across the icy wastes, pulling his own food, losing five stone in body weight, suffering severe frostbite. There are references to the mother of one youngster being 'a cold fish', and someone speaks of the suicide of a young man 'numbing' his key worker.

The worker's internal response was this: 'I find myself cold and aware of the absence of warmth, love, and contact that these workers must encounter with certain young people. That leads me to think about the masochistic doggedness and determination that the explorer of the frozen human soul must endure in order to make contact. The other side of this is perhaps how these workers must deep-freeze their rage at their charges and even turn the fury against themselves. I feel quite helpless and think that I have nothing to offer this team.'

The deputy team leader comes in to say that there are consequences to bad behaviour and that the team should be united in their determination not to accept violence. This brings a painful and angry response from the key worker of the young suicide that, if the team cannot accept and deal with violence, then it is not surprising that the youngsters will turn it on themselves.

The worker decides to intervene at this point to share his feelings of impotence and helplessness at listening to the team's agony, and wonders aloud if such feelings of desperation are perhaps normal and natural in the presence of such human misery as they have to deal with. The worker suggests that if the wish to help another is rebuffed, then the desire to care can become an intolerable burden and, when combined with the struggle not to retaliate, can leave one drained and wanting to keep one's distance.

This intervention seems to strike a chord with members and leads to a discussion centring on the profound difficulties involved in loving and supporting youngsters who behave terribly and appear to kill off the very warmth and contact that they crave. The discussion is marked by a new quality of compassion for themselves in this work and for their charges.

Now, the point of these examples is to show how the worker cannot avoid resonating to the emotional undercurrents in the group and how, rather than ignoring these responses, one can actually use them:

- To reach a deeper empathy with the group
- To identify themes and preoccupations
- To pick out the prevailing feelings
- To develop possible interventions
- To create a context which the group can use

You may see different interventions from those that I made. What is important is how the worker allows the group matrix to enter him in order to empathize and understand. By working in this way the group leader receives the messages and communications of the group but does not get helplessly caught up in them and embodies and models the opportunity offered by groupwork to work together in a way which can transform individual and collective experience.

Here are some questions to ask yourself at difficult points in the group:

- What is happening to me at the moment?
- What do I see going on in the group?
- Why can't I think right now?
- What are people feeling?
- What am I feeling?
- What happened in the group just before this?
- What is trying to emerge right now?
- What does this member/the group need now?

- What do I need now?
- What is missing/being avoided?
- How is the group using me?
- Who am I now for the group?
- What does this remind me of?
- What is the myth/story/film script/song operating here?
- Who is silent? Can they offer anything?

This may seem like a lot of work and some people may feel that it is deserting the group *in extremis*, but there are times when it is vital that the worker step back in order to think about what is happening. The worker is the guide for members and you are modelling very important psychological and social skills. The group will continue while you are deliberating, and your silence and musing will gradually become familiar and the group will internalize this capacity for themselves over time.

By inhibiting your impulse to intervene hurriedly, you can create a space in which to think about some very unthinkable and unspeakable things and prevent yourself responding to an event in a way which justifies the member or group behaving in this manner.

Here are some typical counter-transference reactions that I find repeatedly cropping up in my work:

- *Boredom*: This can result from a mutual avoidance of aggressive or competitive feelings. The attempt to keep such feelings at a distance may lead to an absence of emotional contact. A similar reaction can arise from discomfort with affectionate or erotic feelings on the part of the member or worker or both. Being treated like a thing or object for periods of time by the group can also reduce involvement and stimulate boredom.
- *Sleep*: This has similar origins. It may also represent an attempt to 'kill' or eliminate the worker or a particular member, or keep the group at a distance and protect oneself from intimacy. Sleepiness and profound inertia may also be the group's way of showing an unempathic or demanding worker the power of the unconscious and the difficulty in moving faster.
  The use of stories like *Sleeping Beauty* or *Snow White* can be helpful in generating a context for exploration and inquiry.
- *Devaluing*: Sometimes workers can find that they have disparaging, contemptuous, or derogatory thoughts and feelings about members of the group. This may indicate that the group has projected a devalued self-image onto the worker, who has responded by devaluing the group in turn, instead of thinking about what has happened and using it to open up the aggressive or inadequate feelings.
- *Zealousness*: Workers may behave in a zealous or over-dedicated way with the group. Extending the session time, being unusually active, caring, or committed indicates that the worker is behaving under the influence of demanding or idealizing projections. Alternatively, the group may split off and project their inadequacy, dependency, fear, and vulnerability onto the worker, evoking in him heroic efforts to protect himself against these uncomfortable feelings by his zealous activity. As always, think about what might be happening and discuss with the group.
- *Guilt*: Workers may feel guilt that they do not care enough about the group or are not skilled enough or are not doing enough to help.

This guilt may defend against strong negative and angry feelings about the group being slow or difficult. It is important for the worker to acknowledge this anger to himself in order to deal with its source, which may in fact be the group's own projected aggression. In this way the worker's counter-transference anger can be used to help the group manage their own feelings of hostility and express them appropriately, instead of acting them out by missing sessions, being late, and behaving rudely.

- *Erotic and affectionate feelings*: It is only natural that members in a group will come to have erotic and affectionate feelings for the worker who looks after them through thick and thin, and it is only natural for a worker to have erotic and affectionate feelings when members esteem him. It can be tempting to accept such feelings as one's due instead of using the counter-transference feelings to empathize with how deeply attached the group members wish to be and with how frustrating it must be not to have such desires totally gratified. Other workers may become so threatened by these feelings that they may recoil and withdraw, become unempathic and distant. Such workers need help to understand and permit their loving feelings in order to stay engaged and helpful to their group.

Review

- In order to work more intensively with group experience, the leader must learn how to focus and contexualize
- Focusing is about observing what is happening. Contextualizing is about making sense of what is happening
- The worker represents an investigative attitude and an ethic of exploration and inquiry
- There are a number of contexts in a group which correspond to different types of preoccupation
- The worker can use his own subjective experience of the group to focus on what is happening and generate appropriate contexts

References

1 Sandler, J., Dare. C., and Holder, A. (1979) *The Patient and the Analyst*, chap. 4, 'Transference', London: Maresfield Reprints.
2 Rycroft, C. (1983) *A Critical Dictionary of Psychoanalysis*, London: Penguin, p. 125.
3 Storr, A. (1975) *Jung*, chap. 3, 'Archetypes and the Collective Unconscious', London: Fontana Modern Masters.
4 Foulkes, S.H. (1984) *Therapeutic Group Analysis*, London: Maresfield Reprints, p. 292.
5 Foulkes, S.H. (1984) op. cit., p. 290.
6 Sandler, J. *et al*. (1979) op. cit., chap. 6, 'Counter-transference'.

Chapter 12

Working more synthetically with the group

To the casual observer looking in on the group it appears that a collection of people are interacting, talking, experiencing, and being with each other quite spontaneously. This is true of course, but the more practised observer would see other things occurring. Such an observer would see a spectrum of variegated human preoccupations, concerns, and aspirations refracted through the prism of the group modality.

I have already indicated something of the spectrum of the human soul in my discussion about different contexts for understanding group behaviour and dynamics, but now I want to assert some key principles and concepts which will enable us to explore the spectrum further.

Key principles

Synthesis

Synthesis means the coming together or combining of parts to make a higher-level whole. It is the primary principle which informs the practice of the creative group worker.[1]

You have probably seen and handled the Russian babushka doll which reveals a tiered series of dolls all enfolded inside one large doll.

This is a lovely analogue for a central paradox about groupwork which revolves around the idea of unity and diversity: that groupwork is really about a process which involves multiplicity and union. The group itself is one, but is composed of many members who come together to create an experience which would otherwise be unavailable to a singleton. Group experience is what is felt and lived by the members at any one time but is also pluri-dimensional and composed of many levels. For ease of identification and to enable effective interventions, I suggested that there were five levels or contexts which would make group and individual behaviour comprehensible:

- Explicit context
- Transference context
- Projection context
- Somatic context
- Archetypal context

These contexts are personal and shared, conscious and unconscious, intrapsychic, inter-personal, and transpersonal or archetypal aspects and qualities of the human being. They are interpenetrating and mutually and reciprocally influencing but are fundamentally the expression of this principle of synthesis – the dynamic towards wholeness and emergence out of lower-order and more primitive functioning.

In other words, groupwork is a synthetic activity which includes all the expressions and preoccupations, manifestations and associations of the human being, and shapes and links them powerfully and purposefully into an order, harmony, and beauty which elevates and transforms both the individual and the group.

Identity and the Self

Identity is what marks us out and stamps us as a particular and unique individual. Again there is this paradox of multiplicity and union; we are aware of many aspects and sides to ourselves; we live in many and sometimes contradictory worlds – and yet there is an enduring sense of being a person, of having a core identity or essential Self.

Having an essential Self means that the Self is the essential identity and so the five contexts of experience which we have been looking at are simply ways of describing certain attributes and preoccupations of the Self. The Self that I am:

- Has a body
- Has a psychology
- Is a social being
- Is preoccupied with existential, ethical, and transcendental questions

This knowledge is of profound importance for the group worker, because it makes comprehensible the behaviour of a group in certain circumstances by illuminating the spectrum of motivations and concerns of its members and indicating how group membership serves the needs of the individual.

As we saw in Chapter 3, when discussing Maslow's contribution to our understanding of the motivational impulses in the person, the ultimate need is for Self-actualization – to become everything that one is capable of – although one also has various other needs at varying times. Indeed, the multiplicity of groups exist in order to help individuals deal with different levels of need and so, from a synthetic perspective, different models and schools are not contradictory but complementary. But irrespective of whatever purpose the group has been set up to achieve, one is dealing with whole human beings, and the effective group is one which achieves its goal by appropriately embracing the whole human being.

The effective group fosters a deepening sense of identity and awareness in its members of their essential Self by paying attention to and focusing on:

- *A psychophysical context:* Embodiment – being related to a particular body and environment – what we have called the somatic context.
- *A psychological context:* Subjective experience – consciousness, a sense of agency and intention. Unconsciousness – a sense that some of our experience and responses

emanate from feelings deep within ourselves of which we may be hardly aware – the transference and projection contexts.

- A *psychosocial context:* Relationship – intrinsic involvement in a social medium of meanings, customs, politics, and culture – the explicit context.
- A *psychospiritual context:* Self-awareness, purpose, values, ethics, meaning, intuition, creativity, imagination – the archetypal context

This spectrum of concerns and preoccupations is complicated by the fact that a particular individual or group may generally live and operate in one of these contexts but can experience them all. Most groups, in fact, are set up to explore one of these contexts in detail but it is clear that a person's identity shifts constantly throughout the spectrum and this will intrude on the group. The synthetic group worker must learn to recognize when these contexts are infusing and permeating the group, and how to manage them in order to assist the group move towards its objective. We will turn to this task shortly.

Bifocal vision

Bifocal vision simply means the worker's capacity to see through the surface manifestations of group and individual behaviour and circumstances to the underlying impulse of Self towards wholeness and emergence.

Human development can be viewed as a series of expansions of identity. The core identity is that of Self, and the process is of Self becoming its Self – moving from unconsciousness through consciousness to Self-consciousness or awareness or oneself as an autonomous being capable of intentionality and choice.

The function of the group is to act as an incubator and transformer of human consciousness, and the role of the group worker is to position himself at the appropriate level in the group in order to facilitate the emergence of the next stage of individual and group growth.

Individuals and groups do not grow and develop in a steady process. Growth can be arrested for all sorts of reasons and on occasions groups may seem to regress or revert to earlier stages, patterns, or modes of functioning. This is very common. How often has one heard friends or colleagues speak about their experience of 'one step forward and two steps backward', or had such an experience oneself?

When faced with a challenge or invitation to live and respond in a new way people frequently regress to older and no longer helpful ways of behaving. They may not yet have the necessary skills or confidence and may need to access and rework earlier phases and levels of development in order to facilitate reorganization of their personality along new lines or in new patterns.

It is important for the worker to understand and manage behaviour in the group which appears regressive, because it may herald the dawn of an expansion in identity and self-knowledge and provide opportunities for individual and group development. The synthetic group worker views regression in the group not as something to be eliminated but as presenting a possibility for growth and for the emergence of the essential Self. What enables the worker to reframe regressive behaviour and reach for its emergent potential is the worker's capacity to practise bifocal vision.

Bifocal vision enables the worker to view the group as:

- *A place of formation*: Identity and self-awareness
- *A place of reformation:* Correction, assistance with arrested or malformed identity
- *A place of transformation:* Awakening the Self, evoking compassion, developing a sense of purpose and service

Bifocal vision enables the worker to discriminate between behaviour which is regressive and behaviour which is more obviously emergent:

Regressive behaviour	*Emergent behaviour*
1 Cannot tolerate difference or opposition	Accepts difference and opposition
2 Emphasizes group and mass at expense of individual	Emphasizes right relations between individuals and group
3 Compels and imposes	Negotiates and dialogues
4 Automatic, instinctual	Choice, autonomous
5 Dependent, over-reliant on authority	Self-reliant, co-operative
6 Rivalrous, selfish, violent, suspicious, contemptuous	Generative, altruistic, committed to service, compassionate
7 Façades and images	Authentic and genuine
8 Exclusive, separative, withdrawn, elitist	Inclusive, mutual, reciprocal, shares and contributes
9 Subgroupings, factionalism, tribal, cults	Co-operative view, holistic, community Moral, ethical, growing awareness
10 Ruthless, lacks conscience, rebellious, flouts rules	of social, political issues which affect group life

The will

The will is the direct expression and capacity of an individual to function freely according to his own intrinsic nature rather than under the compulsion of external forces. A conscious act of will is one of the most powerful ways of experiencing oneself as a self-directing being, a free and responsible agent. This involves not being swept up in powerful drives, impulses, attachments, and emotions but developing the capacity to regulate and direct oneself and initiate action rather than submitting passively to it.[2]

The function of the will is to direct and choose. I am not talking here about the Victorian idea of willpower with its connotations of superior force and imposition from above or outside. This is vital for the synthetic group worker to grasp, because it makes all the difference in terms of the quality of group experience and the kind of ethic which informs the practice of groupwork.

The concept of will is intimately linked with moral and ethical questions and the formation of a value system which guides behaviour. One of the essential features which separates the human from other life forms is the human's capacity for rational judgement and planning based on an ability to articulate values and to conduct one's life on the basis of some system of ethical principles. This intentionality and moral agency is the core of human identity and a central pursuit of the group worker.

The worker's constant care is to enable group members to develop mutually agreed, self-generated, and internalized controls and values rather than acquiescing to externally asserted norms and values. From this perspective the group serves the process of individuation – becoming oneself – and the individual, by choosing group membership as a means of expressing and actualizing himself, through belonging to and relating to others, finds himself inevitably in the service of the group goals.

The group moves closer to the ideal of community as autonomous individuals now act out their own will and initiative to come together to express and fulfil their purpose. This invariably involves members re-choosing to be in the group. Power and authority are no longer simply invested in the leader but are functions and rights of membership and the inner experience of the individual. You can see that the group worker seeks every opportunity to activate and foster the members' will and cultivate the intentional and moral capacity of the individual and the group. This allows the worker to include a range of psychosocial, cultural, political, existential, and ethical concerns that many other groupwork models would exclude, reduce, or pathologize.

A definition of synthetic groupwork

Synthetic groupwork refers to the conscious, disciplined, and systematic use of knowledge about the known processes, manifestations, and goals of human behaviour, interaction, and aspiration, in order to intervene in an informed way or promote a desired objective in a group setting. Synthetic groupwork is a helping process designed to correspond to specific instances of individual and group need, based on a view of humans whose core project is expanding their identity by awakening the Self, leading to Self realization and Self actualization.

Let's turn now to consider this spectrum in practice.

Working with the psychophysical dimension of the group

Embodiment is absolutely central to being a person. The body is the vehicle for existing and being in the world and a precious instrument of experience and action. Embodiment also has a psychological and social dimension, because the body is essential as:

- A ground for one's sense of Self and perception of reality
- A vehicle for sensory awareness and emotional responses
- A means of self-expression
- A medium for communication and contact

The body is simply a way of being an incarnate self, and it is the Self in the body which converts sensations and physiological phenomena into significant psychological experience and meaning. Important in this is the total psychological field, current and resonant, in which the sensations are produced.

A group is a rich sensory and psychological field because of the presence of other people and the potential to be publicly shamed, attacked, blamed or affirmed, touched, contacted, and embraced. Add to this environment such factors as spaces which are large, small, private, public, intimate, boring, stressful; changes in scale, lighting, temperature, noise, smells; activities which are verbal, physical, emotional, fast and slow paced, messy and clean – and you can well understand how being in a group with other people can generate somatic and emotional responses.

Groups can amplify and magnify these responses cybernetically, which is why people sometimes avoid or dread groups because of their fears of regression. Group membership involves some loosening of the usual boundaries of the Self in order to participate, and in beginning groups of relative strangers or times of heightened emotion this frequently generates feelings of contagion and invasion accompanied by varying degrees of deper-sonalization or de-individuation. This is why groups sometimes feel 'cold' or anxious, and the worker may use 'icebreakers', 'warm-ups', and 'contact games'.

Of course, temporary loss or suspension of personality can also be a pleasant, even transcendent, feeling and connect us to an ecstatic or tribal and herd experience which may be actively sought out, as when one goes to a rave or pop concert or a football match and the mass experience is spontaneous and uplifting, instinctual and exhilarating.

Here are some manifestations of the psychophysical dimension of the group:

Members report the following:	The worker is aware of:
• Heart thumping • Sweaty palms • Dry mouth • Butterflies in stomach • Difficulty in thinking • Somatic/hypochondriacal symptoms • Pains/aches/nausea/headaches • Back tension • Feelings of deadness/woodenness • The group/other/activity is making me feel this way/putting something into me	• Cold/frozen silences • Stammering • Chattering/repetitiveness • Hysterical laughter • Impulsive behaviour • Greed/aggression/vandalism • Sleepiness, boredom • Blushing/embarrassment/ Shame

The psychophysical quality of group experience means that it is hard to think about and hard to verbalize.

The mindlessness, powerful sensations, and emotions churned up are initially very frightening and the group is prone to impulsive behaviour and acting out. In order to manage such discharges, the worker may decide to think and speak for the group.

Example

It was the second session of a personal development group and the members seemed to take turns to complain about the hardness of the chairs, the coldness of the room, the noise outside the room, their anxiety about my unnerving silence, difficulty speaking, rising panic. Some members would leave their seat, pace around the room, go to the window, go to the toilet, drum their fingers, and tap their feet.

- *Intervention*: I decided to come in as people were getting very anxious, and said that beginnings were often difficult and even traumatic for some people. The birth of a group, like that of an individual, might be such a traumatic experience and one that was hard to bear. I suggested that it might be helpful to view their physical experiences as their way of handling and communicating the discomfort of coming into being as a group.

My intention was to:

- Acknowledge the physicality of the members' early experience of the group
- Normalize this
- Contextualize the material by using the physical metaphor of birth
- Reformulate the physical experience as the basis for reflection, group discussion, and interaction

In other situations the worker may 'contain' the psychophysical experience in the group. This means that the worker makes a space inside himself where he can think about the process of the group's anxieties. Containing the group's psychophysical tension and anxiety when the group is prone to energy discharge and acting out is demanding, and involves the worker's utilizing the counter-transference capacity and skills which we looked at earlier. The worker is empathetically and non-verbally modelling a way of dealing with anxiety which members intuitively relate to and can recognize as different from those occasions when the worker is inattentive, absent, or bored. The template for this is the relaxed and non-anxious mother, of preverbal experience.

The important thing to remember when confronted by psychophysical phenomena and somatizing in the group is not to ignore it but to begin to think about what the group is communicating through this early identity. Reread the earlier section on the worker's use of Self, and try to internalize this mode of thinking and behaving in your group.

Working with the psychological dimension of the group

Each individual in the group has their own idiosyncratic way of being in the world and making sense of that experience. The highly subjective nature of members' perception and modes of relating means that the group process is often highly charged with emotions – anxiety-producing, contradictory, and changeable – and that the group process in turn colours and permeates members' responses. Helping people understand what goes into their subjective experience of an event or phenomenon, clarifying how their response differs or radically diverges from others' experience, and creatively managing the dissonance is an important and ongoing activity for the worker. Helping people think psychologically rather than concretely and literally is vital if the group is learning to work with and manage its own process.

Teaching members to work psychologically involves coaching them to:

> - See and identify patterns, connections, recurring themes/motifs
> - Pause, reflect, ponder, muse, wonder
> - Think imaginatively, symbolically
> - Avoid concrete and literal thought
> - Include feelings and emotions
> - Include intuitions
> - Include somatic communication
> - Bridge between inner and outer worlds of experience
> - Become familiar with the idea of unconscious motives
> - Recognize the contribution of childhood experience to personality formation
> - Become familiar with ideas of repetition and re-enactment of habitual interaction sets
> - Recognize defensive reactions and patterns

Reread the section on page 199 outlining the worker's cultivation of the investigative attitude in the group, and the section on page 205 which gives detailed advice on how to employ the worker's subjective experience to work more intensively with the group. This will confirm what I mean about working more psychologically.

Working with defensive reactions in the group

Defence mechanisms and reactions are attempted 'solutions' to intrapsychic and interpersonal conflicts. They are ways of disguising and distorting shameful, painful, or hidden feelings and desires from oneself and others. The checklists on pages 86, 103 and 116 will give you an idea of how defences manifest in groups.

Defensive reactions are easily stimulated in the group, and must be dealt with sensitively if change is to occur.

Some group workers take the position that defences are 'enemies' which must be overcome, but I believe this to be an archaic and mistaken view, in that to perceive defences thus is to break empathy with the group in a fundamental way and to reinforce the very behaviour which you wish to see changed. The worker's goal is to help group members move from rigid and debilitating ways of behaving to more flexible and appropriate forms of interaction.

Defensive activity in the group originates from three sources:

1   *Defences in the individual member.* There are myriad defences in which individuals will engage, ranging from silence to self-absorption, detachment, cynicism, fault finding, or aggression – anything that will alter the tone, level, or direction of group experience away from intimacy and vulnerability. Watch out for recurrent themes and

repetitive situations which indicate the presence of anxiety and the attempt to defend against it.

The nature of groupwork requires individuals to participate actively if it is to work, and such close proximity can cause anxiety for individuals. Some members will respond with exaggerated independence or feel compelled to be rebellious and destructive. Others may exhibit inappropriate dependence on the leader or be self-harmful.

Managing such reactions involves making explicit the underlying aggression and fear of contact while endeavouring to develop the capacity for concern, mutuality, and interdependence in the group.

2 *Defences of the group as a whole*: Defensive activity may emerge as a response to the needs of the whole group. Reread the example on page 198 which shows how the existing group responded anxiously and defensively to the introduction of new members. You can see how the group is organizing and coping with its anxiety by being attentive to events and phenomena which are significant and carry meaning and anxiety for the collective membership, such as:

- The entry of new members
- The departure of senior members
- Holiday breaks
- Change of venue/time/frequency
- The worker's illness or pregnancy
- The termination of the group
- External events – the Dunblane massacre, the Omagh bomb, Kosovo, Syria, etc.

3 *Defences arising from the worker's counter-transference*: The combined weight of members' expectations, behaviour, and anxiety can exert enormous pressure on a worker psychologically. This regressive pull can tax even the most experienced group worker and undermine objectivity and empathy. When the worker is a novice or is undergoing personal stress, it can happen that the worker withdraws emotionally and avoids or defends against the full impact of the group process. To some degree this is inevitable at some time in every group. See the example given on page 209, where I allowed things to run on inappropriately in the group because I was unwilling to experience myself or present as the final authority.

The defences arise from four underlying fears and anxieties which deter members from reaching out to each other emotionally, and excite protective action:

1 *Fear of impulsivity*: being flooded or overwhelmed by instincts and emotions leads to behaviour which emphasizes control and avoidance.
2 *Fear of abandonment* may provoke exaggerated independence as a form of denial, or it may bring out its opposite – clinging and dependent behaviour and phobic responses.
3 *Fear of merging* or being taken over or engulfed may incite suspicious and hostile behaviour and inappropriate self-reliance.
4 *Fear of vulnerability*: being hurt, humiliated, or revealed as inadequate can generate grandiosity, expressions of disdain and contempt, or lofty and isolated behaviour.

The worker should focus on each member's characteristic style of relating in order to help that person understand the effect and consequences of that style. By examining the biographical events and current triggers in the group, members can come to understand what led to the need to behave so defensively and gradually learn to acquire more appropriate and better ways of protecting and asserting themselves.

Try to demonstrate how the individual or group is behaving and give examples which are difficult to refute. Clarify the motives of the defensive behaviour by identifying the fear which drives it. Determine what is triggering the behaviour now and whether it is an old memory or situation, or a current event which usually can be more easily dealt with.

Working with transference reactions in the group

The presence of others is a powerful stimulant and can enhance the possibility of exposing a variety of relationships and broaden the context in which members' less healthy interactions can be examined.

Groups can promote a situation of regression and provide opportunities for the development of parental transferences to the worker and sibling transferences to peers. The example given on page 209 shows these vertical and horizontal transferences quite clearly, so you might wish to reread this vignette.

It is essential that you understand that transference reactions occur frequently in groups and that they radically influence the nature of group behaviour. Group workers who ignore or misunderstand transference manifestation may seriously misunderstand some transactions and confuse rather than guide the group members.

Recognizing transference reactions

Transference can be simply defined as the experiencing and manifestation of feelings, behaviours, attitudes, fantasies, and defences by one person towards another in the present which do not fit that person but are repetitions of reactions and behaviours originating in relation to significant persons in childhood. So a group member may respond to the worker in the sorts of ways in which they responded to a parent in childhood – looking for help, wanting admiration, rebelling against the rules. Or they may respond to peers in the group as if they were siblings – competing for the worker's attention, bullying each other, creating gangs and subgroups. You can be sure that transference is occurring when you observe behaviour which is:

> - Inappropriate/out of context
> - Repetitious, recurring, cyclical
> - Intense/over the top
> - Ambivalent
> - Tenacious, resistant to explanation

Always give yourself time to observe how members relate to and use each other, how they relate to and use you, and reflect upon your own feelings and process. Gradually you will become aware of how the past is being repeated in the present and enshrouding new possibilities with a sort of archaic psychological cling film.

Here are three tips:

1 *Look for behaviour:*	
a *at a group level*	*b* *at an individual level*
• Dependent behaviour aimed at eliciting protection/security from all-powerful leader • Group is experienced as a skin or body; breast or like mother • Fight–flight behaviour aimed at helping group gain security by battle or escape • Formation of subgroups/gangs which contain safe/unsafe desired, feared parts of member's Self	• Repetitive and reliant questioning • Preoccupation with procedures/tasks • Silence/chattering/superficiality • Withdrawal/self-sufficiency • Hovering/hesitation, sitting on the fence • Clinging/over-dependent behaviour • Exhibitionism, boasting/vandalism/aggression/bullying, expressions of contempt or indifference • Absenteeism, lateness, refusal to join in • Unwillingness to trust/fear of vulnerability/being taken over

2 *Listen to themes in members' discussion:*	
a *People and relationship themes and quality of interaction*	*Implicit message for worker/peers*
• Stories and narratives about activity or intent of employers/bosses, leaders, politicians/authority figures, shop workers/service workers • Stories about work colleagues/team mates/friends/partners, neighbours	• Worker is parental figure who is abusive, interfering, exploitative, deceitful, or, alternatively, loving, helpful, generous, committed, zealous, reliable • Group peers are siblings who are rivals, envious, hostile, belligerent, greedy, deceitful, or, alternatively, loving, generous, compassionate, indispensable

b Places and locations and their qualities	
• Stories about busy bus/rail/ tube stations; dentist's/doctor's waiting room, or descriptions of peaceful/distracting or desired or feared rural/urban/ seaside/mountain settings	• References to quality of group experience, interaction, communication or quality of worker's attention and empathy. May also indicate family re-enactments triggered off by current participation

3 How things work and don't work:	
• Stories about broken cars/ washing machines, dishwashers/ leaking pipes/blocked drains, accounts of unsuccessful/ winning athletic/sports performances, efficient or poorly performing, business/ government/health service	• Reference to how well group opportunity or the worker is functioning or malfunctioning may indicate family re-enactments or early group/school/work/church experiences or current membership of external groups

Example 1

Two new members joined a psychotherapy group and in the next session the older members began to talk about the Irish famine and the role of absentee landlords in deepening the distress and privation of the people. The group therapist quickly realized that the arrival of two new members at the same time might have been too much for the group who were concerned that there might not be enough nourishment for them in the group and they might have to do with less than they were used to. The group therapist put this to the group and they were able to explore their anxieties about sharing the resources of the group. After some discussion the group came to see that more members might actually mean more possibilities for all rather than less. The group therapist then turned to the reference about the absentee landlords and wondered if the group perhaps thought that the therapist might not be attentive enough to the needs of members and had not managed the therapeutic encounter well and could have staggered the entry of the new members. This led to a lively discussion in which the group was able to express their anger with the therapist. After some time it was relatively easy for the therapist to remind the group that they had suffered similar frustrations and disappointments in their original families and they were re-experiencing this in the group but could now choose to deal with this differently and more maturely.

Example 2

A relatively new female member of a psychotherapy group was telling the other members about a recent break-up with her boyfriend. June was met with silence by the group who then moved on to talk about their own issues. A senior member of the group then spoke about her early experiences with her depressed mother and how this had affected her. Some others joined in and there was a good exchange. Then June came in to describe how when she was 11 years old her mother had become depressed after the death of her parents and had withdrawn from the family. She had turned to her father for emotional care and they had become very close. Once again, the group remained silent. After a few minutes the group therapist turned to her and asked, 'Is this what your mother was like?'

She agreed. The therapist was able to engage the group members in examining their response to the newish member and what it stirred up for them. After a time, the therapist wondered with the group if he was becoming like June's father and looking after her since the group mother was withdrawn with her. Again, this generated a useful discussion.

Example 3

A psychotherapy group became very annoyed by the sound of voices and laughter coming from another room. They complained about their quiet space being invaded and outsiders' complete lack of regard for the important work that the group was engaged in. They were angry about poor management and planning of room use by centre organizers. After some time of this the therapist intervened to wonder if the group was really angry with her for not taking enough care of the group. The other group was clearly having fun while this group was struggling with difficult problems. The therapy group did acknowledge envy of the other group and irritation with their therapist. The therapist was able to help the group members think about how in previous sessions they had described being let down by their parents and how they had also struggled with sibling rivalries.

Later the therapist wondered about members' experience of the group and if they feared that other members might sneer or mock or laugh if one speaks or reveals oneself in the group. This led to a lively discussion about what it was like to be in the group and members' hopes and fears. The members were able to talk about how as a consequence of being in the group one's mind could get attacked or invaded by unwelcome thoughts and feelings. One could feel powerless to prevent certain thoughts and feelings coming into one's mind as a result of listening to the experiences of others.

I could give many more examples but I think that you can see how important it is to reflect upon the individual or group behaviour and story and consider the underlying subtext as a communication about transference preoccupations concerning the worker or the other members. Ask yourself: who is the person who is speaking now – adult, adolescent, child? What are they saying about their experience of the group, other members, the worker? What family scenario, sibling or parental relationship is being re-enacted now?

If it appears that the group or individual interaction is immature or inappropriate or repetitious, then you can be sure that you are witnessing transference behaviour. My own approach to dealing with transference in the group is based on identifying whether it is best to intervene at the level of the group as a whole or draw attention to interpersonal or individual patterns and configurations.

Consider the presenting material and assess the group members' ability to examine their functioning in the group, and intervene at the level that will best engage them.

This may mean emphasizing the individual's life and examining the person's biography and character formation for clues as to their typical defences, problem-solving techniques, and ways of regarding and relating to themselves. The next level of intervention is the interpersonal, which points out rational styles and considers what internalized conflicts with siblings, peers, and authority figures is being replayed in the here-and-now interpersonal field. On the collective level, group-as-a-whole dynamics can be explored, illuminating early mother–infant relations as well as including valuable information about the operation of group norms, values, assumptions, and restrictions.

Try to gather evidence and examples of repetitive and therefore irrefutable patterns which you can use to demonstrate the manifestation of transference phenomena. Clarify just what it is about the worker or another member which triggers associations and feelings with significant people and episodes from the past. Explore the feelings and fantasies involved in the transference reaction and try to make a link with the surface interactions and the underlying causes. In this way you can make sense of the transference and help the individual and the group understand what is going on. You will probably have to repeat this activity many times before the transference behaviour will be modified, so don't worry if it recurs.

These patterns were learned a long time ago and take a long time to go away. The important thing is to establish and promote in your group a culture of inquiry and curiosity which engages members in a routine and ongoing examination of their behaviour and motives.

Working with the psychosocial dimension of the group

The idea of a psychosocial dimension in the group is based on the notion that there is an interactional synchrony between the essential self and the relational and social-cultural context in which it emerges, and that this intertwining of self and social context is replicated in the group. The group worker needs to be alert to phenomena and preoccupations which reflect individual and group concerns with important and relevant social and political issues and which can serve the development of the group as a sensitive and responsive instrument for the expansion of individual identity and conscience.

Individual identity is a synthesis of personal experiences and attitudes and social arrangements and institutions. Identity and personhood are socially and culturally organized by access to and experience of these behaviours, practices, and systems:

- Family experiences
- Child-rearing practices
- Kinship systems and social class
- Educational institutions
- Religious upbringing
- Political affiliations
- Gender, sexual identity, sexism
- Marriage and relationship
- Racial and ethnic origins and identity
- Economic systems, markets
- Labour relations, employment, joblessness
- Law, policing, military
- Art, culture, media
- Leisure, entertainment
- Technology, science, medicine
- Ecology, environmental issues
- National and international politics
- Catastrophe, war, terrorism

Since these activities are contained within the individual in the forms of habits, attitudes, and experience, it is inevitable that at times the group will find itself having to confront issues and concerns which mirror debates or dilemmas in the wider society and which enter or permeate the group matrix. Learn to include these concerns imaginatively rather than tell yourself or the group that such issues have nothing to do with the group objective.

Stretching yourself and the group to make space for such reflection and discussion creates an ethos of inclusion and inquiry which can provide an opportunity for a sense of empowerment and engagement with the central issues of the day and, in fact, actually further the group goals – whatever they may be – through direct experiential learning, metaphor, and analogue.

Example 1

The idea that the individual reflects not just a personal but also a collective and even historical identity is, not surprisingly, a daily and permanent feature of my work in Northern Ireland. In the Northern Ireland context there are myriad coded signals which are available and inculturated into the individual from birth and which communicate one's ethnic group, religious background, and likely political allegiance. One's school, address, place of work, and even one's name functions as a potent cultural signal. I recall how in one group a Protestant woman persisted in denying that a significant member for her was a Catholic by consistently calling him Donald when his name was in fact Donal and it was repeatedly pointed out to her. Unconsciously, she had to make him a cultural partner by adjusting the one letter of his name before she could allow him to mean anything to her.

Only as she was able to become aware of this previously unconscious and now unwanted prejudice towards Catholics could she, and subsequently the group, begin to explore how a sheltered and exclusive upbringing might adversely affect a person in many other ways and prevent groups of people from different religious and cultural backgrounds relating honestly and intimately with each other.

Usually these sorts of cultural signifiers and codes are well understood and rarely made explicit. Indeed, one of the recurring difficulties of my work with groups in this type of socio-political context has been exposing the effects and consequences of such implicit and subliminal communication, and making plain the profound denial caused by the fear that the destructive fantasies underpinning much of this communication will invade the group and become 'reality'. Group members will frequently go to great lengths to ensure that the internal cohesion of the group is not threatened by the daily catalogue of terror or grievance in the wider society, or their own role in that society. Despite their best efforts, however, unconscious formations that originate not in individual repression but as expressions of social and cultural conditioning constantly reveal themselves in the group.

Example 2

In the early stages of another group a man came to the session wearing a remembrance poppy. Now, this simple act of remembrance to the dead of two world wars has a particular resonance in Northern Ireland. Few Catholics would wear this poppy. It is associated with certain Protestant and British loyalties and as such could be construed by some as a declaration in favour of the political union with Westminster and therefore anti-nationalist. This member was one of three Protestants in the group, which contained three Catholics and two of other denominations. No one else wore a poppy, and it was not referred to although we were all aware of its significance.

As the session unfolded, two of the Catholic members in this hitherto placid group became increasingly angry with me, condemning me for routinely saying little except to demand something more from them. Gradually other members joined in, criticizing me for wearing a suit which made them feel that I was like an oppressive authority, and commenting on the tension I caused in the group by my unhelpful presence.

In a different culture I might have understood the criticism of me as relating to the beginning anxieties of members and their angry perception of me as a depriving and authoritative parent, and I would have intervened accordingly. However, in a Northern Irish context, an intervention based solely on this insight would have missed the cultural subtext. It was also clear that there was a deep displacement onto me of anger which was really directed at the member who was perceived to distinguish himself by his dress – the wearing of a poppy – as a representative of a hated political authority and rival group.

It was not possible to engage him or the group in those early days in an open discussion of the themes of symbols, allegiances, enemies, and rivalries because of the group's fear that such discussion would invite the possibility of 'war' in the group. My intervention was taken up in part – the political dimension being dropped quickly. But it did not simply disappear. A dimension of members' lives had been acknowledged and an ethos of inquiry had been introduced. As the group developed there was a growing interest in political and cultural differences, and one year later, when the same man wore his poppy to the session, there was a vigorous exchange of political views which was authentic and led to a more mature and ongoing exploration of what it was like to live and interact in a polarized society.

Since 1989 I have been working on a regular basis in England with supervision groups, experiential learning groups, and teaching groups, which include a wide range of ages, sexual orientations, and ethnic and racial backgrounds, and I have found these groups to be identically affected by and resonating to events and issues in their particular socio-political context. At various times I have found that I need to include members' concerns or make references to the dominant issues of the day in order to facilitate a group preoccupied with an external event, or to illustrate how some piece of group process is proceeding along the lines of some structural issue in the wider society.

Example 3

I recall working with a large group of about 80 student psychotherapists in London shortly after the Dunblane massacre, in which a deranged gunman murdered a number of children and their teacher in their school in 1997. My group of students felt shocked and numbed by the tragedy, and experienced a deep sense of helplessness and anxiety that it was impossible to prevent such a thing happening. As students and parents themselves, they felt a deep bond of empathy and affinity with the murdered children and their bereaved parents.

The whole two-hour session was taken up with the group members sensitively and profoundly exploring a whole range of issues and dilemmas to do with living and working in a modern society in which such random and alienated actions occurred. This poignant and sorrowful discussion was a mirror of the same discussion taking place in the wider society, in the media, in workplaces and social meeting points. The group came to no conclusions, of course, but a gathering of some 80 people were enabled to speak about how they were experiencing a major national trauma, and reflect upon and struggle with the sorts of questions and dilemmas it raised for them as members of that society.

I could give innumerable examples similar to this of how the social and cultural context permeates the group and affects members' psychology and relationships.

Here are a few illustrations of how certain events impinged upon and stirred up issues in some of my groups:

Social/cultural/political issues	Members' preoccupations
• Gulf War/Bosnian War/Kosovo/Canary Wharf bombing/IRA terrorism	• National identity; fears of being member of racial or ethnic minority; how groups manage difference, aggression, conflict
• Lowering of age of homosexual consent	• Sexual orientation, homophobia, relations between men and women
• Stephen Lawrence case	• Racial harassment, discrimination of Irish, Blacks, Jews, family experiences of Holocaust, relations with authority, police, teachers, one's internal authority
• Technological/scientific/medical advances, cloning, human genome programme, spare-part surgery	• Fears of Big Brother, helplessness, uncertainty about authority and big business, alienation, worries about not being consulted, illness, ageing, death
• Environmental, ecological disasters/catastrophes, BSE beef crisis, food scares	• Anger about poor responses by authority, lack of empathy, compassion, concern about corporate greed, indifference, impotence, helplessness
• Millennium issues	• How and what to celebrate/remember, secular versus sacred, hopes/fears for future, new beginnings, rituals

This is a brief sample of some of the social issues that have engrossed my groups and the types of discussion which ensued. You can see from the members' preoccupations that there is a correlation between their public and personal response to the issues. Members have emotional and political responses to events and this is the very stuff of group membership and experience. The core issues centre on what it means to be a person in a social world – with the fears, dreads, hopes, and longings this raises. Members have to struggle with the essential group dilemma I described on page 203: how to get close but not too close and how to be separate but not too separate:

- What makes people similar to and different from each other?
- What rights and responsibilities do people have regarding each other?
- What is the relationship between the individual and the group?
- What is the nature of society/community?
- How do groups manage disagreements and conflicts?
- How should a group best organize itself?

Utilizing psychosocial material in the group

Acknowledging the reality of the concerns

Sometimes it can be an indication of emotional well-being and civic responsibility if an individual or a group raises a particular issue. It can indicate a reasonable and appropriate relation with reality and a healthy response to one's actual environment or life circumstances. It would be very worrying to me, for example, if none of my groups which met the week following the Omagh bomb explosion in August 1998 or following the Twin Tower September 11th attack in 2001 had spoken about their shock and horror at atrocities which killed so many people and appalled the world. What members in these groups needed was an opportunity to grieve collectively and to experience the comfort and solidarity of being in the presence of other people who felt exactly as they did.

In other situations – for instance, if a group member or relative has had a serious illness or surgery – their experience of the National Health Service may provoke discussion about the merits and demerits of this system and raise issues about the commitment of political parties to the service. To talk about cuts, economies, and waiting lists may raise legitimate questions about personal values and principles and values in society.

The experience of members or their relatives of police or security forces may reflect actual injustice or discrimination and harassment; this may require space in the group for the reality to be acknowledged that sometimes authority can be oppressive and the law can be an ass. Similarly, individual stories about sexual or gender discrimination at work, accounts of homophobic prejudice and even assault, and racial discrimination and bullying need to be honoured and validated if the group is to prove its worth as a sanctuary and a place where things can be different.

Individuals come to groups with a whole range of concerns and anxieties about what is happening in science and genetics and the internet, with ecological and environmental fears, worries about world debt and ownership of the media, and myriad other social, cultural, and political issues. It is important that the group worker straightforwardly acknowledges and affirms the reality of these preoccupations as a sign of mature and civic responsibility, and endeavours to make the group a place where such discussion contributes to the cohesion and relevance of the group experience in its members' lives.

A fundamental task of any group is to raise members' consciousness of particular issues of concern to them, so including the reality of the world in which members live contributes greatly to their capacity to reflect deeply on the wider social meaning of their problems and struggles.

Opening up the psychological and symbolic level of the material

Often psychosocial events can be used by individuals and groups to communicate some internal and unconscious worries or fears. In the case of the Omagh bomb and Twin Towers attacks, members of my groups continued to speak about the atrocities for a very long time after the event. In some cases people spoke about their sense of evil or hopelessness that the peace process could stay on track and their fears of societal collapse. Now, this was a real danger, since terrorism aims to strike at people's belief and trust that authority can look after them by savagely undercutting the basis of hope and trust in security and civic protection, but these attacks seemed for many to arouse a deeper sense of personal responsibility and culpability.

Members reported feelings of guilt that they had survived when so many had randomly died, a sense of impotence and helplessness to effect change, and a belief that somehow they had contributed to the problem over the years by not more actively renouncing violent groups and politics.

This is a common experience of witnesses and bystanders to traumatic events and catastrophes, both man-made and natural; it requires the group worker to tune into members' distress sensitively and empathically in order to gauge how an external event may mirror some internal anxiety or reawaken some long-dormant dread and worry.

In other situations individuals and groups may use social or cultural issues to protect or defend themselves from the effects of more immediate and personal concerns. The preoccupations with and anger about the state of the Health Service or the government's commitment may, in reality, distract from the individual's personal engagement with their own ageing or illness, or divert the group from having to encounter the pain of finiteness and limitation when struggling to help members with those all too intractable problems.

Similarly, the sense of injustice and experience of victimization reported by members may, in addition to reality factors, contain projections of their own internal bully and victim interactions and unresolved grandiosity, and defend against feelings of inferiority and worthlessness. This may manifest as an exaggerated, even belligerent, advocacy of gay rights, environmental concerns, animal rights, and a host of other assertions. It is important to explore sensitively the underlying feelings of hostility and fears of persecution if the manifest concerns for social justice and fairness are to be given an appropriate and rightful place.

External social events may mirror the group's perception of its own internal arrangements, customs, and experiences. Most group leaders at some point have been compared to Adolf Hitler or Saddam Hussein, and one can readily see the transference projections of the bad father and the cruel, dictatorial group leader who makes demands and imposes rules on the membership. The group's interest in political changes in Eastern Europe, with the demise of communism, the fall of the Berlin Wall, and all the other demographic consequences, may reflect the members' implicit or unconscious longing for more power in the group and a wish to 'overthrow' the leader and usher in a fantasized era of participation and ownership. The important point to remember is that the reference to social and cultural issues may be a psychosocial metaphor or analogue for the individual's or group's preoccupation with its own internal state of mind; the group worker's difficult task is to determine when the reference is reality-based and when it reflects a deeper concern.

Here are some questions to ask when considering psychosocial material:

* What are the social/cultural/political themes in the group?
* Are they current in the external world?
* What currently is happening in the external world?
* How is it impacting on the group?
* How much of the individual/group concern is objective?
* Can I determine subjective elements?
* Why is this theme being discussed now?
* How does it serve the individual/group?
* How is this social theme a metaphor for member–leader interactions?
* Does it represent member–member interactions?

- Does it represent internal configurations within the member?
- Does it represent member/group history/biography?
- What is trying to emerge through this discussion?
- Is there an existential concern here?
- Is there an archetypal/mythic pattern being repeated?
- Does this discussion illuminate values and principles?

The synthetic group worker recognizes the reciprocal interrelationship of personal identity and social context, and endeavours to implement a climate in which members assume a responsible attitude towards the individual, their group, and society, bearing in mind the difficulties and dilemmas involved in interacting and relating to others. The group is a microcosm of the larger collective, and by including and encouraging a psychosocial consciousness in members, the worker enables each person to participate in society and contribute to social change.

Working with the psychospiritual dimension of the group

The idea of the psychospiritual refers to levels of human consciousness that are present and potentially available in all cultures with widely varying content and context. They are concerned with:

- A meaningful philosophy of life
- Creative and purposeful values
- A sense of being a moral being
- Developing our deepest sense of Self and identity
- A sense of place and trustful belonging in the universe
- A relationship with a higher/power/providence/God/divine
- Renewing moments of transcendence
- A sense of the sacred/mystery/wonder/aesthetic and beauty
- A sustaining and creative worldview

The word 'psychospiritual' does not cleanly separate psychology and spirituality but indicates an interface where individuals' mental health and psychological well-being is inextricably intertwined with their spiritual experience and growth. I want at this point to distinguish and differentiate spirituality from religion, which is a specific and organized system of faith, worship, doctrine, and rituals. 'Spirituality' is a word that defies specific definition but is often used to describe the human need for meaning and value in life and the desire for relationship with a transcendent power.

Fukuyama and Sevig report spirituality as

> an innate capacity and tendency to move towards knowledge, love, meaning, hope, transcendence, connectedness and compassion. It includes one's capacity for creativity, growth and the development of a values system. Spirituality encompasses the religious, spiritual and transpersonal.[3]

Clearly, a spiritual dimension enhances personal growth and freedom by promoting a way of being and experiencing:

- Mind
- Body
- Spirit
- Relationships with other beings
- Relationships with nature
- Relationships with work and leisure
- Relationships with organizations and institutions
- Relationships with culture and a worldview
- Relationships with life

I have already indicated that these areas are of constant concern to individuals and groups, and so it follows for me that a psychospiritual perspective and emphasis is a necessary attribute and dimension of groupwork and immensely enriches and expands the opportunity and possibility of group experience and action.

The psychospiritual dimension of the group has two characteristics:

1 An emphasis on awakening the sense of essential Self in each member and with facilitating the manifestations, dilemmas, and preoccupations of this deepest Self and identity.
2 An emphasis on synthesis in the group: harmonizing, integrating, and transmitting collective and interpersonal processes so as to promote an experience of caring and responsive community which endeavours to help members move towards becoming what they are most capable of.

Example

A woman in a group had recurring difficulty in collaborating with other members around issues of mutual concern – when a new member should arrive, changing the time of the meeting to accommodate the others, meeting with the group in the forced absence of the group worker. These and other differences occasioned a great deal of strife between her and other members in the group because it became clear that the woman often had no real objection but was disagreeing out of her biographical history. She was the eldest child and resented her siblings, whom she felt should acknowledge and submit to her priority and authority.

She came from a family which had acquired wealth and felt elevated in a poor community, but also felt insecure about this and anxious about being the object of envy.

It became clear after much discussion over many sessions that the recurring issue for this woman revolved around her difficulty of being separate but not alienated, while being an influential member but not central. These issues of belonging, autonomy, and authority opened up for her and the group important themes to do with what members could expect from each other in terms of rights and responsibilities, issues around respect, power, and privilege, and the nature and limits of self-expression and determination.

Much of the work undertaken by this member and the group involved examining the regressive aspects of this material from a psychological and therapeutic perspective. However, what characterized the psychospiritual nature of the ongoing discussion was the capacity of the participants actively and consciously to include and engage with a sense of the person as a moral being, passionately concerned with principles, ethics, and values to do with the pain and suffering of others and the obligation of social justice. In addition, simple material values and consideration of what was ultimately satisfying were challenged and there was an awareness that self-expression and self-determination must be based on qualities of compassion and ethical considerations if they are not to be ruthless.

This was the focus of debate when the woman member decided to take a holiday during the group term in apparent contravention of the contract to attend each session. It seemed that her will and the will of the group would conflict yet again, but instead there was a sensitive dialogue in which the woman presented a case for her holiday which involved her recognizing the obligations of group membership and asking the group to recognize her autonomy. The difference in the atmosphere of the session and the quality of discussion this time was palpable, and was characterized by a sense of love and tender, authentic relatedness. The woman was willing to surrender to the group's authority and was also negotiating the nature of her identity and relationship to the whole. She was clearly exploring interdependence and connectedness, which was firmly based on her freedom and responsibility and was in no way operating from the old familial compulsions or dynamics.

The group members were flexible and responsive, and willing to encourage creative and innovative behaviour which was motivated by mutually agreed values and principles. This had implications for the group, since it meant modifying existing rules in favour of an individual but it led to an increasing tolerance of diversity and a developing sense of community because the experience of goodwill enabled them to transcend the tendencies towards cultishness and shallow homogenization which lurk in the shadows of every group.

Group rules and norms can shackle individuals and prompt unhealthy individuation and rebellion unless the group and the member can be enabled to work with and connect to the highest values − those emphasizing the dialectic between the emergent and individuating Self and a responsive and self-generating community.

The key to working at psychospiritual levels in the group lies in the capacity of the worker for that bifocal vision which permits both an exploration of regressive phenomena and behaviour where necessary, while recognizing and encouraging the underlying impulse of the essential Self towards relatedness and wholeness. Both individual and group consciousness are consequently transformed and refined. The opportunity to open up the psychospiritual concerns of group members is ever present and can be initiated by individuals as well as by the worker. Here are some examples of situations and events which generated an emphasis on more universal themes in my groups:

Outside the group but affecting members

- War/acts of terrorism/assassinations/bombings/hijackings
- Natural catastrophes − earthquakes, floods, fires
- Political corruption and sleaze
- Food scares
- Medical, technological, and scientific advances

Experience inside the group

- Death of member's relative
- Illness of member
- Presence of clergy as members
- Termination of the group
- Loss of individual's purpose/vision/vocation
- Depression
- Conflict
- Ruthless and selfish behaviour
- Lack of trust
- Cynicism and scepticism

These examples and countless others can often excite in members concerns and preoccupations about:

- The capricious and random nature of life
- Existential isolation[4]
- Anxiety about death
- Fear of freedom[5]
- A loss of meaning[6]
- Awareness of finiteness/limitation/tragedy
- The presence and nature of evil
- The nature of good
- Questioning and searching for spiritual values: idealism, altruism, compassion, justice, mercy, forgiveness, faith, hope, love, peace
- The experience of grace
- The nature of intimacy and sacredness
- The difference between conflict and paradox

These sorts of concerns and questions are the cues which can be used by a sensitive worker to help individuals and groups make meaning out of their suffering and generate new and creative contexts for living. I hardly need stress that a worker does not impose a particular religious or spiritual perspective upon the group but, rather, waits and seeks to stand for and point to a larger context within which group members can locate their dilemmas and preoccupations. This larger context is archetypally derived and spiritually informed and is put forward as a resource for healing and a source of meaning.

The importance of the psychospiritual perspective is that it offers the worker the opportunity to intervene creatively and synthetically:

- *Repair:* The worker can help members deal with their personal wounds by working through the regressive aspects.
- *Individuation:* The worker can help connect and align the member and group to that inherent dynamic towards wholeness within each individual. Inevitably this involves

member and group building a moral and ethical ground and identity which emphasizes agency, intentionality, responsibility, choice autonomy, right relations, and one's
place in the universe.

The key element for the worker is to discern and discriminate where an individual or
group is most identified at any one time. In order to intervene psychospiritually, the
worker seeks to awaken the sense of Self at a deep level or collaborate with the emerging
Self as a free and responsible agent. The question to ask is simple but profound: *Who is this
person most at this moment?*

There are only a few answers possible:

- The person most resembles an angry/hurt/manipulative child
- The person most resembles an idealistic/rebellious/introverted/awkward teenager
- The person is most preoccupied with getting their own way and satisfying their
  ego needs for esteem, power, privilege
- The person most resembles a mature adult concerned with Self-realization and
  Self-actualization

The first three answers give a picture of what most concerns an individual or group at any
one time, and indicate that the correct intervention in group process is to focus on the
psychological and developmental aspects of the difficulty. The last answer paints a portrait
of an individual or group engaged in existential and spiritual inquiry and growth and
indicates to the worker that a psychospiritual intervention is most appropriate.

Types of psychospiritual interventions

There are many forms of intervention that arise out of a particular situation, but here are
four strategies that I find myself consistently using in my groups.

1　Depending on the situation I may recount a story or parable, or make reference to a
myth or fairy tale, which opens up the archetypal context of the group. This engages
imagination, wonder, mystery, and a sense of the numinous to evoke soul qualities like
love, compassion, the tragic, reverence, beauty, which may require acknowledgement
and experiencing if the group is to transcend and transmute its current difficulties.

A good example of such a story is the *Divine Comedy* written by Dante Alighieri.
Dante is the great poet of despair and bliss who plumbed the very depths and heights
of human experience. He describes the deliverance of the human Soul from a spiritually dead and self-centred life and offers a model for transforming despair into
dialogue and hope which is particularly relevant for the modern group worker. The
Divine Comedy is made up of three sections: Hell known as the Inferno is inhabited
by those who have been separated from the social body and are alienated and isolated; Purgatory is a harmonious society in which everyone accepts responsibility for
their actions, behaves socially, and deplores damage to others; in Paradiso the human
is pure spirit devoid of selfishness and constitutes the ideal society. Dante's towering
poem is a medieval draft of a complete and successful group at work. Groupwork

offers the alienated and self-absorbed individual a second chance – an opportunity to engage in ordered and graduated mutual and loving relationships in which desire can be re-educated and appropriately redirected. The sterile isolation and self-congratulatory monologues of Inferno are gradually and with the assistance of a wise guide transmuted into the conversations and mutual ambitions of a developing community so characteristic of Purgatory. And finally, the loving relations of Paradiso mirror a delight and a concern with persons and existences other than ourselves which at times evoke and catalyze experiences of exaltation and transcendence.

2   Frequently I will ask an individual: 'What do you stand for?/What is most important to you?' This is a way of connecting a person to their highest values, and of reminding an individual who they really are and what most motivates them. Often an individual and a group need to articulate what is most essential to them but, surprisingly, many people are able to assert their core values. What is difficult for them is how personality dynamics and biography sabotage the expression of one's deepest desires.

3   It is important to engage and evoke an individual's will. Many people feel determined by their personal history and behave in compulsive ways. I try to remind individuals that they have the power of agency and the capacity for choice even in limiting situations. The exercise of choice is a personal act of creation and involves different aspects of our experience of willing. With some groups and individuals this may require an exploration of the role of purpose and vision as a first step in the act of will.

It may also be important to consider the subsidiary stages of reflection, commitment, planning, responsibility, accountability, and then implementation. Exercises, meditation, affirmation, and, above all, practice in differentiating one's choice and becoming aware of compulsive patterns are ways to encourage autonomy and self-directed behaviour in the group.

4   Affirming the idea of service and responsibility in the world counters narcissistic and unhealthy inward-looking tendencies. Emphasizing the relation of the group experience to the external environment and one's responsibility to others can generate a service ethic which goes beyond members' personal development. Cultivating a sense of compassion in members for themselves and others is essential, as is the building of an experience of community. I look out for any opportunity which can foster and promote goodwill. The goodwill is a will to do good; it is a will that chooses and wants the good and is thus an expression of love and compassion.

A map for the synthetic group worker

I think that by now you may have a sense of what I mean when I speak of synthetic groupwork. This is a method and perspective of practice which seeks to activate and engage group members' will and to cultivate the intentional and moral capacity of the individual and the group.

I have said that the worker does this by discriminating between what is regressive and emergent in group behaviour as a consequence of bringing to bear on phenomena a bifocal vision, which includes a wide range of psychological, psychosocial, existential, and spiritual concerns that many other groupwork models would exclude, reduce, or pathologize. (See figure 12.1.)

Figure 12.1 is an attempt to describe and locate individual and group behaviour in terms of whether it is working towards or away from agreed objectives. The vertical axis

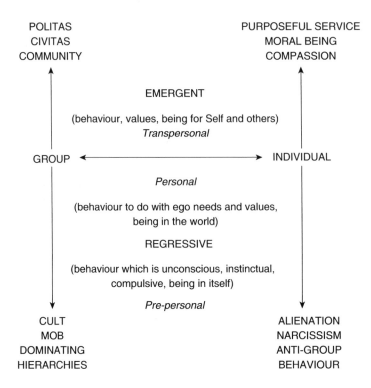

POLITAS   PURPOSEFUL SERVICE
CIVITAS   MORAL BEING
COMMUNITY   COMPASSION

EMERGENT

(behaviour, values, being for Self and others)
Transpersonal

GROUP ←——————————————→ INDIVIDUAL

Personal

(behaviour to do with ego needs and values,
being in the world)

REGRESSIVE

(behaviour which is unconscious, instinctual,
compulsive, being in itself)

Pre-personal

CULT   ALIENATION
MOB   NARCISSISM
DOMINATING   ANTI-GROUP
HIERARCHIES   BEHAVIOUR

Figure 12.1 A bifocal perspective of group concerns

indicates whether behaviour and intention is regressive or emergent. The horizontal axis indicates the relation and tension between individuals and groups. From this it is possible to look at a phenomenon or incident in the group and ask a range of questions and frame possible interventions:

- Does this event involve an individual and/or the group?
- Is the event regressive or emergent?
- Does it propel the group towards engagement with the political/civic/cultural/ spiritual?
- Does the event indicate the presence of cultish, depersonalizing tendencies in the group/subgrouping and dominating hierarchies?
- Does the event motivate the individual to service, purposeful activity, moral responsibility?
- Does the event indicate individual alienation, narcissistic preoccupation, and anti–group behaviour?

Take some time in your group to ponder and ruminate on these sorts of questions. From such considerations you will be able to decide accurately what form of intervention best suits the needs and desires of the individuals and the group at any point in time.

Remember that it takes a lot of practice and experience in groups to feel confident with these sorts of questions and interventions, and be prepared to make mistakes and be corrected by the group. This is no disgrace, and can be the basis of the group's learning that it also has responsibility and accountability for its own development and cannot reasonably expect to stay reliant on you.

Review

- Synthetic groupwork encourages a dynamic towards wholeness and emergence
- Synthetic groupwork emphasizes the expansion of an individual's identity
- The importance of bifocal vision to differentiate between regressive and emergent psychophysical, psychological, psychosocial, and psychospiritual contexts

References

1 Assagioli, R. (1980) *Psychosynthesis: A Collection of Basic Writings*, Wellingborough: Turnstone Press.
2 Assagioli, R. (1980) *The Act of Will*, London: Wildwood House.
3 Fukuyama, M.A. and Sevig, T.D. (1999) *Integrating Spirituality into Multicultural Counselling*, London: Sage, p. 9.
4 Yalom, I.D. (1980) *Existential Psychotherapy*, New York: Basic Books.
5 Fromm, E. (1960) *Fear of Freedom*, London: Routledge & Kegan Paul.
6 Frankl, V. (1963) *Man's Search for Meaning*, New York: Pocket Books.

Chapter 13

Working with different types of groups

As group workers gain in experience and confidence and sometimes reputation, they often find themselves increasingly called upon to operate in a widening range of group settings. They may even find themselves consulting with or supervising less experienced colleagues. In this chapter I want to look at different types of groups that you may be asked to work with and I shall identify some useful operating principles by locating a selection of groups along a continuum that has therapeutic effects on one pole and educational effects on the opposite pole.

I have developed this continuum because I frequently find that group workers get confused about the difference:

- between therapy in a group and the therapeutic effects of group participation
- fail to recognize the relationship between the therapeutic effects of group participation and the educational nature and effects of groupwork and understand that they are two essential sides of the same coin

Sometimes workers want to promote a group whose objective, let's say, is the acquisition of certain social skills. Some workers are frequently anxious about deviating in any way from a set programme and may regard attention to process and maintenance as 'doing therapy'. They do not understand the remedial and corrective possibilities to be derived from involvement and participation in a group and are unable to manage the group experience for maximum benefit of its members. All groupwork has the potential to be therapeutic but not all groupwork is therapy. Other workers might want to develop a more psychological approach to members' problems in groups but may underestimate or even ignore the educational role of the group in generating new possibilities and options and instructing members how to behave in social and interpersonal situations. Effective and creative groups educate their members by increasing their capacity for self-determined choice and expanding their knowledge and skill base. This is different from the formal instruction to be found in the traditional classroom or lecture setting.

The difference between group therapy and the therapeutic effects of group participation

Group therapy has an explicit and agreed purpose. It is to maximize extensive personal change by focusing on recurring intrapsychic conflicts and interpersonal difficulties and assist individuals improve their social functioning and ameliorate their distress. Group therapy is a specialized and purposeful construction and intervention in peoples' lives with their knowledge and agreement.

But whatever their explicit purpose all groups include and offer helpful and therapeutic benefits as a consequence of membership. Participation in any well-managed group can have a therapeutic or remedial effect on individuals who may have had previous negative experiences in groups and can enhance their self-esteem and social confidence.

I have emphasized repeatedly throughout this book that you are bringing people into a work group who may have had traumatic experiences in previous groups or may have social problems which can make group membership difficult or threatening. They are being asked to participate and get involved in a group that can stir up a whole range of anxieties and interpersonal tensions. Almost everyone enters a group of whatever kind with some conflicts and problems around managing relationships. Participation in a group over time generates the desire for intimacy with others, but as these feelings arise members can become anxious about them.

You may recall that I said on page 203 that a core dilemma in groups was how to get close but not too close, and how to be separate but not too separate. To resolve this dilemma, members tend to mobilize their characteristic defences against the disturbing feelings and as part of the process they may stop other people getting close to them and disrupt the work of the group. It is a core task of every group worker to minimize these frustrations and disturbances and provide a satisfying participatory experience for members.

I repeat, this is not the same as doing therapy but is the natural consequence of involvement and participating in a successful working group. You might find it helpful to go back and reread Chapter 8 for a fuller discussion on the helpful characteristics of groups.

Therapeutic characteristics of groups	Educational characteristics of groups
• Normalizing quality of group participation	• New knowledge and skill acquisition
• Universalizing nature of group involvement as a way of dissolving isolation	• Opportunities for rehearsing change
• Capacity of the group to generate, contain and change powerful emotions	• Emphasis on self-determined choices
• Support and relief of peer support and solidarity	• Learning new behavioural strategies
• Opportunities for identification and self-understanding	• Learning to be creative and productive

The effective group worker recognizes that evoking and utilizing the remedial and therapeutic effects of group involvement is a necessary demand of the method and also understands that by encouraging the educational and social training of members the group can promote members' growth and development. The particular purpose of the group will determine whether one dimension is regularly emphasized more than the other but

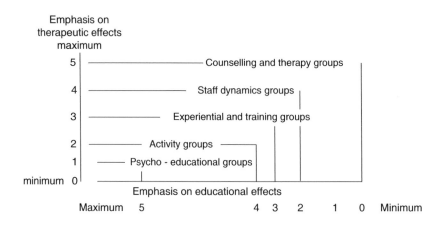

Figure 13.1 A continuum of different groups according to therapeutic and educational effects

attention to both dimensions is the key to successful and creative work with all groups that you are likely to encounter.

In fact it is possible to locate a variety of groups along a continuum with therapeutic effects on one polarity and educational benefits at the other extreme, according to whether one dimension is to be emphasized more than the other in keeping with the explicit group purpose, see Figure 13.1.

The advantage of this diagram is that we can now locate any group in terms of whether we want to achieve a primary objective of emphasizing therapeutic or educational work in a social care or mental health or any other setting. The essential point is to be clear about the purpose of the group and the nature of the basic contract with group members. This will help you decide the type of programme best suited, the style of leadership, and other variables such as number and length of sessions. You might at this point want to turn back to Chapter 1, which looks in detail at planning the group. Let's turn now to think about what is involved in working with these different groups.

Working with the psychoeducational group

A social worker in a mental health setting noted a number of clients on her caseload who suffered from problems of low self-esteem. These vulnerable people also presented with associated difficulties:

- Easily intimidated in social interactions
- Socially isolated with feelings of stigma
- Pronounced feelings of personal inadequacy
- Varied relationship problems
- Difficulties with anger management

The social worker decided to set up a time-limited group for 12 people with a focus on the theme of self-esteem and began to plan the group along psychoeducational lines. The psychoeducational group can take any medical, social, or behavioural theme or concern as its central focus and typically may emphasize:

- Learning about common problems in a group setting
- Mutual help and support
- Information sharing
- Practical solutions to problems or concerns
- Expert presentations on related topics
- Formal group discussions
- Role play and exercises on skill sets
- Creating personalized programmes of improvement
- Setting homework
- Advocacy and consciousness raising
- Liaison with similar interest groups
- Appropriate fund raising
- Development into self-help groups

You can see that such a group will have clear therapeutic benefits for its members in creating commonality and reducing isolation, and enhancing a sense of self-esteem and personal agency, but the basic contract has to do with educating and instructing members by providing information, defining problems, raising consciousness, and acquiring and practising specified skills. The psychoeducational group is leader-directed and sticks closely to a set programme that has been designed in advance and with particular objectives in mind. Good presentation skills and teaching ability are essential in this type of group if you are to keep on track with the material to be covered.

In my example the social worker decided that her self-esteem group should have four objectives:

1   To explain the concept and effects of self-esteem and how it is built and damaged
2   To describe the healing and self-protective strategies required for healthy self-esteem
3   To promote the development of healthy self-esteem through the development of assertive skills and more effective interpersonal communication skills, setting personal boundaries and limits
4   To assist group members to transfer the new skills learned in the group into their real life settings

The social worker designed a programme to achieve these objectives in the group over 18 weekly sessions each lasting 90 minutes. Each session was designed to begin with a short member check-in followed by a simple relaxation exercise led by the worker. The group would then review any homework set in the previous session. This homework was usually a task or reflection relevant to the topic or theme explored in the previous session and that each member was encouraged to practise outside the group. The homework review led to a discussion on what had worked and what didn't and aimed to promote self-awareness and self-responsibility.

The topic for the particular session was introduced and formally taught by the group worker or an arranged guest expert. This didactic input often utilized prepared flip charts or other relevant material. An ensuing group discussion and feedback was useful for encouraging sharing of thoughts and feelings and to ensure that important information was understood.

In the next part of the session an exercise or role-play was offered as a means of acquiring and practising component parts of a skill or an essential behavioural strategy. A short period of individual reflection on the usefulness of practising the skill in everyday life then proved the basis for setting a personal homework which could be reviewed in the next session. A closing exercise was offered that typically revolved around sharing a positive and negative experience of the session.

The group worker arranged the session topics sequentially:

Objective 1. To explain the concept of self-esteem

Session

1	Introductions; purpose of group and setting the group contract
2	The importance of self-esteem
3	Basic principles of building self-esteem
4	Identifying and disrupting self-destructive patterns and habits
5	Emotional healing strategies
6	Positive thinking skills
7	Stress management skills

Objective 2. Developing assertiveness skills and communication skills

Session

1	Introduction to assertiveness
2	Personality types and behavioural patterns
3	Owning our feelings
4	Assertiveness toolbox
5	Refusing and requesting
6	Criticism, feedback, and conflict: giving and receiving criticism
7	Maintaining and developing self-respect and self-esteem

Objective 3. Transferring learning

Session

> 1 Difficult situations in real life
> 2 Taking responsibility for your own self-development
> 3 Where to from here?
> 4 Review of group; appreciations, goodbyes and ending

You can see that this psychoeducational group deliberately utilizes the therapeutic benefits and effects of group membership and participation but is highly structured and emphasizes a clear cognitive and behavioural approach to group learning. It can be highly effective with vulnerable and sensitive people who might benefit from a defined agenda that explores key elements of particular problems or concerns. These groups typically emphasize practical activities and solutions to problems and are less concerned with the meaning of difficulties, so they are appealing to individuals who are both highly motivated to change and conversely are stuck in self-doubt. The psychoeducational group does not require the worker or member to recover traumatic memories or explore the genesis of maladaptive beliefs, as might be the case in a therapy group. Such a process usually needs a longer period of time than many agencies can permit and members can sign up to, and in addition the skill level required of group workers may make this uncovering type of work a more specialist activity. The value of the psychoeducational group is that it is time-limited, focused, and offers a structured opportunity to re-examine core beliefs and experiences and develop appropriate coping strategies whilst availing members of the remedial and corrective benefits of group membership. Many individuals suffer from generalized symptoms and experiences that after involvement in a psychoeducational group can be refined into manageable problems with reasonable solutions.

The advantage for the worker using psychoeducational groups lies in:

- Being able to locate the most relevant concerns for members
- Planning a relevant programme in advance
- Managing and motivating a greater number of members
- Being more systematic and structured
- Providing specific and personalized treatment plans and coping strategies

The disadvantages for the worker may include:

- Not enough time for adequate planning
- Over-preparation resulting in too much material to be covered
- One-sided emphasis on instruction and teaching
- Not being familiar enough with group dynamics
- Not enough time to attend adequately to group process
- Tendency to focus on individuals at expense of group process

Working with activity groups

A wide range of professional disciplines such as teachers, social workers, occupational therapists, nursing staff, and many others who practise in school, hospital, residential, day care, and other settings often utilize activity-based groupwork to achieve educative, thera-peutic, or social change objectives. A diverse spectrum of activity and work groups may be deployed:

- To provide short-term structured groupwork for individuals with particular problems or to achieve specified goals
- To ameliorate long-term or degenerative conditions
- To focus on supporting carers and family members
- To help individuals maintain their independence
- To protect individuals in vulnerable situations and assist them to manage com-plex relationships
- To promote initiative and engage people in their own care

Purposeful and well-managed activity groups have a distinct advantage in that they can engage members experientially in the joy and fun of interactive learning while providing practical and useful development and stimulation. Activity groups use an impressive array of techniques and programmes which require a co-ordination of the different modalities of body, feelings, and mind in order to generate change and growth. Groups may offer activities and experiences to develop and integrate the fundamental capacities and abilities of the human being:

- Physical
- Sensory awareness
- Emotional
- Mental and cognitive
- Social and interpersonal
- Imaginative and creative
- Ethical and volitional
- Aesthetic and beauty
- Transpersonal

Activity based groups provide (i) a content or task which involves and engages people and (ii) a context for individuals to work and grow personally and collectively. Members par-ticipate in and utilize the widest variety of methodologies. Individuals and groups paint, draw, and use clay, play games and sports, discuss topics of interest and share memories, rehearse dramas and act out roles, dance and do yoga, make objects, cook, eat together, and engage in all and any activity that contributes to and promotes a rounded and balanced experience of self.

The nature of action in activity groups

I think that an interesting feature of activity groups is that one has to decide what the action component in such groups is for. I believe that action has an inner dimension and an external dimension. By speaking of an inner action I mean those abilities and capacities that range from the basic functions of consciousness and personal continuity to those that make human existence intentional and meaningful, whereas outer action involves a capacity for agency in the world, modifying our personal environment, and interacting purposefully with other people. Activity groups can be designed to emphasize or preserve an inner action of awareness or develop and promote an outer behavioural action and achieve such action objectives as:

Inner action	*Outer action*
• To inhibit loss of memory	• Inhibit loss or reduction of motor skills
• To assist with disturbance of language use	• Control increased motor activity and agitation
• To diminish perceptual difficulties	• Modify disorganized or impulsive behaviour
• To prevent disorientation	• Enhance social skills and interaction
• To help with difficulties in planning, organizing, sequencing, reasoning	• Develop conversational and communication skills
• To encourage reflection	• Promote socialization and group cohesion
• To develop cognitive and conceptual skills	• Encourage creativity and play
• To stimulate imagination	• Foster alternative occupations and hobbies
• To enhance self-esteem and positive self-image	• Involvement in life of the unit/ centre
• To foster self-acceptance and deepen self-knowledge	• Promote promote self-discipline and concentration
• To refine values and ideals	

Of course there is no distinct cleavage between the two types of action – they are mutually reciprocal, but distinct settings do make particular demands. In an elderly care home the activity group might be utilized more as an instrument of palliative care for memory loss, cognitive deficits, and socialization whereas in a classroom a structured activity group may be a useful informal and creative way of exploring a social and life skills curriculum and engaging boisterous youngsters. Similarly, groupwork with clients who have learning disabilities or are suffering from stroke or brain injuries with attendant limited attention spans and motor skill disorders would benefit from purposefully designed behavioural activity groups. In designing and working with an activity group you will have to consider carefully the client population that you are working with in terms of their therapeutic, remedial, and educative needs and the perceived and desired benefit of group involvement for members. Go back and reread the sections in Chapter 1 that describe creative programme design and activity selection.

The role of the worker in an activity group

Having identified individual and group needs and set appropriate goals the worker has certain responsibilities and duties in an activity group:

> • Determine how these educational/remedial/palliative/therapeutic needs of members are best met by an activity
> • Identify features of an activity that are particularly relevant to your purpose and that might be emphasized or promoted
> • If you cannot explain why you are using a particular activity you shouldn't be using it
> • Where appropriate choose activities that maximize interaction with other members
> • Ensure that the competence levels required for activity suit the mental and physical capacities of the participant members
> • Choose activities that require a minimum of rules, procedures, and structures
> • Recognize your responsibility to adjudicate and arbitrate where appropriate
> • Periodically evaluate and review the activity for utility and satisfaction
> • Remember your responsibility to be a model and example for group members

The advantage for the worker of using activity groups lies in:

> • Being able to engage the most relevant concerns for members in accessible ways
> • Countering individuals' difficulties with language, attention, and dexterity
> • Emphasizing creative, expressive, and action-based modalities
> • Providing specific stimulation and coping strategies
> • Planning a relevant programme in advance
> • Managing and motivating members
> • Being more systematic and structured

The disadvantages for the worker may include:

> • Poor or inappropriate selection of activity
> • One-sided emphasis on activity as an end in itself
> • Failure to provide maturational development
> • Not being familiar enough with group dynamics
> • Not enough time to attend adequately to group process
> • Overemphasis on leader input

Working with experiential and training groups

Increasingly, experiential groups and the laboratory method of process groups or T-groups (training groups) are to be found in organizations and agencies, on a wide range of professional training courses, and as features of many conferences and professional gatherings. These varied groups commonly emphasize heightening awareness and understanding of the complexities of the processes of human group relations and endeavour to promote the development of interpersonal skills and communication. Individuals come together as in a laboratory to study individual and group dynamics by using themselves and each other as the object and subject of their enquiry in a highly experiential participant observation. The group contract is firmly based upon learning from experience and is radically different from traditional didactic and pedagogic cultures.

Some objectives of the experiential group

- Emphasis on the here and now interaction of group and its members
- Learning about group processes and phenomena
- Acquiring leadership skills
- Becoming aware of how others react to one's behaviour
- Learning to gauge the state of relations between other members
- Acquiring skills in appropriately modifying one's behaviour
- Expanding awareness and capacity to choose one's actions
- Developing emotional intelligence and skills
- Refining communication skills and relational styles
- There may be a focus on authority, power, leadership dynamics
- There may be evaluation of roles, tasks, and functions in the group
- Every communication, behaviour, and interaction in the group is available for reflection and consideration

The purpose of the exercise is learning and training not therapy, but of course such a training group is inevitably a very therapeutic experience.

In this section I want to focus particularly on large group sensitivity training, for four reasons:

1   I have personally conducted over a 15-year time period at the Institute of Psychosynthesis, London, a regular large group comprising usually around 60 psychotherapy students but at times numbering up to 90 students meeting monthly for two hours to study inter-individual and large group dynamics as part of their training.

2   I find that increasingly in local and international groupwork conferences and professional gatherings there is a formal slot for large group meetings where mass dynamics can be studied. Indeed the largest such group I have participated in was held at a conference in Dublin in 2008 and comprised 550 people meeting for an hour and a half each day for five consecutive days with no agenda other than to study its own process.

3   Many group workers operate in therapeutic communities and other residential settings where large group meetings of staff and residents are held on a daily and weekly basis to consider and review their interpersonal relations.

4   Recent national and international events indicate that large groupings of individuals are 'moved' to collectively gather to protest, to celebrate, or even to grieve – events beyond any personal relationship. This phenomenon manifests as a force for transformation in a collective sense but is also one where the collective can be manipulated and influenced as in mass movements like fundamentalism and terrorism. It is essential in the modern world to recognize that one is frequently resonating to collective preoccupations and concerns. It is clear that studying and creatively participating in large group trainings provides us with immense analogous learning for understanding and altering the dynamics of organizational life, institutions, society, political culture, and situations of intractable conflict from N. Ireland to the Middle East.

What happens in a large group?

A large group usually consists of more than 30 members and may have only as an upper limit the number of members who can be seated in one room and who can see and hear each other.

> - Typically there is no formal structure or agenda so that members are free to start or join in a discussion or abstain if they wish
> - The usual method of operation is the study of the behaviour of the group and its members' experience as it happens in the 'here and now'
> - There will be one or more leaders who will provide boundaries and may comment at times on what they see happening so as to facilitate learning
> - Members are invited to conceptualize and think about their experience of their current internal and external worlds and put this into exchangeable forms of communication

This is rendered difficult by the multiplicity of differences and subjective perceptions of inequality and the inevitability of some degree of regression and recapitulation triggered by simply being in the presence of so many people. The large group provides these experiences and possibilities because it heightens and highlights one's sense of identity and one's awareness of and relationship with others.[1] This may at times feel regressive and threatening but there is always the possibility of an experience of positive collectivity and transpersonal authenticity. One's experience of oneself may feel tenuous in the face of the mass. One's cultural/religious/ethnic roots and origins – Irish/English/American/Pakistani/Catholic/Jew/Muslim/other may become important in an unanticipated way and the trans-egoic and trans-cultural nature of one's self can be revealed in unexpected ways and thought about – client/professional/Westerner/Third-Worlder/human/social/political/spiritual being.

Because of its mass and form and size, the non-directed nature of the large group experience may generate in many members a sense of unfamiliarity, dread, and strangeness precisely because it is not a concert/football match/religious or political service or any other recognizably familiar crowd situation with familiar roles, behaviours, and expectations.[2] At the same time the large group may equally offer other members experience of euphoria and wonder, creative exploration, and altered states of consciousness, archetypal resonance, and mytho-poetic sensitivity.

Personal identity and the experience of the 'I' takes different forms when confronted in either small or large groups. In small groups the individual is 'known' by its members;

emotional attachments become possible and distinctions are sharpened and refined. In the large group individuality is more fluid and prone to de-differentiation, and in order to belong one is more easily subsumed under some collective identity. The powerful sense of one's smallness, the unpredictable largeness of the group, and the potential to be shamed is a very difficult experience to manage continuously. In any large group setting the struggle to recover the 'I', to stand up and speak, to be recognized, or even to think clearly is a task in itself. To then speak for a value-set that is more than the personal – the political or spiritual – can be threatening and the silence or dissent of others may be very anxiety-making.

The large group resonates with social, political, religious, cultural, spiritual, and intra-psychic and interpersonal attributes and preoccupations. What is determinant is where a member may be personally identified at a particular time – ego/I/Self; group member/staff member; client/professional; smoker/non-smoker; gender or ethnicity, and whether the other large group members accept, tolerate, collude with, or challenge this identi-fication. The member's self-identification, often largely unconscious and defensive but also conscious and value-laden, will determine how each individual member experiences the various group phenomena and interactions. One can feel immersed or submerged, engulfed or exposed, regressed or individuated, and this indicates the educational and therapeutic purpose of the large group.

At the Institute of Psychosynthesis, London, the educational aims and therapeutics of the large group are directed to the recognition and recovery of split-off, repressed, and projected prepersonal potentials; the awakening and actualizing of transpersonal qualities and attrib-utes, and the manifesting of this dialectic in personal and collective dialogue, responsibil-ity, and action. In relation to this, silence or verbal and visible contribution on the part of members of the group may be an expression of prepersonal anxiety or a manifestation of transpersonal awe. In other words, silence on the part of participants can be seen as a pre-personal identification or as a de-individuated response to dread in the context of a large and unnegotiable mass. On other occasions there is no doubt that silence represents the deep inner action of working through complex and multidimensional material.

The collective unconscious manifests in the large group often when space, territory, and identity are threatened or paradoxically when they are celebrated. The complex interrela-tion of personal, social, cultural, and political dynamics and the omnipresent unconscious dynamics may on occasion generate uncertainty as to how to act. In such conditions archetypal motifs and preoccupations appear. The collective unconscious is a source of transpersonal symbols, Archetypes, and emergent potentials for healing and meaning whereby sterile values and cultural mindsets may be transformed. It offers and forms the basis for co-operation and even unification across borders and national boundaries.

The difficulty and task for the large group participant lies in authentically managing a set of complicated relationships in the large group so as to be in relationship and be in dialogue intrapsychically and interpersonally. The complexity of unequal and multiple roles can leave the member 'silenced', 'ambivalent', and questioning but as far as possible members are chal-lenged and encouraged to reflect on both themselves and the group processes in order to:

- Determine ethical priorities and dilemmas
- Select moral choices
- Act and participate responsibly in human relationships thus re-sacralizing the
- ground in which they interact in the world

The large group phenomenon is therefore an opportunity for prepersonal, personal, and transpersonal consciousness and interaction. In other settings large group experiences may have quite different learning outcomes.

An example of the large group at work

A large group of some 60 trainee psychotherapists met for the first session of the new academic year. There was a new group intake and three more advanced year groups present. There were two facilitators. The session began on time but with members talking in twos and threes for some five minutes before a silence gradually emerged. (It is common at the start of sessions for members of most large groups to talk together protractedly as a way of holding onto a safe sense of self and avoiding the anticipated and feared smallness and helplessness of the large group experience.)

After a considerable amount of silence one of the new students commented that the session seemed to him like a Quaker silent meeting and tentatively asked what was the purpose of the large group and could he and his new colleagues be given some direction. This was met with gales of relieved laughter by the older heads and various comments to the effect that the purpose was that there was no purpose and the new people would have to find out for themselves just like senior members.

It seemed to me at this point:

- That the newcomer's desire for direction was appropriate
- That the newcomers' anxiety about the confusing silence was aggressively enjoyed by the senior members who could locate their own discomfort in the inexperienced members
- Senior members were perhaps resentful about these newcomers
- Senior members were withholding leadership or uncertain how to offer direction to these resented ones

After another silence a member of the final fourth year group lamented the exit and loss of the previous final year group who had been so wise and supportive in the large group and remarked on her surprise to find herself now in the final year of training and still unsure what the large group was about. This led to a discussion in which various members identified themselves as belonging to specific year groups and informed the newcomers that they themselves had experienced similar feelings in their time but things would get better as time went on.

I found myself thinking about:

- The feelings of loss and vulnerability generated by the exit of the knowing elders
- The emergence of common feelings of uncertainty and insecurity
- Some attempt to reassure the newcomers
- The way members were using their year group badge as a means of gaining an identity rather than using their personal names and were not yet ready for intimacy

A number of the new members again asked what were the rules of the group, what was permissible, and commented on their nervousness and physical anxiety about speaking before such a large number of people. There were a number of attempts by the newcomers to engage the two leaders in discussion about what was appropriate in the session but these attempts were not responded to in a way that offered solutions.

After a time one of the new members remarked that she had noticed people smoking in the canteen and suggested that the large group might make a rule about making this area a smoke free zone. This generated a lot of discussion and interaction. The smokers in the group protested their rights to smoke and the non-smokers pointed out the unpleasant experience of sharing a smoke filled room. A case was advanced for making an ecological environment; the addictive nature of smoking was discussed as a psychospiritual crisis; a robust debate ensued about human rights and the dilemmas posed for the large group about how to protect everyone's interests; the politics of power and democracy were explored.

It occurred to me that:

- The smoking issue was a way of providing a direction since the leaders weren't going to offer a direction
- The smoking issue offered a means of dealing with the anxiety of powerlessness and the desire for control and order
- It was the experience of the non-structured large group that was unconsciously perceived to be toxic and damaging to emotional health and that needed elimination
- The issue was a way of generating a subgroup identity of smokers and non-smokers since a more personal intimacy was not yet available

I decided to intervene and said that members seemed to believe that participating in this unfamiliar large group was a potentially damaging situation and that in order to make oneself feel safe the members needed an enemy that could be recognized and eliminated or brought under the control of a good and protective group government that one could identify with. I suggested that it might be more helpful to find a way of talking to each other about the experience of being in the large group here and now rather than trying to get rid of what felt like the bad and unacceptable bits of the process by setting up unhelpful and premature group rules.

This intervention appeared to have the soothing and structuring effect of offering a psychological direction that the group might take and emphasized using our own experience as a means of reflection and inquiry without prescribing or prohibiting other possibilities for the large group study. Members did respond to my intervention and began to explore their anxious psychosomatic experience of the group; their desire for leadership and direction; the wish to offer leadership and their fear of being attacked for offering leadership. Shortly the session ended with members beginning to identify themselves by name and reporting a more spontaneous feeling to the group interaction.

The role of the worker in the experiential group

You can see from the example given that the fundamental role of the worker in running an experiential group like a large group or any process group is to help the members learn and understand the nature of intra-group dynamics and relations as they are emerging live in the situation. Invariably different group workers are aligned to a variety of theoretical orientations and may emphasize diverse dimensions of the experiential group but there are common tasks and activities that we can identify for the worker with process groups:

- The worker endeavours to construct a learning situation but does not directly teach
- Actively promotes the value of learning from experience
- Draws attention to what is happening here and now in the group
- Addresses what is not happening or is currently missing in the group
- Does not judge the phenomenon or interaction
- Assists the group to understand its own emerging behaviour
- Does not assume traditional authority role but provides boundary and containment
- Helps the group to formulate appropriate questions
- Encourages members to engage directly with each other
- Emphasizes members' current experience
- Models an attitude of curiosity and reflective inquiry on group life
- Seeks to release the therapeutic potential of the group

Working with a staff dynamics group

There are a range of agency settings such as therapeutic communities, psychiatric units, and diverse residential and other services where the demands on staff are heightened because of the intense emotional stress and particular organizational nature of the work. Staff may be organized into work teams and shifts to perform specific tasks but social and psychological factors may complicate team co-operation and productivity and threaten operational effectiveness. Staff teams can be vulnerable to and affected by a host of difficulties:

Because the list of anxiety-making impingements on team cohesion and performance is inexhaustible, increasingly attention is being paid to the ongoing well-being and professional development of staff teams, and in many places regular meetings of a staff group are held under the facilitation of an outside worker. The objectives of a typical staff dynamics group will include:

- Sharing and talking about the communal anxiety of the staff team
- Detoxifying emotional stresses generated by client contact
- Working through staff-client incidents and crises
- Identifying where clients are impacting on inter-team relations
- Discussing disagreements and conflicts between staff about relations with clients
- Exploring the meaning of pairings and subgroups within the team
- Examining the attitudes and feelings of staff to each other where appropriate
- Evaluating the relationship between the staff team and other teams/head office
- Promoting a culture of honest inquiry
- Identifying suitable theoretical perspectives to understand and discuss the staff dynamics and the staff-client/staff-agency interactions

You can see that working with a staff dynamics group is about utilizing the therapeutic resources of the group and promoting a professional learning culture whose objective is about how to work productively as a team with sometimes difficult clients. Staff dynamics is most definitely not a therapy group. Work with a staff dynamics group is a specialized form of team building: developing the team as a container of its own emotions and promoting its capacity to think about its own processes as a way of cleansing and maintaining itself. A current version of staff dynamics groupwork is called reflective practice groupwork and in the next chapter I will look in detail at how to set up and facilitate a reflective practice group.

Social defence systems in staff dynamics groups

An essential strategy when working with staff dynamics groups involves recognizing and identifying the presence and operation of social defence mechanisms. A social defence system is the way that the members of a group unconsciously collude and combine to organize the structure, culture, and task functioning of the group in order to protect themselves and avoid feelings of guilt, anxiety, and uncertainty generated by the intense demands of their work.

In a classic study Isobel Menzies demonstrated the operation of social defence systems in a hospital where matters of life and death were a constant and everyday source of stress and anxiety.[3] She showed how nursing staff protected themselves from the anxiety of dealing with ill and dying patients by relating to them as parts of the body – 'the liver transplant in bed 6' or 'the broken arm in bed 8' – rather than relate to the patients as whole persons who might get more unwell and distress them. Nurses were trained to follow an extremely rigid task list and discouraged from using their own initiative and discretion as an unconscious way of avoiding the stress of any individual decision making that might cause them anxiety.

A particularly damaging social defence system centred upon the manner in which nursing staff attempted to manage their anxiety about their individual responsibility. It appeared that each nurse experienced an internal conflict between her desire to be professionally responsible and the wish to avoid this heavy burden. The conflict was managed by psychological processes of splitting and projection that converted the internal struggles into interpersonal conflicts within the team. The irresponsible impulse was projected by each nurse into her subordinate or the student nurses who were then universally regarded as careless, irresponsible, and in need of constant supervision and discipline. The strict and responsible part of herself was split off and located in her superiors who were then expected to behave towards her with suspicion and hyper-vigilance.

I have seen exactly these social defence mechanisms at work when training a group of social work supervisors who collectively complained about the poor work ethic of students who were alleged to be unfamiliar with office culture, scruffily dressed, and prone to lateness and inattentiveness due to their preoccupations with constant socializing. The social work supervisors were adamant that the standard of recruit was much higher in their salad days and that they had been more studious and responsible trainees.

In another example, an adult education psychology course was offered by the local university in a school in the evening. The psychology tutor found the attitude of the school authorities to be deleterious to the work of the adult group. Rooms were constantly changed; necessary equipment was unavailable; the working conditions were so poor as to threaten to undermine the group. When the tutor complained to the school authorities he was met with a dismissive attitude and nothing changed. Similarly the university did not support the tutor and expected him to cope with the situation. It was only when the tutor brought the unhealthy situation to his supervision group that the presence of unacknowledged social defence systems could be recognized. It appeared that the hierarchical, authoritarian school culture was threatened by a more creative and informal groupwork model. The school system was organized to deal with unwilling children and was unconsciously envious of the tutor's group who were choosing to be there. The social defence systems activated in the school staff appeared to be based on envy and a desire to spoil the work of the incoming psychology group – composed of volunteers instead of recruits and working informally and creatively instead of formally and rigidly as in the more traditional classroom setting. The university department was seen to be unconsciously inflating itself and devaluing the school by locating its course there and promoting its self-referring standards of excellence at the school's expense. After the supervision experience the tutor was now freed up to think more and react less personally to the school behaviour and began to drop in during the day to speak to some of the relevant teachers as a way of letting them know what he was doing and to see if he could make common ground. Gradually the climate of mutual distrust and envy was lessened to the point where in the following academic year the tutor was allocated a predictable room for his work.

You can see that the operation of these social defence systems weakens the cohesion and smooth functioning of the staff group and causes it to be preoccupied with creating unhealthy forms and interactions as a means of avoiding anxiety generated by the stressful work. The role of the worker in a staff dynamics group is to enable the team members to identify their anxieties and come to terms with the stressful reality of the job. A helpful way of identifying the presence of social defence systems is to consider what the basic assumptions of the staff team might be at any time.

The theory of basic assumptions

This emphasis on social defence systems developed out of the early work of Wilfred Bion who argued that the task of a group could be interrupted by what he called unconscious basic assumptions.[4] Bion argued that in situations of real or imagined stress such as a change in group membership or a trauma to its functioning the group behaves as if certain behaviours are vital to the group's survival. These behaviours are like some unconscious and emotional basic assumption that group members hold in common but never speak about. Bion identified three types of basic assumptions: dependency, fight/flight, and pairing. A fourth basic assumption in which groups mass together in a protective oneness or aggregate as separate individuals has been added recently by Hopper.[5]

You can identify the basic assumption activity of dependency because the group behaves as if its primary task is solely to provide for the needs and wishes of its members.

- The group may act as if it is stupid or incompetent and only the leader has expertise
- The leader or a designated member is seen as having all the answers and is expected to take care of the group
- One can see how charismatic and cult leaders can flourish in this kind of basic assumption dynamic

In the basic assumption activity of fight or flight:

- The group behaves as if there is a danger or an enemy from which it must flee or which it must attack
- The group engages in either fighting (active aggression, scapegoating, physical attack) or flight from the task (withdrawal, passivity, avoidance, ruminating on past history)
- Leadership may be bestowed on the one who either mobilizes the aggressive forces in the group or who helps the group avoid facing the difficulty of the tasks ahead

You can identify the basic assumption activity of pairing because:

- The group behaves as if salvation will come through the pairing of two members within the group
- The group may become inactive as it depends on the pair to do the group's work
- The focus may be on the future as a defence against dealing with the difficulties of the present. Hope for the future (messiah) replaces actual work or facing the group's difficulties in the present

Bion's work demonstrates how groups under threat withdraw from their task and set up structures and interactions to defend against these anxieties. These basic assumptions mean that no meaningful work can be done and the group cannot develop. It is a fairly simple matter for the worker to assess group performance and determine if basic assumptions are influencing group activity and from there identify the social defence systems that the group are locked into.

An example of working with a staff dynamics team

A staff team in an adolescent inpatient psychiatric unit was meeting with a new facilitator after their old facilitator had retired. The new worker had never run a staff dynamics group before and was discomforted when the group members began to query the purpose and usefulness of a staff dynamics group even though they had a long history of meeting for this work. The team complained about their previous facilitator claiming that he had run the staff group like a therapy group and they had often felt scapegoated and singled out. Over the opening sessions with the new worker the attendance was sporadic and the main issue seemed to be concerned with how to be a team together and use these sessions.

Then in one session the team leader reported to the new group facilitator that a female staff member called Susan would be absent today because she had been inappropriately touched by one of the adolescent boys in the unit and that she had gone home suffering from stress. The team leader reproached the present staff members for allowing this to happen and asserted that proper procedures were not followed which had resulted in this incident. Some staff replied that the adolescent should not be allowed to remain in the unit and should be removed to a more secure unit. There was no consideration given to how Susan might be feeling nor was there any disclosure of how this had impacted the staff. Susan returned in the next session and beyond a perfunctory description of what had happened, the incident was not discussed again; nor did the new worker feel able to go into any exploration for fear that she might be seen to be doing therapy like her predecessor.

Over the next few sessions there was a return to the theme of uncertainty about how to work in a staff dynamics group and vague comments about inattentive and inconsistent authority. The facilitator wondered if these comments were aimed at her but did not feel comfortable to raise them with the group. Then in a session the staff members told the new facilitator that the adolescent boy who had inappropriately touched Susan weeks before had been removed from the unit because he had racially abused the Chinese deputy team leader. The facilitator was curious about the different management of the two incidents and wondered to the team why the racial abuse was considered more serious than the sexual impropriety.

The staff members said that the deputy was a mild and somewhat weak person who needed protecting from residents who could be disrespectful of him. They described his management style as soft and not challenging and gave examples of how he wasn't always available to staff in need of help and often didn't adequately give relevant information in shift handovers.

What was going on in this staff dynamics team?

The facilitator brought her difficulties to a supervision group she had just recently joined and in a few sessions was enabled to make some sense of what was going on in the staff dynamics group.

Her supervision group pointed out that there was a fight/flight basic assumption operating in the staff dynamics that was manifesting:

Fight	*Flight*
Team leader's attack on staff	Poor attendance at staff dynamics meetings
Staff attack on previous facilitator	Lack of agreement on purpose of group
New facilitator feeling undermined	Lack of response to Susan's experience
Scapegoating of offending resident	Removal of resident rather than engaging with anxieties of working with difficult adolescents
Scapegoating of deputy team leader	Deputy's passive management style

It was also clear that a second basic assumption of dependency was operating and could be observed in the group's apparent helplessness and acceptance of the team leader's criticisms. It was postulated by the supervision group that the new facilitator was getting caught in the unconscious dynamics of a social defence system that was aimed at keeping hostile and persecutory impulses belonging to the staff at bay. It seemed that the staff team was not processing its angry feelings about the difficult adolescents who kept them up at night, got drunk, self-harmed, and attacked the staff's best efforts to help them, for fear that they might retaliate and attack the adolescents and be attacked in turn, thus generating a spiral of destructive relations in the unit. The violent impulses were split off by staff members and located in the adolescent boy who inappropriately touched Susan and racially abused the weak deputy team leader. This adolescent boy both acted out staff contempt for the deputy who had failed to be a good protective figure and enabled them to get rid of the boy thus satisfying their unconscious desire to retaliate against the adolescent residents.

The 'weak' deputy team leader was unconsciously hated by the staff because he mirrored their feelings of helplessness and impotence and served as a counter to the harsh team leader who acted towards them as they would have wished to act towards the adolescents. The inconsistent management of the two incidents involving Susan and the deputy were part of a social defence system whose aim was to avoid the anxiety and guilt to do with the intense feelings generated by working with a difficult client group.

The facilitator was able to return to her staff dynamics group and gradually engage the members in an exploration of their feelings about their work. Attendance improved markedly and there was no return to the flight from the purpose of the group. Over time the staff group did begin to address the anxieties and stress of their work situation.

Working with the therapy group

The basic contract of a therapy group is personal and extensive therapeutic change and its central focus is on its members' psychological conflicts and interpersonal distress.

Human beings are preoccupied with desire and longing, surrender and loss, love, relationship, and fulfilment. People become ill or troubled because of their experiences with love or lovelessness and because they live in a society that has lost its soul and cannot meet the individual's deepest needs for intimate and authentic relationships. It is my experience that people are wounded and broken and out of alignment with their essential self and each other because they feel unloveable or long for love but dread and mismanage the encounter. They fall into a soul sickness and in some cases cannot go on any longer.

The symptomatic presentations and interactions of the therapy group are therefore nothing more than inarticulate accounts of soullessness and the deep longing for love and transformation. Neurosis is simply the manifestation of difficulties in personal relationships and the debilitating isolation that ensues. Because individual suffering is in essence a fear of entering into loving, co-operative, and interdependent relationships, group therapy with its central emphasis on the creative and transformative power of relationship is, in my view, the treatment of choice for most troubled individuals. Group therapy conducted by trained and sensitive health care professionals can offer unique opportunities to re-engage with issues of intimacy and interdependence. You might find it helpful at this point to return to Chapter 2 and reread the section that details the sorts of anxieties that people frequently encounter and repeat with each other.

Goals for group therapy

* Reducing debilitating personal isolation
* Learning to trust again
* Establishing interpersonal relationships
* Learning to share common problems

- Finding out what one really thinks about things
- Acquiring insight into one's patterns of behaviour
- Identifying and nullifying perverse self-fulfilling prophecies
- Finding out what one really feels about things
- Learning to manage difficult feelings like shame/rage/guilt
- Working on issues to do with intimacy
- Managing aggression
- Learning to assert oneself
- Dealing with trauma/bereavement/illness/ageing
- Questioning and searching for spiritual values: idealism, altruism, compassion, justice, mercy, forgiveness, faith, hope, love, peace
- Exploring the nature of intimacy and sacredness

You can see that this list is really endless because the whole range of human affliction and preoccupation can be explored in sensitive and imaginative group therapy. What is certain however is that the primary objective of group therapy is to establish a safe and contained meeting place where troubled individuals can gradually begin to develop a trusting and confidential relationship with each other and their therapist in which they can discuss and work through issues of personal difficulty. What group therapy provides is a consistent and predictable environment in which members create together an enduring and genuine emotional experience that corrects and replaces their previous experiences and mental templates of the world.

What happens in group therapy?

A therapy group usually consists of no more than eight people and a therapist and the group usually sits in a circle so that everyone is visible to everyone else. Foulkes who developed the therapy model of group analysis likened the group to a 'hall of mirrors'. What he meant was that it was easier to see in others what one could not see in oneself and that over time this mirror-like attribute of the group could result in expanding aware-ness as members came to recognize unwanted aspects of themselves and accept this with-out shame or reproach. Groups may be time limited and start and finish with the same members, or longer-term groups whose membership rotates.

- Typically there is no formal structure or agenda so that members are free to start or join in a discussion or abstain if they wish. Individuals may describe their difficulties and ask the group for help. A common theme may emerge that engages everyone. Sometimes groups may explore a pressing theme over a number of sessions. Some group therapists may draw attention to an item from a previous session and ask the group to work on this.
- Members are invited to think about their experience of their current internal and external worlds and put this into exchangeable forms of communication. This is not easy because members may be caught up in painful life events or experiencing dif-ficulties in relationships that temporarily overwhelm them. Group therapy sessions are often filled with powerful and intense emotions that have been suppressed for a long

time and now find release in a protected and affirming space. All models of group therapy recognize the importance of appropriate expression of feelings and actively encourage emotional catharsis. The psychodynamic oriented group therapy emphasizes that in addition to the expression of painful feelings the group work towards more articulate forms of communication as a way of broadening and deepening the members' range of expression and comprehension.

- Personal disclosure plays an essential part in group therapy. Members are encouraged to reveal material about themselves they would not ordinarily reveal to others. Disclosure of shameful or guilty feelings and behaviours is a risky business for members because they fear being rejected and blamed. But disclosure of emotionally charged and secret material can lead to an experience of release and self-forgiveness and acceptance of one's self because it involves setting aside personal masks and false self-presentations. Successful disclosure generates a culture of trusting and meaningful interactions in the group and intensifies the experience of intimacy and responsibility towards each other. Learning to give feedback to each other in a helpful and positive manner promotes disclosure and similarly deepens the group experience.

- The nature and quality of the interpersonal relations between members is a central focus of group therapy, particularly in psychodynamically oriented group therapy because these relationships frequently imitate important earlier relationships in members' family of origin, and feelings, attitudes, and fantasies about other members are an important means of identifying and exploring how previous experiences continue to distort the present. These transference phenomena typically manifest in member rivalries and intense ambivalent feelings towards the group therapist.

- It follows from this that members do not merely talk about their difficulties but relive and re-enact them in interactions with the group. As a consequence all models of group therapy now emphasize the importance of attending to here and now interactions as a way of highlighting distorted perceptions and relational patterns and promoting change.

- In the humanistic group therapies like Gestalt or psychodrama the group therapist is very active in promoting the interaction of members and usually directs events in a practical and expert way, providing exercises and experiments for members to explore and engage with. In the more psychodynamic group therapies the therapist is much less directive and more inclined to emphasize the importance of the group as the instrument of change. Different theoretical orientations require different activities from the group therapist. Some group therapists may work with the group as a whole and limit their interventions and observation to mass group process remarks. Other workers emphasize individual interaction in the group and regard the group processes as secondary to individual change. My own preference is for the bifocal approach of the group analyst Foulkes who points out the importance of working with both the individual and the group.[6] The group therapist is concerned to assist the group perform its natural remedial functions but is also willing to focus on individual themes and preoccupations.

How change occurs in group therapy

People grow and change in group therapy as a consequence of letting go of dated and limiting self-identifications and expanding their repertoire of possibilities and opportunities.

Participation in a group soon highlights the compulsive and repetitive behaviour of members and therapeutic work can begin. Many people feel determined by their personal history and seem unaware that they have the power of agency and the capacity for choice even in limiting situations. The exercise of choice is a personal act of creation and involves different aspects of our experience of willing.

Group therapy by its emphasis on meaningful and authentic interaction promotes and affirms the necessity of human choice as the only satisfactory way of living and managing the inevitable attendant problems.

Rutan and Stone have identified three other mechanisms of change in group therapy:[7]

- *Imitation.* In group therapy members have the opportunity to observe other relational styles and problem-solving strategies. They can watch how other members manage their intense feelings and learn from them. Group therapy offers multiple opportunities for members to imitate others who display successful, appropriate, and creative ways of thinking and behaving.
- *Identification.* This is a more unconscious process than the more overt imitation of successful members' behaviour. In identification members take on parts or qualities or aspects of another person and modify their behaviour and feelings. Peer identifications are very common but also identifications with the therapist can result in an increased capacity for tolerance of difficult feelings and cultivating a more thoughtful and reflective attitude.
- *Internalization.* This is an integrating process that comes about as a consequence of internal shifts and modifications of members' psychological profile. As members mature in the group they move to a higher and more flexible level of functioning and are no longer as easily disrupted as previously. The result is that members operate more authentically and creatively in their relationships and with increased awareness and choice.

The role of the group therapist

The task of the group therapist is to maximize the opportunities for therapeutic work resulting in lasting change for group members. There are a number of common activities that the therapist will engage in whatever their theoretical orientation. Many of these functions and activities have already been referred to constantly throughout the book, and Chapters 11 and 12 contain detailed descriptions of the worker's tasks which will help you run your therapy group successfully.

An example of a group therapy session

A new therapy group composed of five women and three men had been meeting for 12 sessions in a outpatient psychiatric unit. The group had been listening sympathetically to Joan describing her feelings of grief at the death of her mother-in-law since the last session. After a while John came in to say that he also was feeling sad because today was the fifth anniversary of his friend's death. He had not slept at all last night for thinking about it.

The group did not respond and John moved on to say that he would not grieve if his father died as he hated the man. Mary said that she had long been afraid of a neighbour who had bullied her as a child and she had struggled successfully since to forgive him. Now that she was no longer afraid of him her next step was to speak to him in person. The group continued to talk about experiences of hateful people but without any emotion.

The therapist believed the group were avoiding John's sadness and intervened to ask why they hadn't picked up on what John had said about today being a difficult day because of his friend's death. A number of members said they did not want to upset John more than necessary. The therapist said that John was clearly upset and that perhaps talking about the incident would be more helpful than avoiding it. He wondered if group members were protecting themselves from painful feelings more than they were protecting John.

John then told us the story of how he had been driving a car in which his friend had been a passenger and his excessive speed resulted in an accident and the death of his friend. He had never forgiven himself for his carelessness, nor had his friend's father. As this very moving story was being narrated the group therapist became aware that Mary was unwrapping and preparing to eat a chocolate bar. She had done something similar in the previous two sessions but had not been challenged.

The therapist waited for the group to confront this behaviour but when no one said anything he asked Mary at a suitable point what was it in John's story that made her want to eat. She said that she had wanted to eat since the beginning of the session. The group therapist asked her why she had particularly wanted to eat now and said that he wanted her to think psychologically about the meaning of her behaviour. He wondered if she were behaving in a way that not only had meaning for her but served a group function. Other members now came in and said that they had noticed in the past few sessions that she had started eating crisps and drinking cola. Mary cried and began to disclose that she suffered from an eating disorder and had not told anyone before. The group members now began to think about how eating was a way of managing intense and painful feelings and some of them admitted to using junk food, alcohol, and drugs as a way of dealing with their own unbearable pain. It soon became obvious why the group had skimmed over John's evident distress as it evoked their own feelings of anguish and helplessness. Slowly the group began to explore their unwillingness to speak about emotionally charged experiences for fear that they would be overwhelmed.

This session proved a turning point in the group's ability to get engaged in deep therapeutic work and members began to learn that they could be supported and support each other in working through experiences that they could not manage on their own.

The critical intervention by the group therapist was aimed at both the group resistance to getting involved with John's feelings and also at the individual symptomatic behaviour of Mary. By linking these interactions the therapist was able to get the group thinking about how they avoided intense emotions and how one person's behaviour was something they all contributed to. The healing potential of the group was affirmed and promoted as a therapeutic force that they could all use in the future as needed.

Review

- All groups can have therapeutic and remedial benefits for members
- All groups can offer educational and training benefits for members
- It is possible to locate groups on a spectrum where psychoeducational groups which emphasize the educational and instructional dimension are on one pole and therapy groups which emphasize the therapeutic dimension are on the opposite pole

- The purpose of your group will determine whether the therapeutic or the educational dimension is to be emphasized
- The purpose of the group should always be matched to the need of its members
- Styles of leadership, types of programme, and forms of intervening and processing are determined by the purpose of your group
- Many problems in groups can be avoided if you are clear about the nature of the therapeutic and educational needs and requirements of group members and have geared this to group purpose, activity, and leadership style
- Psychoeducational and activity groups usually have a predetermined programme and are quite leader-directed and often goal-oriented
- Experiential groups and therapy groups usually emphasize exploring and thinking about the spontaneous and emergent here and now interactions of members and are frequently less leader-directed and encourage the expression of emotions
- The less structured the group the more attention you will focus on transference phenomena, personal defences, and social defence systems and mass process interactions
- The more structured the group the less attention you will focus on individual and group processes and the more you will attend to programme relevance, skill acquisition, competency development, and cognitive and behavioural change

References

1 Kreeger, L. (1975) *The Large Group: Dynamics and Therapy*, London: Constable.
2 de Mare, P., Piper, R., and Thompson, S. (1991) *Koinonia: From Hate through Dialogue to Culture in the Large Group*, London: Karnac.
3 Menzies, I. (1970) *The Functioning of Social Systems as a Defence against Anxiety*. London: Tavistock Institute of Human Relations, Centre for Applied Social Research.
4 Bion, W.R. (1968) *Experiences in Groups*. London: Tavistock Publications.
5 Hopper, E. (1997) 'Traumatic experience in the unconscious life of groups: A fourth basic assumption', *Group Analysis*, 34, 1: 439–70.
6 Foulkes, S.H. (1964) *Therapeutic Group Analysis*, London: Maresfield.
7 Rutan, J.S. and Stone, W.N. (1984) *Psychodynamic Group Psychotherapy*, London: Macmillan.

Chapter 14

How to set up and run a reflective practice group

There is an increasing emphasis on the importance of well facilitated reflective practice groups in multidisciplinary settings such as the legal profession, health care, youth work, residential units, psychiatric, forensic, penal, and other institutions as a particular strategy for professional support and development. Reflective practice is a professional competency that involves consideration of the conscious use of the worker's self as a medium of interaction and change and the impact on that professional self and the work team of often demanding and disturbing work dilemmas. Harrison and Wise note that 'Human problems cannot be solved by the simple application of technical solution . . . people's problems are far too complex and messy to be resolved in this way.'[1] Working with a reflective practice group is about utilizing the therapeutic resources of the group and promoting a professional learning culture whose objective is about how to work productively as individual practitioners and as a team with sometimes difficult clients and disturbing situations. The reflective practice group is most definitely not a therapy group. It is a specialized form of team building: developing the team as a container of its own emotions and promoting its capacity to think about its own processes as a way of maintaining itself and promoting best practice.

The most recent interest and increased use of reflective practice groups has its origin in Robert Francis's report into the failings at the Mid Staffordshire NHS Foundation Trust which was published in February 2013. Since then, issues of patient safety, quality of care, and leadership have been in the public eye more than ever. Reflective practice groups are seen by nearly all professional bodies as a way of creating positive organizational cultures to enable the delivery of high-quality care and promote continuous professional development.

Unfortunately, participants and group leaders can frequently experience reflective practice as a management strategy to distract from high workload stress, low staffing rates, and financial restriction, and something that takes them away from 'real work'. There is also for many participants and facilitators an added complication of bewilderment and confusion about the purpose and aim of reflective practice groups arising from their varied experience of reflective practice and process groupwork in their own education and training. However, when reflective practice is genuinely supported by an agency and time and space are made available reflective practice groups are a rewarding means of nurturing and promoting professional learning by encouraging inquiry and engagement with one's work.

What is a reflective practice group?

First, a word about the concept of reflective practice. Reflective practice is drawn from the work of Donald Schon who emphasized the benefits of regular reflection to modify practice and promote continuous learning for those engaged in professional occupations.[2] He believed that reflective practice is a rigorous professional process involving acknowledgement and reflection on uncertainty and complexity in one's practice. Schon identified reflection-in-action when workers think about their practice while doing it and reflection-on-action which may take place after an event or encounter. These two activities are an essential part of the group worker's craft:

Reflection-in-action at the moment the event is happening in the group

- What is happening to me at the moment?
- What do I see going on in the group?
- Why can't I think right now?
- What are people feeling?
- What am I feeling?
- What happened in the group just before this?
- What is trying to emerge right now?
- What does this member/the group need now?
- What do I need now?
- What is missing/being avoided?
- How is the group using me?
- Who am I now for the group?
- What does this remind me of?
- What is the myth/story/film script/song operating here?
- Who is silent? Can they offer anything?

Reflection-on-action after the event in the group

- What exactly happened?
  - o Has it happened before?
  - o How does the event reflect the internal life of the group?
- What was not being spoken about?
- What was not being thought about?
- What was fearsome and to be avoided?
- How were members feeling?
- Why might they be feeling this?
- What might have the anger/silence/depression been about?

- What might the members have been preoccupied with/thinking about?
- Why might the group have got stuck?
- Why is this behaviour/event being repeated?
- What might the loss of creativity mean?
- Why was it difficult to share/trust/decide/work together?
- What was happening between people?
- What was not happening between people?
- What was unfinished?
- What was trying to emerge in the group?

You might wish to read Chapter 11 again to see how these two reflective activities are brought together.

These two activities form the basis and procedure for reflective practice groups which provide a regulated and boundaried forum where clinical and non-clinical staff and workers may come together regularly to discuss the emotional and professional aspects of their work. Reflective practice groups can help staff feel more supported in their jobs, allowing them the time and space to reflect on their roles and think about how they deal with unique and complex situations. Staff who attend these groups report that they feel less stressed and isolated and have increased insight and appreciation for each other's roles and responsibilities. Reflective practice also helps to promote emotional intelligence. According to Daniel Goleman, an American psychologist who was part of the early group who popularized the concept of emotional intelligence, there are five key elements to it:[3]

- Self-awareness
- Self-regulation
- Motivation
- Empathy
- Social skills

These are precisely the skills and culture that the reflective practice group endeavours to promote. Emotional intelligence is the ability to identify and manage your own emotions and the emotions of others. It utilizes skills particularly useful to the professional worker such as emotional awareness; the ability to harness emotions and apply them to tasks like thinking and problem solving; and the ability to manage emotions, which includes regulating your own emotions and empathizing with other people.

You can see how cultivating and developing emotional intelligence is a central part of any professional activity and a core part of the reflective practice group.

There is a wide range of agency settings and other services where the demands on staff are heightened because of the intense emotional stress and particular organizational nature of the work. Staff may be organized into work teams and shifts to perform specific tasks, but social and psychological factors may complicate team co-operation and productivity and threaten operational effectiveness. Staff teams can be vulnerable to and affected by a host of difficulties:

- The frightening and anxiety-making nature of working in crisis situations
- The continual maintenance of disciplined standards and vigilance
- The fear of litigation or professional reprimand
- Intense and inappropriate emotional demands of clients
- Aggressive and violent behaviour directed towards them by their clients
- Violent behaviour between clients in their care
- Death, suicide, and self-harm in clients
- Changes in team personnel
- Anxiety-making life events – illness, retirement, etc. in team
- Diverse levels of competency and ability among staff
- Rivalries and competition in team
- Diverse attitudes towards clients among staff
- Inconsistent and harmful team leadership
- Organizational pressures and demands on staff team
- Public attitudes and expectations of the staff team

The objectives of a typical reflective practice group will include:

- Sharing and talking about the communal anxiety of the staff team
- Detoxifying emotional stresses generated by client contact
- Promoting emotional intelligence
- Working through staff–client incidents and crises
- Identifying where clients are impacting on inter-team relations
- Discussing disagreements and conflicts between staff about relations with clients
- Exploring the meaning of pairings and subgroups within the team
- Examining the attitudes and feelings of staff to each other where appropriate
- Evaluating the relationship between the staff team and other teams/head office/ agency
- Promoting a culture of honest inquiry
- Identifying suitable theoretical perspectives to understand and discuss the staff dynamics and the staff–client/staff–agency interactions

Example of a reflective practice group

A reflective practice group in a residential children's home had been meeting and working well for two years. A particular session started with Michael, one of the care workers describing how recently he had been 'kidnapped' by two of the children and held in a room for an hour. He said that he was fine about it as the children weren't nasty or aggressive and he wasn't disappointed that other staff did not know that it had happened. His colleagues now apologized and spoke about their shock and feelings of inadequacy.

After a while one of the team tried to think about what the children might have been communicating in terms of their experience of being in care. While this was a legitimate intervention the facilitator decided that it was more relevant to talk about Michael's experience and being forced against his will. Michael then did begin to describe his feelings of vulnerability and impotence and his anger at being neglected by his colleagues. This led to a further discussion about the difficult boundary issues involved in engaging very troubled children who did not want to be engaged and the need for staff to soften and sometimes dilute the boundaries which could lead to inconsistency and splitting between workers and anxiety about the right way to behave towards the children. Joan described being assaulted and injured by a child and spoke about how this had led over time to good therapeutic work around remorse for damaging behaviour. The staff spoke of a variety of interactions in which children wanted to paint workers' faces, plait their hair, sprinkle staff with flour and so on. The facilitator said the group was describing play which was fun and enjoyable in the main but sometimes play got too exciting or arousing and a red card was required so things didn't descend into chaos. The facilitator went on to speak about being able to feel angry and even hate the children when play became chaotic and dangerous. This did not mean punishing or retaliating against the children but being able to acknowledge to oneself that one is experiencing painful feelings and to tolerate these emotional reactions in very disturbing situations. The staff found this a very difficult idea to embrace but after a stimulating exchange they came to see that their idea of work was activating in them an unconscious rescuer/messiah/hero complex that they couldn't live up to and which exhausted them. They were constantly being persecuted by their own ideals and left feeling inadequate and not up to the work. The team found this a very helpful discussion and subsequently reported a renewed confidence in their work.

What this example demonstrates is how the reflective practice group can work to identify the emotional stresses generated by client contact that create communal anxiety for the team and how honestly acknowledging this and not ignoring it can lead to a more satisfactory professional self-esteem and confidence. The facilitator was diligent to create emotional awareness around Michael's experience and not have it dismissed or ignored. This led to further discussion where the group was enabled to acknowledge their complicated emotions around the children and then apply them to thinking about practice development.

The aim of the reflective practice group is to offer practitioners a safe and professional space to meet with their colleagues in an environment that is both supportive and challenging. Staff are encouraged to reflect upon the impact of their practice and the work environment on their personal and professional development. They gain experience of and become more comfortable with working together in groups and can experience and reflect and learn how their work difficulties and dilemmas can become enacted in the reflective practice group.

What the reflective practice group is not

We have seen what a reflective practice group is, now let's look at what a reflective practice group most definitely is not. This is important to be aware of because frequently facilitators who are unsure of the purpose of the activity or members who are fearful of the process can allow the group to defensively drift onto more familiar ground.

It is not an experiential group

I facilitate reflective practice groups without a formal agenda and allow themes to emerge as communication in the group develops or as relational dynamics become alive in the group itself. This is not the same as in an experiential group which commonly emphasizes heightening awareness and understanding of the complexities of human relations and developing interpersonal skills and communication. Nor is it like the process groups that many professionals have experienced and had to endure in their training. The task of the reflective practice group is clear and specific. It is to encourage and enable staff to reflect upon the impact on their practice of the work environment in their personal and professional development and learn to manage the associated uncertainty, complexity, and emotional stress in an emotionally intelligent and professional way.

Reflective practice groups that have no formal agenda can be anxiety-provoking at times, particularly at the start when everyone is new to the activity. These anxieties may themselves be worth exploring in the group as they can offer important opportunities for learning about practice for participants. Staff are used to having a specified task and role in their daily work. They are used to meetings which have a structured agenda. It will take time for the group to get used to a new, informal, and unstructured way of working together. While over time most people find that the lack of restrictions characteristic of a reflective practice group provides a freedom that fosters exploration in rich and rewarding ways it is essential that the group is always tightly focused on developing a professional learning culture in which to examine members' professional practice and its impact.

It is not a therapy group

It is important that the reflective practice group is not a cognitive or objective activity but takes fully into account the emotional impact on staff of the frightening and anxiety-making nature of working in crisis situations with difficult clients, terrible suffering, trauma, and the pain of loss and death. Many professionals are trained to be emotionally detached from their clients in order to make objective judgements about care and treatment, but the intensely stressful nature of much professional activity can also result in staff emotionally retreating from their clients as a way of protecting themselves from burnout, compassion fatigue, and emotional exhaustion. The consequence can be in some cases a catastrophic loss of empathy and objectification and depersonalisation of others, as was found to be the case in the terrible Mid Staffordshire NHS Foundation Trust scandal. I consider it to be a primary function of the reflective practice group to help staff recognize that they have inevitable emotional responses to their work and their clients and that acknowledging this and learning to use these reactions is a major part of being a professional. R.D. Hinshelwood warns about 'the professional helper's nonplussed retreat into a scientific mode of understanding . . . in which our humanitarian interest is stymied'.[4] The reflective practice group provides a necessary and useful counter to this.

It is necessary to create a safe and contained space in the reflective practice group where the emotional experience of staff to their clients and each other can be presented and explored and this means that at times members will become upset, tearful, and angry. This is different from a therapy group where the basic contract is personal and extensive therapeutic change, and its central focus is on its members' psychological conflicts and interpersonal distress. The reflective practice group is most definitely not a therapy group. It is a professional learning culture that promotes emotional intelligence in the professional by recognizing the importance of permitting and reflecting on the emotional impact of practice, and helps its members tolerate difficult feelings that they would previously have dismissed and been ashamed of. This takes some getting used to for staff who are more accustomed to presenting a professional persona that appears habitually strong and competent and who are frightened of losing face in front of peers.

It is not a supervision group

Inevitably in a reflective practice group a particular case, event, or interaction in practice will become the focus of attention. It is important in these instances that the event does not become a problem to be solved or supervised. Members are used to working on a task and may find the unstructured activity of the reflective practice group difficult. They may resort to presenting cases as a way of making the group more familiar and less threatening. Of course, it is entirely legitimate that members may wish to think about how a different approach might have worked or offered other possibilities. Reviewing a situation can address ongoing problems or issues and can offer insight to improve practice in the future, but it is important that the reflective practice group does not defensively meander off into becoming a supervision group or engage in case formulations. The emphasis must be firmly maintained on the members' processes, decision making, feelings, and actions at the time of the event so as to promote staff's capacity to tolerate feelings of inadequacy, vulnerability, and uncertainty. This is much more important than trying to resolve a situation. Indeed, I would go so far as to say that you should not look for resolution in a reflective practice group but rather keep in mind the opportunities for promoting the emotional and professional well-being and practice of members.

On occasion I will offer a limited theoretical contribution that I judge may help members to make sense of a situation they have struggled with but as I have said before this is not to introduce a technical rationality but more to emphasize that experience creates reusable knowledge and that value conflicts are a central part of professional practice.

It is not a training group

A reflective practice group will invariably examine client–worker interactions and other events and seek to evaluate how things might go better in the future. This may require learning new skills and integrating new ideas into practice, but this is not the primary purpose of the reflective practice group. The aim of the reflective practice group is to offer practitioners an opportunity to meet with colleagues in an environment that is both supportive and challenging and reflect upon the impact of their practice and the work environment on their personal and professional development. Skill gaps and the need for theoretical orientation may be identified but that task is best carried out in a dedicated training session. It is your job to ensure the reflective practice group does not slide into a training group. I recall one supervision group where the facilitator was unsure of the purpose of her reflective practice group and anxious that she could hold the group to task. She did not want the group to turn into 'a whingeing match about management' so she allowed the reflective practice group to turn into a training session and actively introduced some role-play to work on a case that the group came up with. I took some time to demonstrate to her that an attack on management might be more appropriately considered in terms of the client's anger at their worker's lack of perfect care of them due to the ubiquity of restricted resources and high demand for service. The worker might then unconsciously blame management for putting them in the face of this attack and be angry with apparent management indifference to the complex and stressful nature of their work. Exploring these client–worker–agency dynamics and value conflicts is a very different activity from carrying out a training session.

Setting up the reflective practice group

There are a number of important tasks that need to be carefully considered if the reflective practice group is to operate successfully:

- Becoming aware of the need or problem
- Negotiating with the agency
- Administration of the reflective practice group
- Thinking about leadership
- The framework of the reflective practice group
- Introducing the reflective practice group to members
- The first session
- Establishing the professional learning culture of the reflective practice group
- Managing the typical problems and resistances in reflective practice groups

Becoming aware of the need or problem

The first point to consider is how the demand for the reflective practice group comes to your attention. The reflective practice group always inhabits a professional context and is continually impacted by that fact. Increasingly professional associations and bodies are promoting reflective practice and agency management is sensitive to this trend. They may decide that the provision of reflective practice is an important activity in a residential children's home or a hospital ward and is now a requirement of your job and you may be expected to facilitate a team. In many situations, an agency may view reflective practice as a response to a crisis; a staff team may be struggling with internal tensions as a consequence of inconsistent leadership or members may have been disciplined or removed from the team because of safeguarding incidents with clients and an agency representative may approach you as an outside facilitator to help rebuild confidence and institute a reflective practice dimension. The quality and depth of agency attitude and support for reflective practice is critical for the success of the group and must be a part of your decision to work with the group.

Occasionally a team itself may decide that reflective practice is an important addition to its professional life and may approach you as an outside facilitator. Considering how the demand for groupwork comes to your attention is essential because it raises some important points:

- Who makes the application?
- For whom?
- Why?
- What do they want?
- What do the beneficiaries of the reflective practice group actually need?
- Will the agency properly support the reflective practice group?

If you think for a moment you will realize that there are many people who did not originally request help but who are now receiving it and occasionally the demand for a reflective practice group represents more the needs of workers or an organization to be seen to provide certain services than it does the real needs of potential group members. This is a recurring factor in why some groups just don't work and will be explored more fully in Chapter 15.

In other circumstances people can ask for help with no real understanding of an agency's services or obligations and then staff can find themselves caught up in a reflective practice group that they are unwilling to be involved in. The point is this, by carefully and thoughtfully assessing how and why you became aware of a particular demand for a reflective practice group service you can:

- Begin to establish the motivations of yourself and colleagues to offer a reflective practice group
- Decide that there really is a need that can be met by groupwork and which justifies time, resource, and expenditure
- Gather preliminary information about the history of the group
- Make it easier for people to participate in the group
- Highlight the range and functions of agency provisions and the consequences of involvement
- Negotiate an appropriate contract with the commissioning agency to support the reflective practice group

Example of an agency request for a reflective practice group

An external facilitator was contacted by the head of a children's residential care service to provide reflective practice to a particular children's residential home. In discussion it emerged that there were interpersonal tensions between staff members as a consequence of the rigid leadership style practised by the manager of the home and which had resulted in the formation of competitive subgroups. The head of service was prepared if necessary to split up the team and redeploy members as a last resort but decided that a reflective practice group should be set up to solve the team's problems with power and authority and the team reluctantly agreed to the measure rather than be dissolved.

The external facilitator met with the team in the children's home for an initial consultation and explained what reflective practice was and agreed a contract to work for an initial six sessions and then review.

In the next session it soon became clear that there were tensions that had not been explored or talked about in a meaningful way. Susan wanted to talk about them but did not yet feel ready and did not know how to proceed. Ann adopted the position that she had never done anything like this before and didn't talk about her feelings ever. John, the only male worker, was quite articulate about the 'darkness' of working in the children's home and the impact on his personal life. The team seemed to rely on him a lot to manage the difficult interfaces with each other. Mary was a trainee care worker and gave a positive version of the team. Three other female staff and April, the team manager said nothing throughout the session.

In the following session April was absent on leave. Initially there was a lengthy silence eventually broken by John who asked the facilitator how the team could protect themselves from the stress of the work. The facilitator asked what was the work that the team needed protection from. Other members came in to describe the emotional impact of having to work with disturbed and abused children and reading files where abuse and negligence leaped off the page. After a time, Jean, who had not spoken until now, said that the work with the children was difficult but not as difficult as the 'office politics' and referred darkly to tensions and problems in the team. The facilitator said that tensions were a normal part of team life and if talked about could be understood and managed. Gradually some members spoke about feeling bullied and hurt in various ways by April. Sheila then described being in dispute with April for over two years now and was depressed that the team was fragile and no longer able to be fixed. There was some more talk about April's managerial style and Sheila said that she was uncomfortable talking in April's absence. The facilitator said that the team could think about how to tell April in the next session what they had been talking about. The facilitator then went on to speak about how the children in their care came from dysfunctional families with poor parenting and that perhaps this was being replicated unconsciously in the team. The tensions in the team and the struggles with authority might reflect the children's experience which was so awful for the staff to bear. The facilitator wondered if by unconsciously turning away from the emotional pain of the children the team had merely imported the distress into their ranks. This intervention seemed to settle the team and gave a context for understanding what their interpersonal tensions might really be about. Sheila said that she was still anxious that the team could not be fixed. The facilitator suggested that they might have to renegotiate their relationships and spoke about the importance of roles when relationships were strained.

In the next session April was present and the team started with expressions of how 'together' and 'creative' the team had been recently. Then Sheila said that she might be redeployed and began to cry. The team became flustered and tried to help her practically. The facilitator asked Sheila to talk about what redeployment meant for her. She continued to cry and asked for others to talk. After a long silence John asked the facilitator how they could help Sheila. The facilitator said that as a start the team could express their thoughts and feelings about Sheila being redeployed. Jean agreed and immediately spoke at length about Sheila's contribution and collegiality and how much she valued her. Then April the manager spoke glowingly about the high quality of Sheila's work and how in awe she had been of her. Sheila said that she valued this, and it would have been good to know this before now as she felt that April treated her differently from the others in the team and often blamed her. April said that this was not intentional and talked about a blame culture and how management was often blamed. The facilitator asked how this might occur in the group and April said that she thought the team might blame her for everything that went wrong. The facilitator asked the group if this were true and they disagreed. April then spoke about having had a complaint made about her by a past team member which was untrue but resulted in a painful investigation. She had never shared this with the team as she was ashamed and as a result had become quite distanced from the team. There were some supportive exchanges around this and the facilitator pointed out that there were now two hurt and pained team members. Some members said that they had never thought about the stress that April had been under and began to talk about how hurtful and draining their work was. After a time, the facilitator again pointed out how important it was to think about the team dynamics in terms of the difficult work they did and how it might reflect the children's experiences more than simple personality clashes.

In subsequent sessions the team was able to think more psychologically about how their own interactions with agency management and authority also mirrored the children's relationship with their parents and authority figures, and the blame culture really reflected client and worker and agency disappointment and frustration with imperfect human relations. Focusing on the client–worker–agency dynamics enabled the staff to think differently about their interactions and the pressures of the workplace. Sheila was not redeployed and remained a valued member of the team. April noticeably softened and was more involved in the team life and less separate.

What this example shows is how the agency saw reflective practice as a way of solving a difficult problem and not as an important, necessary, and ongoing part of team life. Reflective practice was really about regaining management control of a team that was struggling with disappointments around power and authority rather than creating shared responsibility for the work and practice of the team. The agency had to be seen to be doing something to respond to a crisis that was increasingly challenging organizational standards and did not understand that it was also part of the problem. Accustomed to having to split up dysfunctional families and take children into care the agency was considering splitting up the staff 'family' and putting some members into another residential home.

The team itself viewed reflective practice initially as something that was to be done to them because they were dysfunctional and were reluctant conscripts to the group. They were like the children that they worked with who had to be put into care/treatment because of their personal and family problems. The facilitator was aware of these different agendas and was at pains to present the team tensions as more than personality clashes. By re-contextualizing the interpersonal tensions as reflective of the emotionally painful nature of their work the facilitator was able to encourage the team to concentrate less on their relationships as faulty and consider the difficulties in appreciating and interacting with each other as indicative of the histories of their charges and the nature of the agency's professional task. Reflective practice was repositioned as a way of thinking about and managing staff reactions to disturbed and disturbing work demands and an ongoing feature of professional practice and team life.

Administration of the reflective practice group

Negotiating with the agency

As we have just seen the first task of importance in the administration of the reflective practice group concerns the relationship of the group to the agency, institution, or community of which it is a part. Whitaker suggests that, 'There are many settings in which it is not prudent to undertake groupwork until after one has thoroughly explored one's plans with one's colleagues.'[5] There are good reasons for this. It is important that you talk with the appropriate management level in the agency in order to determine what their view of reflective practice is and how they see it fitting in with the policies, procedures, and ethos of the organization. The members of the reflective practice group are going to leave the ward, the office, institution for a period of time on a regular and continuing basis. That means working out important logistical issues to do with cover for staff, necessary financial compensations, time in lieu and a host of other issues to do with meeting place, supervision, and debriefing time for the facilitators and so on. The agency needs to be fully aware of what is involved and genuinely signed up if reflective practice groups are to succeed and take their place in organizational culture.

One way of securing the support of senior colleagues is to demonstrate to them that the involvement of staff members in a reflective practice group can actually contribute to and enhance their work. To do this you can gather some data and published evidence about reflective practice groups in similar agencies for management to think about and talk over with you. There are organizations like the King's Fund which is an independent charity or the Point of Care Foundation who work to improve health and care and can furnish you with suitable and convincing evidence.[6]

Ensure that the general aim and the goals for your reflective practice group are compatible with agency objectives. You should identify the agency's actual operational concerns in relation to potential group members and establish what the priorities are. Try to work out the contribution your group can make to the service being offered by the agency and pinpoint where the group will enhance, back-up, or confirm the work of colleagues.

The contract with the agency will cover:

- Reflective practice groups' support for agency policies and ethos
- The agency supports reflective practice groups as a way of promoting best practice and staff care
- Agreement that reflective practice groups are an important activity for professional staff teams
- Reflective practice groups are seen as part of a permanent organizational culture
- The groups will be financially supported
- Meeting venues, time off for staff, and any other reasonable resources will be guaranteed
- Facilitators will be supported with supervision

With the genuine support and understanding of the agency you can now move to the next task of administration.

Thinking about leadership

The dilemmas thrown up by dual roles

I frequently see situations where a member of a multidisciplinary team such as a social worker or psychologist is expected to provide leadership and facilitation for their own team because they are presumed to have some technical expertise. Rarely do they see it that way and all too often they are inhibited in front of peers who know them.

These reluctant facilitators report being fearful of being seen to be incompetent or inadequate in front of peers. This is more of a dread with their professional peers than it is with their patient caseloads. They describe their fear of not being an expert with groups and are terrified of making a 'mistake' that might follow them around when they meet with peers or liaise outside the group in professional contexts. Dual roles are sometimes multiplied when facilitators are a member of the multidisciplinary team, may provide consultation and case formulation to other members, and then have to lead the reflective practice group.

Such situations often reveal the poverty of real consideration by agency management about the role of reflective practice groups in their service. Management may be going along with the trend for reflective practice in a reactive manner and not really sitting down to consider what is involved in supporting best practice. I advocate that facilitators should not be members of their own teams and should decline to act in this role. They are unable to stay separate from issues in their work teams in such a way as to facilitate reflection. They are 'contaminated' in that they are a part of the team and have their own experience and feelings about the issues discussed by their group. They may even be part of an interpersonal tension that clouds the group. As far as possible avoid acting as a facilitator for your own team. Offer to swap with another team who can then provide a facilitator for your own team. The better practice would be that heads of service would agree that a facilitator from one team would provide reflective practice for another team in the service in a reciprocal way. This means taking oversight of the needs of the whole service and intentionally deciding on the time factors, financial considerations, and other requirements to genuinely support the development of a reflective practice culture in the organization. Ideally this would take place in your discussions with your agency about the role and place of reflective practice groups in the organizational culture. A lot of confusion and bad experience in reflective practice groups would be eliminated and a mature and professional approach to practice would be instituted.

Co-facilitation

Are you going to co-facilitate the group with a colleague? Why is this? What is your rationale for this? Why are you not going to facilitate the group on your own? It is important to address these questions because often the arguments advanced for co-working are in fact based on fears about the group. The idea of mutual support offered by co-facilitation frequently masks an us/workers and them/group split. Turn back to the section on co-leading in Chapter 2 for a full exploration of the anxieties that can be hidden in the decision to co-facilitate.

Co-facilitating a group is a sophisticated practice and not one for beginners and yet surprisingly it is often where new group workers do in fact begin. Is it best for your reflective practice group to be facilitated by two new anxious workers? I would advocate that the reflective practice group is best facilitated by one person who then endeavours to make the group her co-worker. What I mean by this is that the worker explicitly adopts an attitude and demeanour which actively makes the group itself a partner in the work. The group has many more resources and capacities than one person and it is the job of the facilitator to continually activate and access these potentials. The facilitator seeks to constantly to engage the group in a developing culture of curiosity and inquiry. If, however you do decide to co-facilitate then you must ensure that:

- Both co-workers should be clear and in agreement about the purpose of the group
- Each co-worker should be clear why their agency wants them present and what the agency hopes to contribute to and get from the group project
- Each co-worker is aware of the contribution of the other, values this, and believes in it

- Each co-worker needs to be very clear about her own role and responsibility
- Both co-workers should be prepared to fully discuss the conflicts, tensions, and feelings aroused in them by joint work and group experience
- Each co-worker should be willing to permit and invite differences in perception, style, and approach as long as there is agreement about purpose
- Each co-worker needs to collaborate, share, trust, talk to the other, in and out of the group. The ability of the group to share their practice, and deal with conflict and interpersonal issues is directly related to how effective co-leaders are at this
- Co-workers must ensure that they have negotiated agency agreement that sufficient time can be set aside for preparation and debriefing and that adequate supervision of practice is available

Co-facilitation is a difficult but worthwhile collaboration when the pair are willing to be open about the problems and pitfalls involved. Recognizing the potential for rivalry between the pair, splitting of the pair by the group, the ever present shadow of inadequacy and shame between workers, fear of difference and so on, and being able to honestly discuss this will ensure that your co-facilitation of the reflective practice group is of a high standard. Chapter 2 contains a full examination of the typical problems to be found in co-leading groups.

EXAMPLE OF A CO-FACILITATED REFLECTIVE PRACTICE GROUP

A reflective practice group for trainee doctors was co-facilitated by a male social worker John and a female nurse Jane and had been meeting for the past seven monthly sessions. In this particular session it was a hot day and the small room felt unusually overcrowded. There was a long silence at the start of the session which was ended when Jane said to her co-facilitator that she felt as if the group was very full today and perhaps that made it difficult to talk. John agreed with her and said that perhaps something was baking in the mind of the group. After a few minutes one of the participants, Susan said that she felt overwhelmed by so much work that she had to do and her sense that she needed to be superhuman. She began to cry quietly. The members empathized with her and another member Mary said that she wished she could be superhuman as she felt redundant and useless much of the time. The other members gradually came in to speak about their feelings of inadequacy, being disempowered and made impotent by the demands of patients and the limitations of the service.

After a time, Jane intervened to wonder if some part of the worker self was feeling persecuted by unrealistic internal ideals colliding with an external, brutal, and sometimes deadly reality. There was a long silence and then her co-facilitator said to Jane that it seemed she had got things wrong and he wondered how she was feeling about this. Jane acknowledged to him that in a part of herself she felt useless that her intervention hadn't helped and perhaps this was how the group members often felt. At this Mary agreed and said she loved the work that she did but it was very hard and often made her feel bad. Her colleagues agreed with her and there was some discussion about how the thing that was loved could also be persecutory and brought them up against brutal limitations. Mary spoke about a consultation just yesterday in which she was not the knowledgeable medic she wished to be but could only listen to and affirm her patient. The female co-facilitator suggested that perhaps there might be something useful in the opportunities to be more limited and good enough. The group agreed that this was something to seriously think about. John then said to his co-facilitator that he thought this was an interesting suggestion and he wondered how this idea of a useful limitation might operate here in the group. Jane asked the group if they thought the facilitators were perhaps limited and not good enough.

The members then said that they had at first found it difficult that the co-facilitators did not always seem to agree with each other and sometimes disagreed but they had come to see that usually the co-facilitators were actually both right more often than not and were really emphasizing different ways to see the same thing. The group said this gave them confidence that not everything needed to be black and white. The session ended shortly after that with members leaving feeling they had really learned something about how their internal ideals could actually get in the way of more realistic work.

What this example demonstrates is a mature pair of co-facilitators who know well how to use each other to engage the reflective practice group in a more emotionally intelligent relationship with their work. The co-facilitators knew that their relationship could catch and resonate with the group's unspoken and unthought emotional preoccupations and were willing to talk to each other about their internal experience of the group with this perspective in mind. They were able to harness their emotions and apply them to tasks like thinking and problem solving for the benefit of the group. The group members were then able to internalize the co-facilitators in their mind as a more mature and less critical model of professional authority.

The framework of the reflective practice group

The reflective practice group needs to meet in a suitable place. It needs to meet regularly and predictably and securely. This is what I mean by the framework of the reflective practice group and there are serious implications to consider. If you do not pay attention to creating and protecting the framework of the group you will find all sorts of resistances developing that could and should have been avoided. On first thought the room where the group meets once booked is hardly worth mentioning but in practice it can assume a great importance. Many reflective practice groups will meet on site. This has disadvantages if the room cannot be secured and boundaried. I can think of groups which meet in a children's home and are continually interrupted by children walking in, wondering what staff are doing, looking for a particular staff member, and so on. Staff who cannot be at the group because of duties may also intrude looking for files or a telephone number. In another residential unit the group takes place in a side room of a locked ward. If an alarm sounds indicating that there is an emergency with a patient staff are obliged to leave the group room to assist colleagues. This means that staff are never fully separated from the potential anxieties of their workplace and free to reflect but are partly concentrating on what may be occurring outside the room. Another group used to meet next to the morgue in a hospital as the only available room. You can imagine how this influenced the group discussions.

In some NHS trusts it seems difficult if not impossible to secure the same room running. Reflective practice groups may have to meet in different rooms, occasionally in different locations. Inevitably there are all sorts of problems with lateness and absenteeism. So, you can see why it is important that you should think ahead about the group room and anticipate any problems. Reflective practice groups are anxiety-making enough for staff without magnifying the emotional resistances and defences to them or allowing the venue to become the medium of resistance to the group. As far as possible the group should meet off site but that can make for other problems because of increased time away from work and transport difficulties. If the group does meet on site, try to secure a room that will not allow for intrusion and will not inhibit the work of the group.

Another part of the framework of the reflective practice group has to do with the time duration and frequency of sessions. Some groups may run for an hour, but I run my groups for an hour and a half. I find that the slightly longer time allows for a deepening of communication and reflection. Many groups meet monthly and others meet every two months. The usual argument here has to do with staff shortages, work demands, and other restrictions. Whatever frequency and time you decide upon you must stick with it as the reflective practice group in particular requires predictability and consistency. Set the schedule for the year ahead so that everyone knows exactly when the group meets. There can be a temptation to vary the schedule if approached by a team leader pleading a reduced staff on a particular day. I cannot state strongly enough that you must not rearrange or cancel the session as this will inevitably become the basis of confusion and resistance. Sit in the room on your own if you have to and thereby model the importance of protecting and preserving the reflective space. Arrange your own holiday leave so as not to conflict with group meetings.

Set the length of the session and the date and stick to it as far as possible. Another complication may arise with summer arrangements for the group. I do not think it is advisable to cancel the group because of staff holidays and leave. It can be hard to start up again in the autumn if the group has not met over the summer. Even if the group meets with reduced staff this can still be interesting and different for members.

A final consideration with the time of the group meeting has to do with what comes before or after the session. Sometimes the reflective practice group meets on a day when a team has a regular meeting planned and most staff are available. If the group convenes after a team meeting there may be a tea break or lunch slot. This has important implications for the group starting on time and not having its opening period taken up with a defensive focus on food. Try to ensure sufficient space between the reflective practice group and any other activity coming before or after it otherwise you are certain to encounter resistance and intrusions into the group time.

Key elements of the framework

- Ensure that the venue and meeting room is secure
- Check for potential disruptions and intrusions into the group meeting
- Use a regular and predictable room
- Decide on a suitable length of time for the group to work in a session
- Determine the frequency of the sessions
- Create an agreed calendar in advance for group meetings
- Do not change or cancel sessions for any reason
- Consider what activities come before and after the group session

Introducing the reflective practice group to members

The prospect of a reflective practice group will probably have been mooted at a team meeting so members will know that it is going to happen. If you are the facilitator and a member of the team it is important to monitor your thoughts and feelings about the proposed group as the team know you and will clearly pick up on your attitude and it will influence their behaviour and expectations accordingly. You may be anxious about performing in front of your peers but try to remember that you really do not need to be the expert. At its simplest your task is to open and close the meeting. Make the group your co-worker and engage them in reflecting on their practice. Keep out of the way and be as curious as possible rather than trying to make interesting observations and interventions. Whether you are a member of the team appointed to facilitate the group or in the much sounder position of being an external facilitator there are some early tasks to accomplish. It can be helpful to circulate a written piece about reflective practice that covers basic information about its purpose, procedure, and benefits. Keep this concise and jargon free. It is simply to stimulate thinking and prepare the ground so that members have an idea of what they can expect. It may also be helpful to ask for a slot at a team meeting to have a brief discussion about the group and how people might use it.

- Identify the background history to the proposed reflective practice group
- Indicate the purpose, goals, and objectives for the group
- Discuss the agency perception and outcomes for the group
- Consider the issues that might be brought up in the group
- Speak about the facilitator's role
- Discuss membership, time, date, venue, duration of group, length and frequency of session
- Try to anticipate with members any possible difficulties that may arise

---

Before the first session spend time thinking about how people might view groups in general and a reflective practice group in particular. It really is important for you to keep constantly in mind that you are bringing people into a work group who may have had difficult experiences in previous groups or may have social anxieties that can make group membership uncomfortable or threatening. They are being asked to participate and get involved in a group that can stir up a whole range of anxieties and interpersonal tensions. The group is a very public space with multiple opportunities for blaming and shaming to take place and this can agitate and trigger anxieties and concerns to do with loss of face, criticism, rejection, scapegoating, competition, rivalry, envy, and a plethora of social tensions and emotions. For now, be aware that the invitation to join the group and make a commitment to attend and not to flee the threatening relationships, as previously they might have done, activates members' anxieties and sets off their typical devices for avoiding intimacy and sabotaging relationships. Have another look at Chapter 2 for a fuller discussion of this. So much of your work in the first session is to be mindful of members' anxieties and concentrate on making the experience as safe and non-threatening as possible.

The first session

> - First experience of the reflective practice group
> - Different form of contact with other members in this new group context
> - First contact with facilitator in new group context
> - Different way of sharing one's practice
> - Opportunity to reveal/expose self, behaviour, attitudes, etc.
> - An opportunity to hurt or be hurt
> - An opportunity to enjoy the new group
> - First opportunity for worker to establish climate and engage members in work

With a little reflection, you can extend this list. The important point to grasp is that the first session is the beginning of familiarization, association, and commitment by individuals to the reflective practice group ethos and culture.

Example of a first session in a reflective practice group

A single facilitator met with a hospital ward team working with children who were ill with cancer to initiate a reflective practice group. The facilitator introduced herself and stated that she was here because management had decided to invest in this reflective practice group, recognizing it as a positive way of promoting staff care and professional development and learning. The agency was committed to ensuring that the group had the necessary time and resources to enable staff to use the opportunity. She then asked the various staff to introduce themselves and describe their jobs and roles on the ward. It became apparent that the staff team comprised a variety of different professional disciplines. The facilitator then offered a preliminary working definition of reflective practice which stated that in her experience the aim of the reflective practice group was to offer practitioners a safe and professional space to meet with their colleagues in an environment that was both supportive and challenging. Staff could use the group to reflect upon the impact of their practice and the work environment on their personal and professional development.

The facilitator then asked the participants about their experience and understanding of reflective practice. A number of staff warily described being familiar with keeping reflective journals from their training. Some staff said these journals were also used as evidence of competent practice. The facilitator immediately recognized that members might be anxious about the reflective group being used by the agency management for purposes of monitoring and surveillance and moved to address this fear. She said that the reflective practice group was not a form of accountability and no record would be kept or information about the group discussion shared with anyone. She also stated that no one would be asked to keep a journal or do 'homework' but that what she had in mind was a more collaborative and shared practice. This had the effect of lightening the mood and members continued to discuss what they thought reflective practice might offer. Their contributions still focused on a more cognitive and skills-based approach so the facilitator wondered how the reflective practice group might be different from just thinking about practice.

Some staff then began to describe their emotional reactions to working with very ill and dying children and how it was hard to switch off after an emotionally gruelling shift. They described how impossible it would be to do the work if they didn't support each other informally during the working time. The facilitator acknowledged that the group could also be very helpful in creating a safe space in which staff could share their painful experiences and think about the personal and professional impact of this terrible work on their capacity for empathy and compassion as an example. Some staff expressed anxiety about breaking down in the group and the facilitator stated that feelings of vulnerability, sadness, and inadequacy were inevitable in their work and were signs of a healthy professional and not in any way evidence that the carer was unsuitable for the work. She emphasized that the reflective practice group was not a therapy group and again restated the premise of the reflective practice group as a safe place to reflect upon the impact of their practice and the work environment on their personal and professional development. She said that the group was for reflection and support and was not a place for interrogation, shaming, or blaming. She then asked the participants what they might need to make the group a safe place. After some more discussion which drew up a varied list of requirements the facilitator suggested that it would be helpful to make a group contract to include these requests and delineate what members could expect from the group and each other. They quickly agreed a contract that covered a now mutually agreed purpose and agenda for the group, times and frequency of meetings, and expectations of and commitments to each other. The purpose of the group explicitly ruled that the reflective practice group was not a vehicle for therapy, supervision, or training and positively focused on the building and development of a professional learning culture for the ward team. The contract also made provision for participants to alter the direction of group exchanges if they did not like or agree with what was happening or if the group strayed from its task, thus engaging the group in its own authority.

The facilitator now directly asked the team for the first time what it was like to work on the ward and members began to describe their jobs and responsibilities and their work with sick children and their distressed families. They spoke about a child who had suddenly died on the ward recently and movingly described their sorrow and loss and sense of helplessness. The facilitator sympathetically listened and did not try to reassure or make things better but simply allowed the team to talk about this recent harrowing event. The team seemed relieved to be able to talk openly about how this had affected them and how they tried to be strong and carry on for the sake of the ward and the other children and families. Some members were off duty when this child had died and while they too were affected they had a little more emotional distance to support and witness those who had been present at the time.

At an appropriate point the facilitator indicated that the group would have to stop and suggested that the members take turns to check out and say how they had found the session and what they had learned about reflective practice and what they were taking away. Each member summarized their experience and expressed relief that the group was not the fearful and potentially shaming thing they had anticipated but actually had been very surprising and helpful. They eagerly agreed to meet again the following month.

This example illustrates a number of important points:

- The facilitator carefully anticipated participants' fears about shame, exposure, being monitored and looked to address them early in the group
- She set the scene by giving agency sanction and commitment for the group thus locating it in a professional context and normalizing the enterprise

- She offered her own vision of the group without imposing it on members as a means of introducing possibilities for the group
- She then invited participants' views of reflective practice and shaped and deepened them into a mutually agreeable purpose
- She looked to the participants to determine their safety in the group and set boundaries and limitations
- She negotiated a mutually agreed contract for work
- She entered into a first experience of how the group might work
- She instituted a checkout procedure that enabled members to psychologically exit from the group and re-enter the workplace
- She managed the time boundaries to set the culture of the group and demonstrate containment

Establishing the professional learning culture of the reflective practice group

A group culture builds over time and describes the characteristic attitudes, norms and behaviours, values, ideas, and customs that prevail in the group. New members joining the group quickly adapt to the established culture but of course they can also modify it with the new and different experience they bring in. This helps avoid conformity and the phenomenon of 'groupthink'. Establishing and developing a culture in the reflective practice group is an important task because it will shape and affirm the activities, procedures, and work of the group. The culture that you want to inculcate in the group involves privileging certain values and activities. Cultivating and developing emotional intelligence is a central part of any professional activity and a core part of the reflective practice group and so it is a primary function of the reflective practice group to help staff recognize that they have inevitable emotional responses to their work and their clients and that acknowledging this and learning to use these reactions is a major part of being a professional.

In the course of interacting with each other to achieve the goals of the reflective practice group members will gradually develop a value system which refers to beliefs about which activities and behaviours are good and bad, desirable and undesirable. In a reflective practice group values will emerge which will include an emphasis on thoughtfulness, inquiry, honesty, tolerance of emotional reactions to the work, trust, confidentiality, caring, and respect, among many others. The values of the group will reflect its goals and purposes and play an important and often decisive part in determining individual behaviour. So, it is important that you give some thought as to what sort of values you want to promote in the group. It is also a good idea to discuss this with the group.

In order to ensure that members behave in accordance with agreed group values and goals, certain rules or norms will become established which prescribe those actions in particular circumstances which are correct and proper, and those behaviours which are improper. Norms are values expressed in behavioural terms. The acceptance of norms by members depends upon their appropriateness to individual and group concerns, the cohesiveness of the group, and the nature of norm enforcement.

Norms are enforced by sanctions which will require or persuade individuals to conform to group values and beliefs. These sanctions will punish members who fail to conform to group norms or reward them if they do so adequately. The group's impulse to create norms and behavioural controls can be of great benefit to you when working with the group. Most beginning workers seek to establish personal control over the group fairly early on. They fail to realize that the most effective means of control within any group is that based on establishing norms of behaviour which are acceptable to all and identifying and using those norms which already exist. By trying to develop and make satisfying and rewarding existent norms, you will find that you are likely to be more successful than trying to control the group externally.

Here are some values and norms that you might want to discuss with the group and promote:

- Reflective practice is a professional activity and an essential part of continuing professional development
- Individuals and group can reflect on practice and the work environment
- Promoting curiosity
- Promoting enquiry
- Cultivating emotional intelligence and learning how to tolerate and manage difficult feelings
- Harnessing emotions to think and problem solve
- Respect for silence as a means of gathering thoughts
- Developing empathy
- Encouraging team collaboration and co-operation
- Constant monitoring of the interactional synchrony of team dynamics and agency and client contact

Managing the typical problems and resistances in reflective practice groups

Reluctant conscripts

Probably the first difficulty you will encounter is a group of staff who have been told by their management to turn up in a room at a particular time for a reflective practice group. They are reluctant conscripts! In the worst case there has been some crisis in the unit and someone on high has decided that a reflective practice group is the answer. In the minds of staff, you and the group may be conjoined as a rebuke for their incompetence or inadequacy. The staff may feel shamed and resentful at being obliged to attend and be unwilling to engage with the group task. Look for any opportunity to address this early.

I recall a first session in one group where staff straggled into the session in twos and threes over a period of 30 minutes. I commented on this as staff showing me how little control they had over their schedules and how random and unpredictable their work was. They were surprised at this and agreed with me. I was then able to wonder about their motivation to attend this group and the members grumbled that it was an additional stress on an under-staffed team. I suggested that it could be a support rather than a stress. It would only be a stress if they got nothing out of the group or it didn't work. I pointed out that the agency had allocated the time for the reflective practice group in the knowledge that the team was under pressure and in the belief that this resource could help staff think about and protect their practice in a stressful work environment. I asked members what they might like to get out of this time since it had been made available. Since there was not much response to this I reflected that the staff were somewhat in the position of their clients who were obliged to interact with them reluctantly and staff might be experiencing some of the feelings they had to contend with in clients who didn't wish to engage with their agency service. This parallel resonated with the team and evoked their interest. It stimulated the team to talk about the difficulties they regularly encountered with resistant and ambivalent clients. After a more enthusiastic discussion ensued I asked the members if it might be helpful to have this time and space to reflect on how their practice threw up all sorts of similar complex and difficult issues for them and if the group could be used as a place to talk about and look for support in dealing with the uncertain and disturbing situations they faced on a regular basis. There was a very different and more positive response from members now and a recognition that their work was demanding of them personally and professionally. We were now able to talk about their willingness to take responsibility for the quality of the mandated reflective group experience rather than simply passively and compliantly attending the session. The staff members shared their understanding of what the reflective practice group might mean and what it might offer them. We concluded the session by negotiating a contract that gave them power over the purpose and task of the group.

You can see from this vignette that it is important with reluctant conscripts to acknowledge and address their resentment if it is not to become a real impediment. You do yourself and the group no favours at all to ignore it and simply postpone the eventual reckoning because it will manifest in lateness, absenteeism, and superficial conversations. Locate members' resentment in a parallel with their experience of worker-client dynamics and they will recognize this and be professionally stimulated. From here you can go on to engage their will by showing them how they have full power to make this a helpful experience or a dull and inert obligation.

Fluctuating membership

Many work settings such as residential homes and ward environments have to operate 24/7 shift patterns of work and this has an important consequence for the reflective practice group. It usually means that the group is unable to host a regular returning membership and the group has a more open and changeable quality to its operation. Participants may only be able to attend every other group session at best or only one in three or four sessions at worst. Night staff must be highly motivated to attend reflective sessions held in the day time. The constant modification of group culture inevitably makes the group less stable and more unpredictable. This can result in less depth and intimacy in reflection and discussion because the membership fluctuates over time and the group is inhibited in its ability to predict how other members will respond to each other in this new situation. There is more of a tendency to form subgroups, cliques, and alliances based on status, hierarchy, and shift colleagues. These subgroups often coalesce around boundaries which demarcate the qualified and unqualified staff. Among the qualified staff further subgrouping may occur as similar ranks and grades seek each other out. The subgroups will usually physically congregate together. The result is that the group is harder to balance and integrate. It is important to discuss this with the group and endeavour to acknowledge and utilize the differences rather than ignore them or attempt to work around them. As facilitator you might try to promote the advantages of the greater variety of experience, resource, and skill to give a more accurate and plural perspective on the team's work and challenges. This can be greatly helpful as different disciplines and ranks get to hear about each other's difficulties and work dilemmas. It may also highlight envious and rivalrous feelings between unqualified staff who often have more hands-on responsibilities and interactions with clients than qualified staff who may have more accountability and governance responsibilities and who complain about the mountains of paperwork and administrative tasks. Learning about each other's onerous responsibilities and challenges can dissolve misunderstandings and assumptions and foster a more shared sense of the collaborative nature of the team's work.

The fluctuating membership may be more preoccupied with issues to do with change and adaptability than other reflective practice groups who have a regular membership. Again, as facilitator your job is to utilize this by highlighting how the fluctuating membership can give good insights into initiating and terminating relationships with clients and perspectives on inclusion, separation, and termination as staff come and go that can be valuable in understanding some of the dynamics of client work.

A difficulty with fluctuating membership in a reflective practice group is that unqualified staff are more likely to be rostered to attend than qualified staff and this has important implications for your facilitation style. Because unqualified staff are unlikely to have previously experienced anything like reflective practice the more usual pauses and silences found in the unstructured session can be extremely off-putting and stressful for them. It is not helpful to leave them to make something of the encounter as you might with qualified and more experienced staff. You will find that it is best to ditch the non-directive style in favour of something more conversational in which you try to engage staff in exploring and thinking about their work. This more Socratic method involves questioning staff in a systematic and calibrated manner while trying to develop and concentrate on basic concepts, values, principles, issues, or problems in their practice. Starting from a spontaneous discussion you can ask a series of questions in order to help staff

- Explore the origin of their thinking
- Identify and separate fantasy and rumour from reality
- Clarify their thinking
- Challenge assumptions
- Consider alternative viewpoints
- Reflect on implications and consequences
- Think about value conflicts and dilemmas
- Discuss basic concepts and principles
- Model the reflective and questioning strategies
- Enjoy practice opportunities to improve their reflective capacities

Perhaps the best response you can have with these more fluid groups is to take a very long-term view. This means thinking more about embedding the idea of reflective practice sessions as a regular and ongoing part of the team's life rather than worrying overly about the undoubted challenge of the fluctuating membership. It is important to acknowledge your frustration, but it is more important that you consciously choose to embody the value of reflective practice and demonstrate your commitment to it. That means getting along to every session irrespective of low or volatile numbers and despite the team leader's offer to cancel so that you can make better use of your time because there are only one or two staff available! The team is permanent. The reflective practice group is a part of the team's life. Staff come and go, transfer to other positions, go on holiday, retire, and so on. The best that you can do is to attend each designated session, thereby embedding reflective practice as part of the team's life so that over time the expectation is built up that whatever staff are available will attend and use the reflective practice group experience.

Management bashing

A recurring fear for team leaders and the agency is that the reflective practice group simply becomes a moaning session where staff ventilate their frustrations and resentments about their management. As a consequence team leaders tend to absent themselves from the group under the guise of creating a free space for staff to talk without fear of censure or retaliation. Such a situation is based on a misunderstanding of reflective practice. We have asserted that reflective practice is a professional strategy for thinking about and managing staff reactions to disturbed and disturbing work demands and should be an ongoing feature of professional practice and team life. Thus, interpersonal tensions in the teams or problems with authority should as equally be seen as reflective of the emotionally painful nature of their work with clients as limitations or perceived machinations on the part of management. The facilitator must be able to encourage the team to concentrate less on their relationships with each other and with management as faulty and inadequate and consider the difficulties in appreciating and interacting with each other as also indicative of the disturbing demands of client work and the nature of the agency's professional task. Rather than simply permit a session of management bashing your job as facilitator is to inquire a bit more deeply into staff frustration with authority and perceive if there is a psychological resonance for staff with their clients and patients that might be fruitfully explored. The idea here is that staff will sometimes respond and relate to management as an unhelpful or negligent parental authority just as they might be seen by their clients as indifferent or incompetent helpers. The powerful emotions aroused in these client–staff relationships can become conflated and entangled with staff–management dynamics and relationships and need to be unpicked and thought about. This raises awareness of the limitations of the helping relationship and agency responsibilities and may be uncomfortable in itself for those concerned but it is a more mature position than simply blaming each other for a lack of perfect care and limitless attention. Where staff–management relationships are inadequate then they do need genuine consideration but at an appropriate point these dynamics can be suitably repositioned to consider ongoing staff–client interactions.

Fear of being shamed or blamed in the reflective practice group

A major task for the facilitator has to do with managing participants' fear of being blamed or shamed in the reflective practice group. It is part of everyone's social conditioning starting in the family and continuing through school, one's peer group, workplace, and so on. It has its roots in one of the oldest forms of social control and is at the emotional centre of the scapegoat phenomenon (see page 203). The very public nature of the group means that members fear loss of face and demotion of status and prestige and so they will go to great lengths to protect their professional and social standing and self-esteem. The nature of the reflective practice group means that each member's professional practice is on display at some point. This can be extremely anxiety-making and participants are alert to criticism and depreciation from the facilitator and peers and so are sensitive to the possibility of being made out to be in the wrong or somehow mocked and made to feel contemptible.

Based on their sometimes negative previous experiences of training and supervision members may fear joining the reflective practice group and they may voice their concerns about being found out or stripped bare by the others. This often takes the form of an explicit fear of 'breakdown' and being vulnerable. Many professionals pride themselves on their capacity to 'just get on with it' in the face of disturbing client interactions and fear displaying anything that might possibly reveal them to peers as incompetent or inadequate. Most professionals have a great deal of their self-image and worth bound up in their work and so they may also fear that exploring their emotional reactions to their work could reveal personal material about themselves that could lead to them being found wanting or stigmatized in some way. They are afraid of something being discovered or revealed about them that could lead to being shamed or rejected and may worry about the consequent damage to their self-esteem. Deeper feelings of being unloveable or unworthy may surface at this time and it is vital to take time and explore and soothe these fears if possible. The anxiety to do with somehow being unacceptable and the dread of rejection are at the basis of much initial resistance to exploring any emotional dimension of the work setting in the group. Voluntarily making oneself vulnerable to the reaction and control of others can be a terrifying and extremely off-putting fantasy.

The best way of dealing with these core anxieties is to remind the worried members that everyone else is in the same situation and that getting to know other people's professional struggles and how they respond to the emotional demands of the work is going to take time, and until they feel comfortable they should not take unnecessary risks. It is important to emphasize the generally supportive nature of groups and highlight the benefits of belonging to a group whose members takes seriously their responsibility and obligation to one another. Be clear with the members that if anything like their fear of being blamed or shamed or rejected occurs that you will support them and require the group to explore what is going on and not just behave according to the member's past experience. Point out how important these opportunities are for personal and professional growth and development and that you will protect such possibilities to the best of your ability. By showing willingness to take seriously the members' fears you can encourage an emotional bonding that can be helpful for them in the early stages of the group's life, and you will find that as the members grow in confidence with the group they will naturally reduce their dependence on you.

Fear of vulnerability or breaking down in the reflective practice group

As we have already seen many professionals have a great deal of their self-image and worth bound up in their work and so they may fear that exploring their emotional reactions to their work could reveal something about themselves that could lead to them being seen as inadequate or wanting in some way. Members of the reflective practice group may keep a tight rein on their feelings because they are afraid things will get out of control or because they see expression of feeling as weak and immature or unprofessional. These members do not trust feelings and try to avoid them either by consciously suppressing or unconsciously repressing them. However, unwanted feelings do not just disappear. They continue to try to enter awareness and behaviour directly or covertly and they often encounter more opposition. The result may be an unhealthy group with a flat, dead feel, or a tense, anxious group may be poorly or inappropriately expressed. Difficult or irrational feelings do not go away by being censored or denied. They go away by being recognized, accepted, and worked through so an important part of your facilitation involves helping staff recognize that experiencing feelings and emotions is an integral part of being human and professional. No one has to apologize for having feelings. It is really how we act and behave around our feelings that makes them negative or positive, and a core competency of being a professional is developing emotional intelligence. A particular and recurring task of your facilitation involves cultivating and developing emotional intelligence as a central part of any professional activity and a core part of the reflective practice group.

There is always some risk for members expressing feelings in the group because they can never be sure how others will react. However, if you have encouraged people to be more aware and accepting of their feelings you have reduced much of the risk and unpredictability and members will be more likely to express their feelings in an appropriate fashion. In some ways feelings are the common denominator between people in a group setting. Unconsciously each member is preoccupied with feeling states: wanting to feel happy, good, approved of, and well-regarded; feeling bad or rejected and wanting to change that. Much of the colour, diversity, and richness of group life is provided by the feeling tone of members' interactions. Try and encourage staff to become more comfortable with feelings by emphasizing the importance of expressivity in determining the quality of group experience and helping them learn how to deal with difficult and emotional client encounters. Remind members that behind every feeling, conflict, and disturbance is an unfulfilled need that the person is trying to meet through her emotional responses and behaviour. This is not only important for the individual but has major consequences for the reflective practice group. It is in the group's interest to allow and respond to the feelings of its members. If the group and the person can become conscious of what is really needed when angry, depressed, or tearful then they can consider options and make choices to meet the need, which will be more constructive and will enhance group and personal experience. If someone does become emotional don't leave them exposed or alone. Create bridges to other members by asking if others have ever felt like this. In this way you can promote togetherness and solidarity. Always keep the work context in mind and point out the inevitable emotional reactions generated by uncertain and often disturbing work scenarios. Consistently remind staff that this is a reflective practice group and not a therapy group.

Working with the unrealistic worker self-image

Since most professionals have a great deal of their self-image and worth bound up in their work it is a consequence that many staff have an inflated professional self-image of how they should operate and what they can do which has severe and damaging repercussions for them. A great deal of the work in a reflective practice group inevitably centres upon exploring this sensitive subject. In Chapter 8 we saw three characteristics of this over-blown professional self-image:

- The wish to be all powerful – omnipotence
- The wish to be all knowing – omniscience
- The wish to be all loving – benevolence

From what was said earlier we might identify the other dimension of the worker self as a devalued and reduced professional self-image characterized by:

- The dread of helplessness – impotence
- The dread of confusion and not knowing – incompetence
- The dread of anger and hatred – malevolence

You can see how professionals can find themselves in demanding work situations where they become unconsciously persecuted by their own impossible ideals. Look again at the example of the reflective practice group on page 268 to see how this happens and how you can facilitate staff to explore this.

Modifying a grandiose professional self-image and replacing it with a realistic worker self is an ongoing and essential task of the reflective practice group. It requires a willingness and courage in members to engage in self-examination and a desire to cultivate reflective qualities and attributes that will serve the work and not just one's own need to protect oneself from the emotional rigours of the work. It is equally a delicate and central task for the group facilitator who must be vigilant for the scenarios and narratives which indicate that staff are struggling because of inflated demands on themselves or overly self-critical and harsh judgements about their work. It is important to grasp and explore these scenarios early in the group life in order that it becomes a normal and unexceptional feature of reflective practice for group members. The facilitator must endeavour to reflect and mirror back members' own capacities and individuality with compassion and understanding whilst encouraging and promoting the idea that staff are frequently making inappropriate and impossible demands of themselves.

Food as a resistance in the reflective practice group

Eating food in reflective practice groups is a commonly reported behaviour by facilitators that also *eats up valuable time*. Sometimes the group is arranged on a day when a team has a regular meeting planned and most staff are available. If the group convenes after a team meeting there may be a tea break or lunch slot. This has important implications for the group starting on time and not having its opening period taken up with a defensive focus on food. A group may easily spend 20 minutes of a one hour or one and a half hour reflective session on its lunch and casual conversation if you do not take charge of this important boundary. Another group can suggest that the cake and buns are a way of affirming the team and doing something nice together.

Remind the participants that this is a work group and wonder with them if they have anxieties that the reflective practice group may not be nourishing enough or cannot nurture them. Make the eating behaviour into a psychological communication about the sort of meal that might be served up in the reflective practice group from the members that can be thought about and talked about. Are they afraid that the group might be sour or not sweet enough? Might it be hard to stomach or digest? Will it be lean fare or a strange diet? The important thing is to take the eating behaviour seriously as a communication and potential resistance and not simply and passively accept it. Offer the behaviour to the group to talk about and share as food for thought.

Try to ensure sufficient space between the reflective practice group and any other activity coming before or after it otherwise you are certain to encounter resistance and intrusions into the group time.

Power and authority issues in the reflective practice group

An important consideration for the facilitator involves the presence of the team leader. Some reflective practice groups do not include the team leader for a variety of reasons, the most common being the idea that this will make for a freer experience for the team members. I do not consider this to be a valid rationale. Not surprisingly this often comes from a team leader who may be anxious that staff will use the opportunity to blame or criticize management style and authority. Sometimes staff will wish the team leader to absent themselves for fear of losing perks or being retaliated against in some way if they raise issues about management. The reflective practice group should have as far as possible all the relevant members present and the nature and operation of power and authority in the team can then be fully and properly explored.

In the usual staff team, power and authority manifests in a pyramidical structure with tops, middles, and bottoms in order for the task of the team to be carried out. In the reflective practice group, the participants work together in a circular model in which each member is equally responsible for the purpose of the group which is reflection about the impact of the client work and agency environment on their personal and professional practice. The team leader and staff members are all co-equal and responsible for this process and the manifestations and dynamics of power and authority can be reflected upon by all. The usual power hierarchies and leadership roles are temporarily suspended in order for their effect to be thought about. It is important for you as facilitator to have this distinction in your mind at all times. In its daily activity the staff team has traditional leadership functions and responsibilities while in the reflective practice group the task of the group is to reflect upon how power and authority issues may reflect worker–client dynamics and agency–worker–client difficulties and misunderstandings.

As facilitator much of your understanding and handling of criticism of the agency or management might be more appropriately considered, for example, in terms of the client's anger at their worker's lack of perfect care of them due to the ubiquity of restricted resources and high demand for service. In a parallel process the worker might then unconsciously blame management for putting them in the face of this attack and be angry with apparent management indifference to the complex and stressful nature of their work. Staff management may react to this criticism defensively thereby getting caught in a spiral of discontent and reaction. Exploring these client–worker–agency dynamics and power and authority conflicts is an essential part of the reflective practice group. It is vital for the relevant staff authorities to be present. The team leader is not there to be attacked or to defend herself but to be part of a collaborative process in which all members can reflect on how their power interactions and differentials catch and reflect their relationships with clients and the agency.

Another manifestation of how power and authority can impact on the group is frequently found in a recurring fear on the part of the facilitator that they might harm the group. This usually manifests as the facilitator's fear that too much silence will be painful for the group to bear and so she may be more active than needed in order to protect the members. The facilitator may be anxious that undue silence will disturb participants and cause them to avoid or abstain from the group. It is not an unreasonable fear as staff are used to having a specified task and role in their daily work. They are used to meetings which have a structured agenda, and group meetings that have no formal agenda can be anxiety-provoking at times particularly at the start when everyone is new to the activity. The facilitator can internally dread the painful silences but really might be better to consider this experience and think about how she could use this for the benefit of the group. She could remind the group that the task is to reflect and reflection means getting used to pauses and silences as a means of gathering and collecting one's thoughts. The facilitator has authority and power to run the group in a particular manner and must accept that allowing silences is a part of the process and not something that they are imposing needlessly on the group. Professional staff are usually very active and busy people with little time to pause and think about their work. Many in fact prefer this. As a consequence, silences can bring back disturbing feelings about client encounters and members may wish to remain busy rather that consider these occasions and the emotional responses triggered. The facilitator might remember this and reflect on their fear that they are harming the group by re-contextualizing this anxiety for the group as an unwillingness to return to difficult and painful experiences that might rise up in the silence. Rather than accept that they are doing something unpleasant to participants the facilitator might also consider the possibility that a parallel might be occurring in which staff are unconsciously re-enacting a scenario in which clients might feel coerced in some way by staff. These anxieties are worth exploring in the group as they can offer important opportunities for learning about practice for participants. It will take time for the group to get used to a new, informal, and unstructured way of working together and the facilitator must not be afraid of her authority to run the group as she thinks best.

Conclusion

The aim of the reflective practice group is to offer practitioners a safe and professional space to meet with their colleagues in an environment that is both supportive and challenging. Staff are encouraged to reflect upon the impact of their practice and the work environment on their personal and professional development. They gain experience of and become more comfortable with working together in groups and can experience and reflect and learn how their work difficulties and dilemmas can become enacted in the reflective practice group. At its best the reflective practice group is a way of thinking about and managing staff reactions to disturbed and disturbing work situations and an ongoing feature of professional practice and team life that promotes emotional intelligence as a core professional competency. Setting up and running a reflective practice groups makes many demands on a facilitator and it is necessary to spend time thinking about the complex issues that have to be confronted in the group. The particular difficulties of the reflective practice group involve a careful and ongoing attention to the dynamic administration of the group – who to involve; possible membership problems due to shift systems; establishing a professional learning culture; relations with agency, facilitator roles; and learning to manage the inevitable anxieties and resistances created for staff by working in a different and unfamiliar group setting.

The psychological tasks of running a reflective practice group are immense and require an understanding of how to place team conflicts in the context of worker–client–agency interaction.

Review

- The reflective practice group utilizes the resources of the group to promote a professional learning culture whose objective is to think about how to work productively as individual practitioners and as a team with sometimes difficult clients and disturbing situations
- It constantly monitors the interactional synchrony of team dynamics and agency and client contact
- It promotes emotional intelligence as a professional competency
- It is not a therapy group
- It is not a supervision group
- It is not a training group
- When setting up the reflective practice group consider how you became aware of the need
- Negotiate with the agency
- Consider whether to work solo or with a co-facilitator
- Establish a framework for the reflective practice group
- Think about the first session
- Establish the professional learning culture
- Consider the typical problems and resistances that might occur

References

1 Harrison, R. and Wise, C. (2005) *Working with Young People*, London: Sage, p. 196.
2 Schon, D.A. (1983) *The Reflective Practitioner: How Professionals Think in Action*, London: Temple Smith.
3 Goleman, D. (1996) *Emotional Intelligence: Why It Can Matter More Than I.Q.*, London: Bloomsbury.
4 Hinshelwood, R.D. (1999) 'The difficult patient', *British Journal of Psychiatry*, 174:189.
5 Whitaker, D.S. (1976) 'Some conditions for effective work in groups', *British Journal of Social Work*, 5, 4: 249.
6 See Kingsfund.org.uk and also pointofcarefoundation.org.uk

Chapter 15

Setting up and running a supervisory group

There are many settings such as residential institutions, therapeutic communities, day centres, hospital, clinic, and social work departments where groupwork is a major method of service delivery or there are a number of workers running a variety of groups. These workers may be required to attend a supervisory group or it may be that a more experienced worker is called upon to offer guidance and assistance to less experienced workers. Initiating and running a group to help two or a number of group workers think about their work and develop their skills can appear to be a daunting task, so in this chapter I want to put forward a model for group supervision which presents the essential elements and tasks of the supervisory process.

In Chapter 17 I will distinguish between the consultant as one who is voluntarily sought out by an individual group worker to help support and develop practice and the supervisor who has some responsibility for overseeing the worker's practice. What I have in mind in this chapter is a form of group supervision where two or more group workers meet regularly with a designated supervisor for an hour or more to consider and share the dynamics and dilemmas generated by their work.

Different features and qualities of supervision in individual and group settings

Individual setting	Group setting
Personal and undivided attention	Team sharing, multiplicity of feedback, ideas, experiences
Lack of peer rivalry and competition	Peer rivalry can be used to reflect dynamics of work group
Greater transparency and disclosure	Issues of trust, fear of shame, blame, competence, exhibitionism may be amplified and require attention but can be used in relation to the work group
Identification with supervisor	Opportunities for multiple identifications and mirroring by peers
Individual transference to supervisor	Multiple peer transferences
Limited perspectives	More creativity and capacity to tackle complex problems and learn about groups in a group setting; ethnic and cultural diversity in group can generate a wider cross-cultural perspective

You can see from this that individual supervision provides undiluted personal attention, support, and intimacy and eliminates the anxieties and vulnerabilities to do with exposing one's work to the scrutiny of others. On the other hand the group supervision setting provides an unparalleled opportunity to learn about working with groups by consciously working in a group with all the complexity and creativity the collective offers. For the group supervisor, running a supervision group is just like working with any other group with the added tasks of teaching the method and monitoring practitioners' progress.

Different types of group supervision

Brigid Proctor has identified a spectrum of types of group supervision that may interest and appeal to a variety of participants.[1] She does not see types of group supervision as hierarchical or one as better than another. Different supervisees may prefer one type of supervision group at different times and according to their experience and interests. I have included her typology with a slight tweak of my own.

- *Type 1 Authoritative group supervision:*   Supervision *in* a group

  o   The supervisor is an expert and the group is more like a master class. The supervisor works with each member in turn and manages the group.

- *Type 2 Participative group supervision:*   Supervision *with* the group

  o   The supervisor is responsible for supervising and managing the group. Participants are expected to act as co-supervisees.

- *Type 3 Co-operative group supervision:*   Supervision *by* the group

  o   The supervisor is a group facilitator and supervision monitor who agrees with the participants that they will actively co-supervise and develop a supervising group.

- *Type 4 Peer group supervision:*   Supervision *as* a group

  o   There is no designated person responsible for supervision but a group of colleagues or peers come together to take shared responsibility for supervising each other and being supervised.

While Proctor does not see these types of supervision groups as hierarchical, my own sense is that they probably do reflect most practitioners' professional journey as they gain in experience and move from being supervised by an expert to joining with a peer group of seasoned colleagues. Of course, experienced professionals can also enjoy periodic involvement with a type 1 supervision group, say at a conference, and peer groups do not have to be made up of greybeards to be useful! The emphasis in this chapter will be on the type of group supervision in which an individual is designated as the responsible supervisor even though they may not see themselves in any way as an expert.

The environment in which group supervision takes place

When thinking about setting up or taking on an existing supervision group it is important to consider the implications and consequences of the context in which the work will take place. A training context for example may require supervision to adhere to a particular theoretical orientation or groupwork model and will be different from, say, a supervision group made up of social workers running a variety of community based work groups and who might be less preoccupied with the specifics of theory. Some environments are group friendly whilst others are less so; do try to think about the institutional culture and consider what impact it is likely to make on your supervisees' work groups and on your supervision group.

Becoming aware of the need

The first point to consider is *how the demand* for group supervision *comes to your attention.* Is it a *request* from an already existing group for help? Consider why the previous supervisor has left and what this may mean for you taking over the existing group. You may find that there are criticisms of the previous supervisor or that the individual was highly esteemed. This might mean that the group or a sponsoring agency may have certain expectations of you which you need to think about and possibly discuss with members if you are not to find yourself being unhelpfully compared with or even unnecessarily competing with the previous incumbent.

Perhaps the provision of group supervision is a *requirement* of your job. You may be expected to manage the quality of a groupwork service, ensure accountability, and promote the professional development of your staff or trainees. Is the idea of group supervision a *response* on your part to emerging worker needs or recognized themes in team, office, agency workload? Considering how the demand for group supervision comes to your attention and the environment in which it is to occur is important because it raises some fundamental points and helps you focus and tune in:

- Who makes the application?
- For whom?
- Why?
- What do they want?
- What do the beneficiaries of the group supervision actually need?
- What are the expectations of an agency or training team or department?

By carefully and thoughtfully assessing how and why you became aware of a particular demand for group supervision you can:

- Begin to establish the motivations of yourself and colleagues to offer group supervision
- Decide that there really is a need that can be met by group supervision and which justifies time, resource, and expenditure

- Gather preliminary information about possible goals and tasks for the supervision group
- Make it easier for people to participate
- Highlight the range and functions of agency provisions and the consequences of involvement
- Anticipate potential dynamics and problems in the supervision group

Different contexts for group supervision will make different demands on the supervisor and the group but I think that the three key elements to consider are:

- Accountability
- Recording
- Evaluation and reporting on supervisees

If you are providing group supervision for an agency or are part of a training team teaching groupwork methods these responsibilities will be a primary task for you as a supervisor. On the other hand the increasing requirements of accreditation to professional bodies means that group workers may seek out, on a voluntary basis, membership of a supervisory group to refine and develop their professional skills, and you may find that these responsibilities while still present are far less demanding.

Accountability of the group supervisor

Much of this will have been worked out when the leader examines the requirements of the context in which group supervision occurs. Some of the important issues to be clarified here are:

- To whom is the group supervisor accountable?
- What are the procedures and protocols to be followed if the group supervisor has concerns about clinical practice or ethical issues?
- Has this been explained to the supervision group?
- Who needs to be informed about what is going on in the group supervision?
- How much and what do they need to know?
- What kind of recording is required?
- Where will it be kept and who will have access to it?
- Who will guide, monitor, or supervise the group supervisor's practice?
- Identify agency requirements around meetings, referral procedures, and third party communications.
- Make certain that professional insurance and legal requirements are met and up to date if appropriate.

It is important to have clear and explicit agreements or contracts governing all these issues, particularly in the sensitive areas relating to communication with colleagues and other third party agencies with an interest in the group supervision.

Recording the group supervision

A lot depends on the purpose of the recording, so ask yourself:

- Who is the recording for – agency, colleagues, supervisor's use, supervisee's use?
- What do these people need to know?
- What is the minimum material to be recorded – individual and group behaviour, supervisee performance, interaction; particular incidents; supervisee's interventions, use of theory, capacity to use the supervision sessions?
- Who will have access to the recordings?
- Where will records be kept?

Have a look again at Chapter 17 for a fuller discussion on how and what to record.

Evaluating and reporting on supervisee's professional development

Depending on the context in which the group supervision is taking place you may be called upon to evaluate the progress of the supervisee or trainee in managing their group to a suitable or required standard. Think about how to assess:

- The supervisee's or trainee's acquisition and development of skills
- The supervisee's learning targets
- The supervisee's knowledge base and use of theory
- The development of the supervisee's professional self-image
- How the supervisee uses the group supervision
- How the supervisee makes use of suggested interventions and advice
- The overall functioning of the group supervision
- To determine if objectives and goals are being achieved
- To assess whether the group is tackling priority needs
- To ensure the group is using resources effectively or identify necessary skills and facilities
- To provide further material for supervision
- To influence policy making
- To validate the group and ensure its survival and funding

Reporting on the supervisee's or trainee's progress and development is a sensitive issue and in my view one best managed with the individual's and supervision group's involvement. I find that it is useful to institute periodic internal reviews with the group that can form the basis of more official reports later if needed. Many of the reporting issues are similar to the accountability issues discussed earlier.

Aims and objectives of group supervision

1   The primary objective of group supervision is to enable the supervisee to become a group worker or become a better group worker. This means developing and polishing a whole range of skills in the supervisee such as the planning and setting up of their work group; focusing on building the supervisee's capacity to recognize themes and patterns in their work group; helping them understand the stages in the life cycle of the group and know where to direct their attention and how to intervene effectively.
2   Group supervision can be very effective in helping the supervisee learn to tolerate and manage their emotional response to their work group. Groups can evoke a mix of powerful emotions in their leaders that can be disturbing. Being able to explore these counter-transference responses in a supportive atmosphere with knowledgeable and caring peers is essential if the supervisee is to understand and actively utilize the emotional communications that characterize their work group.
3   Group supervision provides exciting opportunities to understand the underlying dynamics and process issues in the supervisees's work groups and to consider suitable interventions and acquire technical ability.
4   A fourth objective has to do with promoting an appropriate and realistic professional self-image whose central aim is to serve their group (see Chapter 8 for a full discussion of this).
5   Group supervision provides support and containment for supervisees trying to manage a work group going through a difficult crisis. Supervision can also contain supervisees experiencing some personal crisis of their own that may impinge on their work groups.

The group supervisor's tasks

The first task of the group supervisor has to be to create a predictable and consistent space and promote a learning culture in which supervision can take place. This regulated and boundaried space in the work life emphasizes the primacy of thought and reflection and provides experiences of mutual attunement, expansion, and creativity. Seek every opportunity to promote a culture of inquiry and curiosity and constantly underline the importance of being thoughtful and reflective about one's groupwork and especially emphasize how the experiences and events in the supervision group might illuminate the dynamics and processes of the supervisees' work groups.

The public arena of the group will inevitably excite a range of inclusion issues that need to be dealt with, and the emotional response of supervisees or trainees to exposing their work will evoke feelings of shame to do with perceived mistakes, feelings of incompetence, and competitiveness with other supervisees. These anxieties need to be sensitively addressed by the supervisor but it is vital to remember that the purpose of a supervision group is supervision and not therapy. You can explore with supervisees the sorts of feelings that get excited in them by the process of supervision but you must locate the rationale for this in emphasizing the ubiquitous power of groups to generate similar feelings and look for ways of helping them manage these themes in their own work groups. Keeping aligned to the context and purpose of the supervision group is essential when dealing with the subjective and personal experiences of the supervisees.

Gradually the supervision group comes into being as a definite place in time and space with a distinct culture of reflectivity where one may think and share with others the challenges and pressures of working with groups. You may wish to accelerate the establishment of the supervision culture by offering a flexible structure in which supervisees take turns in presenting material about their groups and consider allocating an end period of time for anyone needing assistance with a crisis. I have also found that an initial period of time spent reflecting on the characteristics of healthy and unhealthy group experiences in the supervisees' history is helpful in enabling group members to attach positively to this current group opportunity.

Once a distinct space and learning culture is established the work of the supervision group intensifies and deepens and now the next task of the supervisor more clearly emerges. You are a teacher of the groupwork method. You have knowledge and expertise in the method and authority to transmit this body of experience.

The important question here is about teaching style. At times a more didactic or pedagogic style is required and the supervisor will describe some theoretical concept that speaks to a particular set of circumstances in a supervisee's work group or give references to suitable literature that the supervisee may read. There may be time set aside occasionally in the supervision group to discuss an appropriate theoretical paper or article that might inform or illuminate a matter of technique or intervention. You may suggest a particular intervention in a supervisee's work group or offer advice based on your own experience in similar situations and perhaps even set up a short role-play to demonstrate a technical or strategic intervention.

More often a collaborative style of teaching begins to prevail in the supervision group in which you endeavour to harness the multiplicity of perspectives and feedback to elucidate the intricacies and dynamics of an unusual or difficult group event. This collaborative style aims to bond the supervision group into a team and make the team the supervisory instrument rather than relying solely and permanently on you as expert. It is also a marvellous way of inculcating in supervisees the ethic and culture of groupwork.

At other times you may find it important to include a more therapeutic or pastoral dimension in your teaching style. This does not mean that you are doing therapy with supervisees as I cautioned above. What it means is that you need to pay attention to the emotional and developing professional well-being of the supervision group members if they are to be sufficiently engaged and motivated to be willing to disclose their learning needs and anxieties. Attunement to the supervisees' feelings and experiences of self-doubt, frustration, and shame will enable you to determine their capacity for tolerating vulnerability and uncertainty and help you decide how supervision may be most useful.

Supervisees will need your help to soothe and contain their feelings of inadequacy or calm their anxiety about turbulent periods in their work groups. This is perfectly appropriate since a vulnerable supervisee will not be able to focus on their work group effectively and may even feel frightened or angry or avoidant about their work group or more disastrously, the supervision group.

Again, the modelling offered by your capacity to contain difficult feelings and experiences in the supervision group, and in supervisees' work groups, and make them comprehensible, becomes an intrinsic core of the supervisees' skill set. The constant integrative and affirming aspect of your attitude and stance is essential in teaching supervisees that making mistakes and making them meaningful is a necessary part of learning to become a group worker. In this way the necessary criticism that is part of supervision is experienced as helpful and creative, and damage and injury to self-esteem is minimized and reframed as the endurable and natural process of professional identification.

On occasion personal events in a supervisee's life may impact on their work and on the supervision group and require your attention. Such events may involve a bereavement or personal illness or may have to do with the supervisee's family. It could involve impending surgery or a pregnancy or be as simple as the supervisee moving to a new job. It is important to remember your role as a group supervisor and to avoid becoming a therapist. As always stick to the context and purpose of the supervision group and you will not go wrong. You have to decide how best to manage such painful disclosures without compromising the work and purpose of the supervision group. Your responsibilities are to the supervision group, the supervisee, and their work group so it is essential to determine the extent of the emergency or traumatic event and the potential impact on the supervisee and their work group and the supervision group, in that order.

Supervision groups have a huge capacity to contain difficult and painful events in the life of a supervisee so don't be afraid to give time for this and be confident in the opportunity to model the management of such events in a manner that can be transposed into the supervisees' work groups. An appropriate time can be set aside to deal with the group's reaction to the disclosure of a difficult life event. Management strategies for the supervisee and their work group can be considered and when the immediate impact has been prepared for them it might prove helpful for the other supervisees to think about how they might in future manage similar events in their own lives and work groups.

A third important task for the group supervisor involves knowing where and when and what to focus attention on when a supervisee presents group material.

- You may focus attention on the group process and dynamics, history, and stage in the life cycle aiming to elucidate the underlying needs and conflicts and communications. This might mean zooming in on a particular work group member's behaviour or thinking about a certain subgroup or identifying a conflict or worry in the work group.
- You may draw attention to the supervisee's counter-transference reactions as a way of understanding deeper issues and communications in the group and consider strategies and interventions.
- You may focus on the supervisory experience itself, on the relationships and reactions between the supervisees or between you and the supervisees as indicative and reflective of phenomena in the work group being presented. This is called a parallel process event and is an important and regularly recurring part of supervisory work. Parallel process re-enactments require particular skills on the part of the group supervisor because they are unconscious phenomena which invade the supervision group and make it a replica of the work group from which they originate. Conflicts and difficulties in the supervisee's work group elicit strong feelings of shame, inadequacy, anger, and helplessness and stuckness, and these get re-enacted in the supervision group sweeping everyone present into the emotional drama and making it hard to be objective and reflective. Sudden intense eruptions of emotion or unusual feelings of boredom or impasse in an otherwise reasonably co-operative supervision group are the indicators of the presence of parallel process phenomena and the sorts of intrusions that it is essential you pay attention to.

Some examples of parallel process re-enactment in group supervision

Example 1

An inexperienced female group worker presented to her supervision group a narrative about the early stages of her work group. In this work group a particular man would continually endeavour to get her attention by any means, fair or foul, to the exclusion of the rest of the group members. The group worker was finding herself increasingly fed up with this man's behaviour and angry about the passivity of her group whom she wished would intervene more on her behalf to curb his unhealthy activity. She described her frustration with the situation with such mounting irritation and tearful anxiety that the group supervisor felt compelled to intervene to try to calm her so that the situation could be more thoughtfully examined. Somewhat intimidated by the intense emotional atmosphere of the supervision session the other three supervisees in the group offered no comments and accordingly the group supervisor made a number of suggestions to the anxious group worker about how the situation in her group might be dealt with.

It was only after the supervision session that the group supervisor was struck by the similarity of what took place in the supervision group to the description of what continually occurred in the supervisee's work group. It seemed evident that the forceful dyadic interaction between a group member and the group leader resulting in the exclusion of the other group members was identical in each situation. In other words there was a clear parallel re-enactment of the process of the work group now taking place in the supervision group.

In the next supervision session the group supervisor briefly returned to and highlighted this parallel process and invited the group to examine their experience of the last session in order to see what had occurred and whether this might reflect some of the dynamics in the work group and even perhaps suggest an appropriate intervention. The group worker spoke about her feelings of inadequacy in managing her group and her fear of seeming incompetent in front of her peers. The other three supervisees spoke about similar feelings of helplessness and uncertainty as to know how to assist her that left them with a desire to remain uninvolved. It soon became evident that this was exactly the process in the work group where there were feelings of inadequacy and hesitation to do with unacknowledged inclusion and dependency issues for members. The group supervisor was able to locate the troublesome dynamics of the work group in the context of the beginning stages of a group and a number of interventions were arrived at by the supervision group that were successfully carried out by the less anxious group worker in subsequent sessions with her group.

Example 2

A male group worker presented an account of his work with elderly people in a day centre. He had started a group to engage these clients in reminiscence work and social interaction but was frustrated that his group members only wanted to play bingo in the sessions and were reluctant to try the other activities in his programme. The other members of the supervision group offered ideas as to what might be going on, to do with the elderly people's fears of revealing frailties and vulnerabilities and suggested that perhaps the group worker might talk to his members about what they felt capable of and design a more appropriate programme. The group worker insisted that he had attempted to talk to his group about the problem but they wouldn't engage with this and wanted to play bingo. He believed that it was important that they do this at other times in the centre and concentrate on what a reminiscence group could offer them in terms of slowing dementia and providing social therapy.

Very quickly an impasse occurred in the supervision group with the group worker and the other supervisees disagreeing about the priority of the elderly people's needs and the type of programme best suited for them. The group supervisor soon realized that a parallel process re-enactment was occurring in the supervision group. The presenting group worker was at odds with his peers and everyone was frustrated and locked into an unsatisfying impasse. This was identical to the work group where the group leader and members were not communicating in a healthy manner and were frustrated by each other's attempts both to hold onto a traditional activity and introduce a change.

The group supervisor pointed out the possibility of a parallel process re-enactment and invited the supervision group to set the discussion aside and reflect on their current experience. The presenting group worker described his feelings of impatience with his colleagues' apparent difficulty in understanding his motivations and settling for easy options while his peers described their frustration at not being heard and their dissatisfaction with what they regarded as his single-mindedness.

The supervisor asked the group worker to talk about his motivations and aspirations for his group and in the course of this it became apparent that the centre where he worked wanted to urgently extend its service programmes in order to protect itself from threatened cutbacks in agency funding. The group worker had come under management pressure to offer more intensive activities and this was the reason for his insistence on the reminiscence work. When this was made explicit both he and the other supervisees experienced some relief and were able to see that the anxiety operating in the day centre had permeated and polluted the worker's relationship with the elderly group and had additionally invaded the supervision group.

It was then a relatively simple matter to think about a strategic intervention that offered an inclusive solution rather than the previous either/or approach. The supervision group suggested that the worker return to his group and talk to the elderly people about their willingness to have group sessions which included a reasonable warm-up period of bingo and then focused on the reminiscence work. The group worker was pleased to do this and no one in the supervision group was subsequently surprised when the worker later reported that his group was successfully engaged in the new expanded programme.

Example 3

A female group worker presented her therapy group for supervision. The therapy group was composed of people suffering from depression and was frequently a difficult group to work with. The worker described a particular session where one member complained about the negligence and inattention of various authorities to intervene appropriately and early enough with children in dysfunctional families. The member had demanded that the worker explain the existence of evil in the world and why there was no goodness. When other group members supported these ideas the emotional tone of the session became very low and the worker quickly felt helpless and inadequate to respond.

In the supervision group the worker queried the usefulness of groupwork with such severely depressed people and wondered if she had made a mistake in offering group treatment when they perhaps really needed individual attention and additional social support and financial assistance. For a time the supervisees discussed this and tried to be encouraging but nothing was forthcoming that might prove helpful for the worker with her group. Indeed the supervisees became increasingly morose about the limitations of group therapy and looked to the supervisor to produce an effective rationale and creative interventions. When the supervisor's suggestions were subsequently found wanting or thought to be too abstract the supervisor himself felt inadequate and unable to sustain the supervision group.

It was at this point that the supervisor realized that a parallel process re-enactment was occurring in the supervision group. The depressed member in the therapy group had undermined the group worker's confidence in the value of the group and her own competence and this was repeating in the supervision group. The group supervisor asked the group to consider the possibility of a parallel process re-enactment operating and invited reflection and comment from the supervisees on their here and now experience.

After a period it became apparent that they were indeed resonating to the dynamics of the therapy group and it emerged that an unconscious attack on the group therapist was at the core of the disturbance and was being re-enacted in the supervision group. It seemed that the dynamics of this had to do with transference feelings towards the therapist displaced onto critiques of authority, God, and society, and which were based on an infantile rage against neglectful and abandoning parental figures. The therapist was also unconsciously envied for her goodness and supposed freedom from personal difficulties.

The supervision group were soon able to consider a range of interventions that the therapist could offer, such as helping the depressed member of the therapy group to think about her own particular family circumstances and failures rather than focusing on generalized critiques of authority. The group therapist was also enabled to direct her group's attention both to their envy of her and their need to find her a reliable and strong object who could withstand their attacks and not retaliate or collapse as had been their experience with parental figures in the past. She was also able to affirm the usefulness of the group opportunity and promote it as an alternative to previous disastrous group experiences.

Discussion of the examples

You can see from these examples that a central task of the group supervisor is to maintain constant vigilance about the supervision group's interaction and monitor both one's own and the group's subjective experience. Parallel process re-enactments are both ubiquitous and inevitable and are a rich source of communication and information about the underlying dynamics and preoccupations of the work group presented which do not come across in the conscious and verbal descriptions and narratives.

The supervisee's tasks

The primary task for the supervisee is to present their last group session or a particular difficulty as fully and honestly as possible so that everyone can think about it with them. This is not an easy thing to do because the supervisee has an investment in not appearing inadequate or incompetent in front of their peers and previous experiences in public learning situations may make them prone to shame and fear. Tendencies to exhibitionism and a desire for status and admiration may also get excited.

So material presented by the supervisee may be unconsciously edited or deleted or exaggerated and may skew what actually occurred. Supervisees need to be continually encouraged to take responsibility for their own learning which means actively cultivating a receptive attitude to appropriate criticism, differences of opinion, and theoretical orientations. The supervisee also needs to realize that they are expected to be responsible for actively contributing to generating cohesion and creative collaboration in the supervision group if they and the others are to profit from the supervisory experience.

You can facilitate this ethos by spending some time in the early sessions considering with the supervision group members their experience of helpful and unhelpful learning situations and drawing out features which might obstruct this occasion and others which would make it maximally useful. This is time well spent.

Decide with the supervisees the simplest format for presenting group material. This initially may involve them giving a brief pen picture of their work group members, their roles in the group, alliances, and subgroups. The supervisee should describe the institutional context and purpose for the group and then go on to narrate the particular session or circumstances to be considered and their interventions as accurately as can be recalled. Finally the supervisee should be encouraged to describe their emotional responses and counter-transference reactions.

The next task for the supervisee is to reflect on their presentation. Often in telling the story of a particular session a supervisee will make a comment about what they now see was going on in the group but missed in vivo, or gain insight as to why they intervened as they did. This capacity to listen in on oneself while simultaneously being in the process is an important attribute to be acquired by the group worker and should be actively encouraged and practised in the supervision group.

The other members of the supervision group can be asked for their responses and comments and again the supervisee must be encouraged to learn to set aside their desire to inappropriately preserve self-esteem and really listen to and hear what is being said to them. The transfer of this learning to the work group by the supervisee can be great. The other supervisees may offer opinions and describe their own experiences and again the presenting supervisee may learn how to discriminate and select suitable insights and weave a satisfying basis for understanding what went on and how to suitably intervene next time.

Building these reflective skills is the basis of enabling the supervisee to engage with a third task of synthesizing the supervisory experience in such a way that results in modifying technical activities and performance. The object of this is to acquire a competence and awareness about how to work with groups. Throughout the whole of the presentation the supervisee learns how to move between past and present preoccupations and gains facility with 'here and now' and 'there and then' thinking which is an important skill to bring to their work. The supervisee internalizes the emphasis on multiple focusing of attention on the individual members of the work group and the group as a whole and learns to distinguish process issues and how to think about them.

Typical problems in the supervision group

I have already noted that the supervisory experience is a difficult one for both the supervisee and the supervisor. The supervisee is required to exhibit and expose their work with the inevitable background fear that it is their very self that is being scrutinized and judged. Similarly the supervisor has to balance precariously between avoiding injurious criticism and being inappropriately therapeutic.

But other problems can arise with the supervision group because of:

> • Difficulties with the composition of the supervision group
> • Supervisor–supervisee relations
> • Internal group dynamics
> • Difficulties in the environment of the supervision group
> • Cultural, ethnic, social, and political conflicts and issues

The composition of the supervision group is important to consider. Sometimes the supervisor can select members for the supervision group while at other times the composition of the group is already fixed. An obvious difficulty has to do with the degree of heterogeneity and diversity. Problems may arise if there is too much difference in the professional backgrounds of supervisees. A supervision group made up of youth and community workers, group therapists, teachers, and social care workers for example may strain to find enough common ground to sustain each other's interest in their groups or the value of supervision. The divergence in their client populations, their professional trainings and assumptions, and the wide differences in the types of groupwork interventions may make it difficult for such disparate professionals to be of much help to each other and may in fact only create an unsatisfying supervisory Tower of Babel. Some members may drop out through lack of common ground, and participation and attendance among the rest may be at best unreliable or compromised.

Another factor to consider in setting up and running a supervision group has to do with the relative levels of experience and seniority among members. There are arguments that can be made for mixing levels of experience so that beginners learn from more experienced colleagues and seasoned workers can revisit and revise basic perspectives and skills, but I think this is at best a temporary phenomenon and soon the needs and priorities of the different constituencies will create oppositional dynamics and tendencies. It is also probable that more experienced and senior group workers will have an investment in not losing face or being shamed in front of neophytes and that an inevitable pecking hierarchy will emerge that will undermine inquiry and adventurousness and creativity.

The supervision group's chance of success will be enhanced if it is composed of members who share similar professional backgrounds and client groups and who operate with broadly similar objectives and strategies. A homogenous supervision group is to be preferred to a heterogenous grouping.

More common are the difficulties that arise from tensions between the group supervisor and the supervisee which are misunderstood or poorly handled. There are two central things to bear in mind with seemingly personal affections and relationships. A supervisor will invariably get drawn into antagonistic and hostile relationships with the group or individuals if s/he does not understand the nature of transference and counter-transference phenomena and actively seeks to correctly set troublesome relations in this context.

The authoritative nature of the supervisor–supervisee relationship and the group dimension will invariably activate parental and familial dynamics that will permeate and disrupt the work of the group. Supervisees are prone to experiencing shame because of their blind spots and inadequacies or as a result of mishandling their groups and making mistakes. They may overcompensate by exaggerating their competency or competing with their peers. The group supervisor who is too controlling or too critical of individual or group exhibitionism and rivalries will induce shame or angry and rebellious responses in supervisees, triggering a mutually distrustful cycle of uneasy relations. It is important for the group supervisor to ensure that s/he does not mistakenly and inappropriately personalize relationships that really need to be understood and contextualized in a transference paradigm.

There are two easily recognizable types of supervisees among the many personalities that you may encounter. The first type of supervisee may be described as psychologically immature, vulnerable, and dependent. They may seek a lot of approval and affirmation from the group supervisor and their neediness often ensures that they can get caught up with issues more to do with supervision and their relationship with peers and the supervisor than to do with their groupwork. The second type of supervisee may seem more independent and may on occasion compete with the supervisor or try to impress with superior knowledge. These supervisees are more aggressive and preoccupied with issues of control and autonomy. Both types of supervisees may feel criticized and misunderstood by the supervisor who can get caught in a seemingly difficult and problematic personal circumstance. If the group supervisor is to be effective it is vital to recognize and differentiate supervisee transference reactions to the supervisor and counter-transference responses from apparent conflicts in personal relations and re-contextualize these interactions in the supervisee's work group if possible.

Equally important is the care with which the supervisor translates apparently personal difficulties in the network of supervisory relationships into the language of parallel process repetitions where appropriate. Many problems in supervision groups could be easily avoided if more supervisors were aware of this phenomenon whereby the supervisees' own relations with their groups become re-enacted in the supervision group. The supervisor who is perceptive will not be needlessly therapeutic or carelessly dismissive but will recognize the opportunities provided in parallel process occurrences to correct disturbances in relations and model thoughtful means of intervention and mediation.

Supervision groups have exactly the same stages of development and internal dynamics as every other sort of group and since you will have to pay attention to these it is worthwhile reading over the earlier chapters dealing with these issues.

The supervisory work can be compromised if the supervisor is careless around time boundaries and permits some individuals getting more attention. This encourages grabbing and greedy presentations and intensifies rivalries and subgroupings.

Rivalries and cliques may also constellate around certain theoretical orientations and the supervision group risks getting caught in unhelpful doctrinal disputes. Whilst encouraging theoretical debate be mindful that diversity can be a breeding ground for unhealthy rivalries in an unbalanced supervision group.

New members entering the supervision group and valued older members leaving generate anxious feelings that have to be addressed and always you must monitor the group for avoidant, unassertive, or quiet supervisees who need encouragement.

Punctuality and attendance are good indicators of cohesion in the supervision group and the transparency of presentations and quality of criticism offered and received will tell you about the internal dynamics of the group. The environment in which the supervision group takes place can pose difficulties just as the supervisees may similarly struggle with their own environmental obstacles and frustrations. Be alert to how problems in one setting may get replicated in the other. The setting and venue for the supervision group will influence the atmosphere and quality of work depending on whether it is a neutral, removed site or is in the work premises. There may be competition or conflict for a suitable room that can be guaranteed and protected from outside interferences and interruptions. It will be difficult to ensure the appropriate safety and privacy for the supervision group if telephones constantly disturb or patients enter without warning. Ensure that the room is set up for the group and you do not have to move furniture around.

If you are working in an institutional context it is important that you negotiate clear agreements about reporting arrangements, referral procedures, purpose, and time-scales for groups. Agency managers will have different priorities and conflicts about funding, staffing, and other resources that may adversely impact the supervision group. Attitudes to groupwork may pose difficulties and this has consequences for attendance and adequate attention to supervision. Groupwork may be perceived erroneously as an economic means of service provision or may be suspiciously regarded as a frivolous activity or worse as a luxury.

Consider how your supervision group which emphasizes professional development may collide with other supervisory requirements which focus on case allocation or other more service delivery oriented management issues. If there are potential conflicts of interest minimize them as best as possible or else try to live with them if you can whilst acknowledging the frustration. Not everyone will share your enthusiasm for groupwork or understand the need for a reflective space to think about the work so be aware that your supervision group may excite envy and irritation in others that can impinge on your efforts. Be vigilant for unhealthy splits that set the supervision group apart from its environment or get carried into the group as a type of zeal or superior knowledge possessed by the supervisees.

Cultural, ethnic, gender, and political complexities can influence the creative working of the supervision group and need sympathetic and delicate attention. The ratios of ethnic groups and genders may be a given but you need to monitor proceedings for any evidence of careless or unconscious stereotyping that may cause offence or resentment. Female supervisees may be allocated nurturing stereotypes, for example, and the male supervisees may privilege management of conflict or exercise of authority. Such unhelpful caricatures need instant examination and dismantling if they are not to undermine the group. Ethnic and cultural differences may fuel disturbances in the group as a consequence of difficulties understanding accents or unfamiliarity with the shared language. It is important that you model an inclusive attitude which places a premium on understanding and respect for the different and unfamiliar. Over time different cultural perspectives in the supervision group can enhance and deepen understanding of common work group problems and offer new and creative solutions. Political rivalries and historical complexities are similarly best addressed if they show disruptive potentials in the supervision group.

Remember you do not have to resolve any cultural or ethnic or gender conflict. You are not responsible for past injustices or current vulnerabilities. You are responsible for the smooth operating of the supervision group and as such it is your obligation to engage members in any examination of their interaction and process that threatens to disrupt the group. It is a simple matter for you to point out how interactions that induce shame and resentment cripple the supervision group and must be dealt with sensitively and without blame. The relevance to the supervisees' work groups can be suitably emphasized.

Review

- Group supervision offers advantages over individual supervision
- The group is the primary supervisory instrument
- The group supervisor aims to create a reflective space and a learning culture
- The group supervisor provides education and instruction, therapeutic support, and co-creative opportunities
- Anxieties about shameful exposure, competency, inadequacy, status, and competition and rivalry are normal features of a supervision group
- A central norm of the supervision group is that mistakes, errors, and weaknesses are the stuff for learning, development, and transformation
- Participating in a well-run supervision group is a way of practising and internalizing an effective model of groupwork
- It is essential to look out for transference and counter-transference phenomena and not react to so-called personal difficulties that require re-contextualizing
- Parallel process re-enactments are a central feature of group supervision
- It is vital that you check your accountability as a supervisor and consider the demands and requirements of the setting and context that you operate in

---

Reference

1 Proctor, B. (2008) *Group Supervision: A Guide to Creative Practice, 2nd ed.*, chap. 3, London: Sage.

Chapter 16

Why some groups don't work and what you might do about it

Groupwork offers members a participative and shared experience that is unique and powerful and is increasingly used by a multitude of agencies today for a variety of reasons. Youth workers, nurses, social workers, psychologists, and others are expected to run groups to provide guidance and assistance across the community and health and social care system – cancer care, diabetes, mental health, looked-after children, learning difficulties, and so on.

Many groups work well and deliver the planned objectives and benefits for their members. However, some groups just don't work because they are so poorly planned or represent more the needs of workers or an organization to maintain its grant-aid or be seen to provide certain services than it does the real needs of potential group members. In other circumstances people can ask for help with no real understanding of an agency's services or obligations and then find themselves caught up in a programme they are unwilling to be involved in. Increasingly multidisciplinary professionals are expected to work together in a group programme and may struggle to work as a group themselves.

Agencies may rightly view a group service as an economy involving fewer staff and maximum client numbers in a well thought-out programme but in many other situations agencies have no real strategy for developing a groupwork programme beyond reducing weighty caseloads or managing staff shortages. The essential point is that no group is a closed system but operates within a set of intermeshing contexts that need to be thought about and taken into account because there is a multiplicity of factors that impact on the group if it is to be successful, productive, and efficient. Let's consider some examples of groups that don't work.

A group that never got off the ground

A head of service was anxious about the perceived status of her core staff and decided to improve their professional profile with colleagues in allied but different professions. At a senior inter-agency management meeting she unilaterally offered her staff to set up and run a group supervision service to help workers in the other agencies improve their practice. While her colleagues initially agreed that this might be a good idea no working party was set up to advance and administer the idea. The head of service instructed her staff to initiate the group supervision, but as they were uncomfortable with their competence to run such groups she contracted an external facilitator to provide a short training course in group supervision. This was to be supported by a series of six consecutive monthly supervision sessions for the five potential supervisors who would themselves have an experience of group supervision in which their own practice of group supervision could be developed and refined.

The short training course went ahead and the supervision groups began. In the first supervision group two of the members were absent on leave despite the dates for the groups having been agreed in advance. In the second supervision group it emerged that none of the proposed recipients of the anticipated group supervision programme had responded or could be contacted to set up the service. They simply did not answer any communications. In the third supervision group two different members were absent on another training course. The external trainer began to suspect that all was far from collaborative and wondered with the group if there were some problems impeding the implementation of the offer of providing the group supervision service. The recipients of the proposed group were not responding and the group supervisors were not regularly attending the training. It was clear that something was not working and that people were not signed up to the idea.

Gradually it emerged that the staff who were expected to provide the group supervision had been instructed to offer this service but did not feel confident in providing it because they believed that it required skills and competencies that they did not possess. Further, the service planned was in addition to their normal full-time duties and there was no consideration of a reduction or restructuring of their work schedules to include this extra responsibility. It became apparent that the potential group supervisors were reacting to the plan in the same way as the proposed recipients and refusing to co-operate by absenting themselves. They did not feel confident in putting their objections to the idea to their boss and simply undermined the idea. The training of the group supervisors became irrelevant in these circumstances and the course ended as a complete failure. No group supervision was initiated for other professional colleagues and time, money, and resource was needlessly wasted.

What this example illustrates is a sort of *professional imperialism* and a failure to create an agreed and shared context and strategic vision for groupwork. A particular agency anxious about its profile decided to boost its image and status by offering a groupwork service to colleagues in other disciplines. This was a unilateral offer of help and was not sought out by other agencies who undoubtedly resented the idea that someone outside their sphere of influence had decided to improve their professional practice on their behalf. One can imagine that consciously or unconsciously they deeply resented being made to feel like the recipients of aid and wisdom from a superior external elite and simply decided not to co-operate with the imperial power. Similarly, the potential supervisors were not consulted and engaged in the proposal but instructed to perform a duty they were not confident in and which was an addition to their normal responsibilities. The result: a group that didn't work, couldn't work, and never got off the ground. There was a failure to model effective groupwork from the beginning in which the various stakeholders might be engaged in discussion and dialogue and encouraged to take responsibility and ownership of the project.

What was wrong:

- The decision to offer groupwork did not arise from any request or recognized need
- Management anxiety about profile of the service

- Groupwork seen as a solution to solving management anxiety and promoting profile of the service
- No coherent strategy or context for the groupwork programme
- A lack of consensus and collaboration with other heads of service
- Subsequent failure to engage other agencies
- Absence of a monitoring party that could reflect on emerging difficulties and revision
- Failure to engage the supervising staff
- Lack of planning and rescheduling for increased workloads of supervising staff
- Not listening to their anxieties
- Lack of dialogue and feedback all round
- Excuses and resistance

A group that kept losing members

An agency was faced with static caseloads and long waiting lists. It was considered that a psychoeducational group might meet client needs and could be an economy of service. Staff were encouraged to scan their caseloads and refer potential members to two workers who were randomly designated by the agency to run a group each. Neither of the workers met with the potential members before the groups commenced nor was there any preparation of the members by the referring staff. The clients were told that the group service was a more suitable treatment and support for them than individual treatment.

The groups were to consist of 15 members each but only six people in one group and seven in the other turned up for the first of 12 sessions. The absent members were not followed up and were deemed to have removed themselves from the service and agency responsibility. By the third session one group had been reduced to two members and could no longer function and was ended. The other group ended prematurely after five sessions because of reduced numbers. The agency regularly reported a 75% dropout rate in subsequent groups and discontinued its groupwork service.

What this example demonstrates is that:

- The group service was really designed to meet agency needs and not client needs
- The groups were seen as an economy but lacked any strategy or context beyond reducing waiting lists
- There was no preparation of members by referring staff
- Members were not seen beforehand by the group workers so no positive treatment alliance was established or individual goals and objectives agreed
- The group offer was impersonal and industrial and members perceived this and acted accordingly
- 50% of potential members never attended the first session and there was no follow-up to ascertain why

- Remaining members decided that the group service was not for them and ended prematurely
- There was no provision for reflection by staff or agency as to why the groups didn't work
- There was a lack of responsibility and accountability within the agency and its professional staff
- Action was more important than vision
- As a consequence the groups were poorly planned and bound to fail

The Tower of Babel or a confusion of tongues

Increasingly multidisciplinary professionals work together in a group programme with a common client population. In one instance a number of different agencies working with young people aged 16–19 years, not in education, employment, or training (NEET), decided to come together to provide a programme that might engage these young people more effectively in line with governmental directives. The teachers had observed that the young people were not motivated in the classroom and were failing in basic learning. A number of these young people were involved with social workers and were also known to local youth workers. The young people had variously:

- Encountered a negative experience of education
- Been bullied at school
- Had literacy and numeracy problems
- Had problems with parents
- Been in care or on the edge of care
- Been involved with drug and alcohol abuse
- A physical disability/learning disability
- Committed a crime
- Had a mental illness

At a senior management level, the three agencies got together and decided to pool resources and create a special programme aimed at motivating the young people and enabling them to achieve certain set educational and social targets. These targets involved literacy and numeracy programmes, issue based and conflict management groupwork to promote ongoing awareness of the effects of antisocial behaviour and community safety, and help for young people solve their conflicts and problems in more positive ways.

It was decided to locate the programme in the school classroom and the youth workers and social workers would work alongside the teachers to deliver a more creative and inspiring curriculum and deal with the most challenging pupils by providing more interactive sessions. A particular school was identified as a test pilot and a team made up of the three disciplines was designated to work with a group of difficult young people.

However, the interagency team soon encountered difficulties with each other that impacted on their work and reduced effectiveness:

- A teacher was required to be present at each session in the classroom even though they may have had no particular role in that session. This discomforted the youth worker and social worker who felt observed and judged by the teacher who had more authority than they possessed.
- The teachers were less tolerant of rowdy behaviour than the youth worker or social worker who were more used to informal groups of clients and could accept and manage boundary infringements more readily.
- The various professionals had different attitudes to discipline, control, authority, sanction, and reward, and different ideas about how to work with groups based on their training.
- The youth workers found having to work with more prescriptive programmes difficult and less satisfying than their more usual process-oriented groups.
- Similarly, the teachers found the more interactive process groups more difficult than their usual content-driven teaching sessions.
- Confidentiality and reporting was a problem as each discipline had different statutory responsibilities and duties.
- Increasingly the workers became confused as to their roles and contributions and confused each other.
- There was no joint supervision for the three disciplines that might have helped them deal with the discomfort of moving beyond familiar practices and begin to work as a team.
- There seemed to be a hierarchy of professional status in which the teachers esteemed themselves ahead of the social workers and the youth workers who felt least esteemed.

This example demonstrates how just as in the biblical story of the Tower of Babel a joint endeavour became disrupted because different professional languages and assumptions unfortunately prevailed to the detriment of the groupwork programme. The laudable aim of bringing together different professional groups to pool their unique skills and perspectives in order to serve a disadvantaged group of young people effectively foundered because not enough consideration was given to the very fact of their differences and how these might help and where they might hinder collaboration. Since professional groups distinguish themselves through their language differentiation and their worldviews, operational philosophies, and value systems, a multi-agency project must invest time, energy, and oversight to ensure that:

- Each worker is aware of the contribution of the other, values this, and believes in it
- Each worker needs to be very clear about her own role and contribution
- All workers should be clear and in agreement about the purpose of the group project
- Each worker should be clear why their agency wants them present and what the agency hopes to contribute to and get from the group project

- All workers should be prepared to fully discuss the conflicts, tensions, and feelings aroused in them by joint work and group experience
- All workers should be willing to permit and invite differences in perception, style, and approach as long as there is agreement about purpose
- All workers need to collaborate, share, trust, talk to each other, in and out of the group. The ability of the group to share, deal with conflict and interpersonal issues is directly related to how effective co-leaders are at this
- This requires that all workers have negotiated agency agreement that sufficient time can be set aside for preparation and debriefing and that adequate supervision of practice is available
- An essential inter-agency objective should be to ensure that the co-workers become an effective and productive group if they are to work successfully with client groups

In this example the inter-agency desire to respond to governmental directives to work with NEETs started from a poor foundation that failed to emphasize the importance of the different professionals working to become a team/group themselves. The lack of joint supervision for the professionals contributed to the failure to develop a collaborative ethos and resulted in an unhelpful and ultimately divisive hierarchy of status. The workers continued to differentiate themselves into familiar professional bunkers and the nature of the difficult work they faced reinforced their prejudices.

The primary role of the agency in failing groups

A lack of a systemic perspective that leads to an unnecessary culture clash

I have given these examples because in my experience the main reason why some groups don't work is because of the failure of the agency to fully understand the nature of group-work and take the appropriate steps to establish a group partnership in which all the stakeholders are encouraged and enabled to participate and collaborate actively and effectively. This can be summed up simply as the failure or inability of the agency management to think systemically.

A central and recurring reason for this lies in the professional culture and operational philosophy of most contemporary agencies and organizations. In nearly all agencies power and authority manifests throughout a *pyramidical* structure with tops, middles, and bottoms in order for the task of the organization to be carried out. This reflects wider societal group structures such as family, school, church, and business which are traditionally and historically based on obedience and submission to authority and have given rise to one set of ideas and attitudes about how human interaction might be organized. Individuals have responsibility and power to lead and compel groups and teams. Rarely are such individuals trained to work with groups and teams but are appointed or assume responsibility for the group. Often such leaders may practise a style of authority unconsciously informed by earlier experience in family and school but not necessarily suited to working with adults.

Agencies are socially structured and culturally patterned so power and authority is based on hierarchy and status in a typical model of domination rather than collaboration and collectivism. There is usually an emphasis on control of complex processes. Concepts such as ownership and partnership so familiar to the group worker may be far removed from everyday organizational experience because not every member or worker has equal power and authority and participates fractionally in the agency. The more facilitative style of leadership practised by the group worker is different to the control and directive leadership found in most agencies and may not be easily understood by management.

Since most agencies provide specialized services to their clients they require professional expert workers to provide largely individualized practice and interventions. Agencies tend to operate on principles based on individualism even when they provide services to families and groups. Agencies and workers are not trained to think or practise systemically. The result, in my experience, is that there is an unconscious culture clash when it comes to many agencies creating and operating groupwork programmes. The pyramidical or triangular model of most organizations is often at odds with the *circular* model of effective and creative groupwork where the concepts of ownership, partnership, and active participation are promoted and encouraged and members are expected to be equally responsible for the success of the group. Communication and decision making operates differently in the linear agency model based on the individual's need to know and act, whereas in the group all members equally witness and share in the communal experience. Agency management tends to approach and view groupwork through an individualist perspective rather than a group-centred lens. It is not in any way an intentional disregard for groupwork but rather an untutored bias for unexamined individualist assumptions. Management usually has little understanding of the complexities of the groupwork modality or what is required to support it in practice. Management sees its task as managing a plethora of demanding variables, risks, and needs and delivering services. This is quite a different task from facilitation or enabling as practised in the group and the different tasks generate different operational philosophies and cultures.

There is of course no need for a culture clash if more management were trained or practised group workers, or were emboldened to simply adopt a philosophy of authentically shared partnership that informed and supported collaborative practice. In the absence of such a culture, however, an essential task of the intending group worker is to recognize that the agency may lack the ability to think systemically about the relationship of the group to its host organization and may need coaching and assistance to adopt the most helpful attitude to the group. This requires you as the group worker to be proactive and identify the agency's actual operational concerns in relation to potential group members and establish what the priorities are. Try to work out the contribution your group can make to the service being offered by the agency and pinpoint where the group will enhance, back up, or confirm the work of colleagues. It is vital that you link up with an appropriate manager who can authorize the necessary strategy, resources, and conditions to ensure the success of the group. This may mean that you have to be more insistent with the agency than you would normally be but remember that you are the professional facilitating the group and its success will be determined by your ability and willingness to engage the agency in a more systemic approach to the project. This requires a sizeable and courageous shift in perspective and confidence on your part to move from working for the agency to working alongside and with the agency to help it fulfil its objectives and discharge its obligations.

Poor infrastructure

The failure to think systemically can lead some agencies to provide inadequate infrastructures for their groupwork programmes. These are basic physical and organizational structures and facilities that need to be thought about and taken into account because there is a multiplicity of factors that impact on the group if it is to be successful, productive, and efficient. The agency needs to formulate a coherent context for the group. The context is the circumstances that form the setting for the group idea and state the terms in which it can be fully understood and justified as an agency priority. The context determines that:

- There is a clearly demonstrable group need or problem
- Groupwork can achieve gains for these potential members
- The reasons why the group setting is more effective than the one-to-one setting
- There is not another medium or form of intervention that can achieve the desired outcome as well as the group
- The groupwork programme is commensurate and compatible with agency operational objectives

Having a context for the group focuses thinking and makes it easier to locate relevant literature and research or talk to other group leaders who have worked in this area, in order to obtain a better understanding of the needs of the group and learn about more effective and appropriate ways of working. The context for the group can now be operationalized in a *strategy* which is a plan of action designed to achieve the long-term or overall aim of the group. It will typically cover these areas:

- What is the purpose of the group?
- What special properties of the group will be emphasized?
- How will the group meet members' needs?
- What are the specific outcomes desired?
- How will these be achieved?
- Can reasonable estimates of time involved, type of programme, cost, resource, supervision be made?
- What difficulties can be foreseen?
- Who will facilitate the group?
- How many workers? What are their roles, responsibilities, accountability?
- Is there provision for adequate supervision and preparation time?
- Who will manage/supervise them?
- Are other agencies to be involved?
- Can the objectives of different agencies be synchronized?
- What are the roles, responsibilities, inputs, share of costs, resources of different agencies?
- How are workers from different agencies to be managed/supervised?
- How will inter-agency oversight operate?
- How will the group project be evaluated?

Without a coherent context and realistic strategy that will set achievable goals, mobilize and ensure the appropriate resources, and engage the agency collaboratively your group simply will not work.

If at all possible I would recommend that you should be part of setting the context and strategy for the group alongside senior management from the beginning so that you can advise and assist as much as possible. This may mean asking to join the planning group or liaising regularly with appropriate seniors and will ensure that the foundation for the group will be solid and the necessary infrastructures in place. This is not an unreasonable request and can be presented in a respectful manner as providing the planning group with valuable expertise. It may be that the context and strategy for the group is determined at a senior level and much of the planning of the group is left in your hands. It is still important that you reflect on the context and strategy and seek an input where you believe that there are unreasonable expectations on the part of the agency about what groupwork can provide or if there is inadequate provision for supervision or issues involving inter-agency co-operation. You must take responsibility as a professional person and expect to be consulted and not instructed.

Agency desire for a standardized programme

Agency management is fearful of risk and always alert to the possibility of limiting exposure to danger or the possibility that something unpleasant or unwelcome will happen. This means usually that the agency is preoccupied with control and will prefer predictable and manageable group projects particularly for use with difficult or disadvantaged client groups. There are nowadays many standardized and manualized groupwork programmes that can be purchased and rolled out in a variety of client situations. These programmes derive from cognitive-behavioural origins and are skills based and involve taught material. They have a series of tightly structured sessions and planned activity and often involve homework for members. Organizational management can be attracted to these manualized groupwork programmes because they are scripted and do not require much groupwork skill or experience from facilitators who just have to follow the plan. They can be attractive to agencies who do not have the time or finance to train personnel to run groups. They are replicable and can be used again and again.

There can be some difficulties with these types of groupwork. A common report is that absenteeism and dropout rates can be higher than expected because members are expected to possess literacy and numeracy skills to engage in sessional work and homework. Difficulties with members' literacy and numeracy may not be foreseen and only surface after the group has started. Another problem is that members often prefer to talk together about their experiences but the scripted programme doesn't allow for much free verbal interaction. This can be frustrating for members and workers who are obliged to cut short interesting conversations in order to keep to a timeline and content plan. For workers who like to work at more of a process level with groups these structured groupwork programmes are tedious. Other workers report being intimidated by the degree of structure involved and may feel inadequate if they cannot achieve the session objectives in the time set.

But you can see why agencies like these safe and predictable group programmes. No one is going to get emotional or break down. The groups are unlikely to get out of control. They are manageable, conservative, and can be replicated across a service. The problem is that sometimes they are plain boring for workers and members alike! Where you do find yourself operating such a group it is important that you do not allow yourself to be persecuted by the ideals and stated outcomes of the programme. You can easily allow more time for reflection and conversation arising out of the thematic content and you will find participation in the group is more enthusiastic and energetic. Beginning group workers may feel more comfortable with these scripted group programmes initially but it is important to experiment a little and try to engage the group more, or all involved will feel like they are back in the classroom with obvious consequences that will produce reduced motivation and lessened participation.

Misunderstandings about the group as an economy

Increasingly financial constraints and austerity means that agencies see groupwork as a very useful economy involving fewer staff and maximum client numbers to deal with staff shortages and growing waiting lists. There is no doubt that a well-planned group service is an economy but only if it is supported by the appropriate infrastructure. An economy is not a shortcut.

A group can offer:

- Good value for money
- Careful use and management of available resources
- A service to a greater number of clients by fewer staff
- A potentially richer resource than individual casework
- The stimulating nature of group participation and interaction
- The support and relief of peer support and solidarity
- The opportunity to extend and highlight the range and functions of agency provisions
- Better and more effective engagement with an agency's services

These are some of the valid reasons that might encourage an agency to consider including and initiating more group programmes, but if groupwork is to be productive the agency must ensure that the group has maximum opportunity for success. There can be no reason to reduce planning or skimp on providing resources and support. The agency should formulate a clear and coherent context that indicates that there is a clearly demonstrable group need or problem and that groupwork can achieve gains for potential members. The context for the group can now be operationalized in a strategic plan of action designed to achieve the long-term or overall aim of the group. The group facilitators must ensure that the purpose of the group is clear and achievable and should be in agreement with the agency objectives. It is essential that workers know what their roles, responsibilities, and accountability are and have secured provision for adequate supervision and preparation time. Clear and accessible lines of management and supervision should be put in place.

I cannot emphasize enough or repeat enough that an agency must invest properly if the group is to be an effective economy. You cannot throw a group at a problem! The agency must act professionally, honourably, and realistically. Your job as the group worker is to ensure this is the case as much as possible.

The role of the group worker in failing groups

The importance of cultivating a systemic and group centred perspective

Group workers need to know specifically how to think about the necessary conditions for successful groupwork practice and how to engage with their agencies and with their groups to ensure them. I have written about this throughout this text but I think increasingly group workers need help to develop a group-centred perspective that runs from a macro agency level through a range of perspectives to the micro level of the proposed group. This is a systemic way of thinking that is absent in the training of many professionals. To help us with this I want to consider again the definition of groupwork that I offered in the introduction to this text.

> Groupwork practice refers to the conscious, disciplined, and systematic use of knowledge about the processes of collective human interaction, in order to intervene in an informed way, or promote some desired objective in a group setting. In the sense that it is used in this book, groupwork practice is a helping process designed to correspond to specific instances of individual and group need, based on a view of human beings as in constant interaction and relationship with others. Groupwork is a productive, healthy, and creative experience, carried out on the basis of explicit agreements, openly pursued and clearly arrived at, about the purpose and task of the group and the rights and responsibilities of members.

What is essential in this definition is how it offers the group worker a way to think about groups and make effective plans. It is clear that no group is a closed or separate system.

- The essence of the human being is social, not individual
- The essence of the group is shared experience
- The individual is part of a network of social processes (family, occupational, political, religious, etc.)
- Disturbance in these networks can be re-enacted in the current group
- The current group can help individuals become aware of their unhelpful patterns of social disturbance and make new choices
- Groupwork is based on explicit agreements and contracts

These insights require the group worker to think in relational and systemic terms. Your clients are biologically individual and separate but are psychologically conditioned and defined by membership of a variety of groups. These groups interpenetrate and influence each other and shape and structure the lives of their members. The effective group worker recognizes the interplay of these different groups and keeps this constantly in mind. The word individual derives from the Latin word *individuus* which actually means indivisible. The individual is not a separate singleton but is indivisible from the group networks that form and support her. The group worker looks at the person and sees the influence and presence of their group networks.

The worker is the embodiment of an ethic which is based on the idea that the essence of group membership is shared experience and that anything which might inhibit this development requires thoughtful examination, discussion, and correction.

Many group workers get into difficulties with their agencies and with their group members because they do not consciously cultivate a perspective that enables them to think systemically and relate to a system. The map below indicates the picture of the group that the worker must keep in mind. It illustrates the point that a group is a complex subsystem operating in and influenced by a wider system. The group is a part of a network of social processes that must be considered and planned for. Thinking of the group systemically is a central preoccupation for the worker and an extremely demanding task. It is the primary requirement for ensuring the group is productive and successful. With this perspective firmly in mind the intending group worker can approach the planning and preparation of the group and generate an appropriate strategy for effective and successful practice.

This map enables the group worker to picture in their mind the influences that impact on the group and its membership and to consider their significance. The worker can now systematically think about the matrix in which the group operates and plan how to utilize each variable favourably so as to effect a successful outcome for the group. The group is

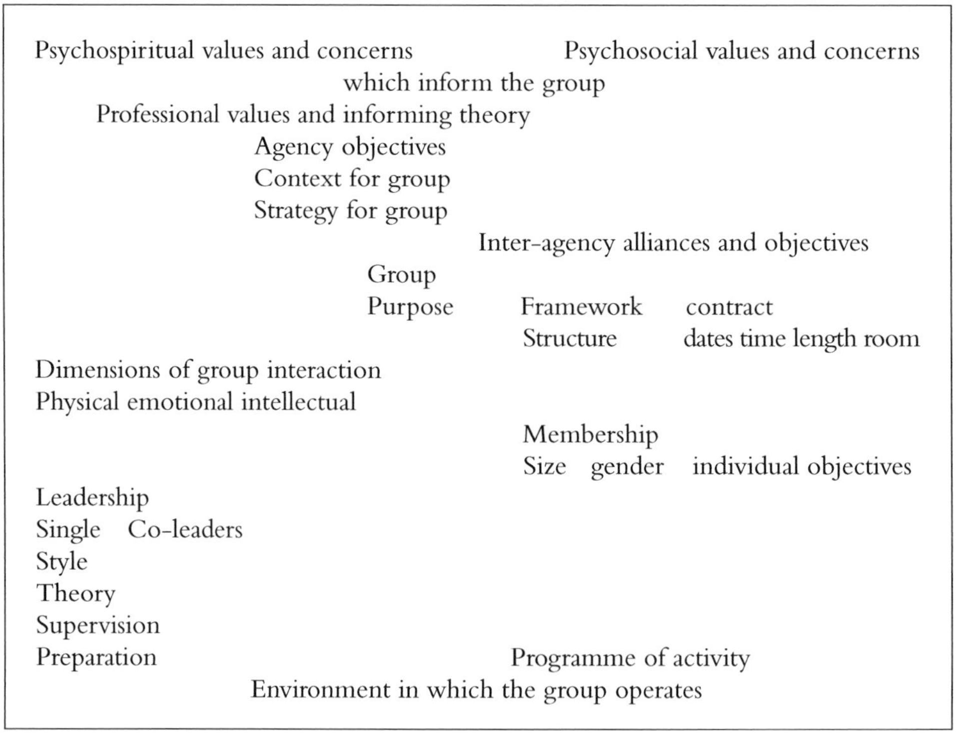

Psychospiritual values and concerns   Psychosocial values and concerns
which inform the group
Professional values and informing theory
Agency objectives
Context for group
Strategy for group
Inter-agency alliances and objectives
Group
Purpose   Framework   contract
Structure   dates time length room
Dimensions of group interaction
Physical emotional intellectual
Membership
Size   gender   individual objectives
Leadership
Single   Co-leaders
Style
Theory
Supervision
Preparation   Programme of activity
Environment in which the group operates

Figure 16.1 A systemic representation of the group and the environment in which it operates

embedded within a wider group of processes and is not a closed system. Practise thinking systemically!

Here then is your systemic checklist for planning your group to ensure success.

The group in relation to the agency

> - How has the proposal for a group come to your attention?
> - What do you believe is the motivation of the proposer?
> - Is it compatible with your professional values?
> - Is the proposal for a group in line with agency objectives?
> - What social or cultural values might inform and impact on the group?
> - What research is there on this type of group response?
> - Is there a demonstrable need for the group?
> - Will it meet client need?
> - Will clients be seen and respected in the context of their wider social influences and networks?
> - Is there a clear agency context for the group?
> - Is there a clear agency strategy for the group that provides appropriate resources, funds, supervision?
> - Are other agencies to be involved?
> - Is there a clear context for inter-agency work?
> - Is there a clear strategy for inter-agency work?

Administration of the group

> - Is there a clear, realistic, and agreed purpose for the group?
> - Will it meet client need?
> - How will this be evaluated?
> - What form of leadership is required?
> - What does research say about leadership for this type of group?
> - Single or co-leaders?
> - If working with facilitators from other agencies how will different professional perspectives be understood, accommodated, and managed?
> - Is there adequate supervision?
> - Consider membership issues.
> - Meet prospective members beforehand to assess their suitability, set individual goals, and form an alliance with you
> - Consider programming issues
> - Does the programme cater for the physical, emotional, intellectual, spiritual concerns of members?

Working in the group

- What theoretical model informs your leadership and interventions?
- If co-working, does everyone understand and agree their role, responsibility?
- What are the potential frictions and problems?
- How will different theoretical models and styles of work be accommodated?
- Are members seen in the context of their wider social influences and networks?
- Consider behaviour or an incident as a communication from the group about the group
- Understand that the group has some investment in the problem
- Remember that groupwork is based on explicit agreements and contracts
- Make the group your co-worker and ask them for help with the problem
- Expect and encourage the group to take responsibility to manage its own behaviour and experience

It is important that you can think about each element on this checklist. If you cannot be clear about these issues or see how they fit together to define the group it is likely that your group will fail. See the time spent in reflecting on the relationship of your group to its wider systems as time wisely and well spent!

The importance of thinking systemically about difficult behaviour in the group

Not many group facilitators are specifically trained to work with a group. Frequently some workers are directed or instructed to run groups as a part of their job and may not feel comfortable. They have been trained in traditional casework approaches and are used to working with individual clients. The agency may offer a variety of group services to its client population and expect staff to run these groups without considering that they will need training, supervision, and monitoring. As a consequence, group workers often need help managing what they call difficult members. Managing these difficult members is covered at length throughout the text but the essential point here is that many groups fail because group workers are unused to making difficult and challenging behaviour a communal problem.

I have said above that the essence of the human being is social, not individual and the essence of the group is shared experience. This gives us the key to working with difficult behaviour and challenging members. If the group worker can cultivate a group-centred perspective then she will not allow an individual to be seen as a problem. An individual's behaviour can be reframed as occurring with the permission or collusion of the group and as having important consequences for the group. The behaviour is thus seen as some sort of communication about the group and therefore as something that needs to be examined and thought about by the group. From this group-centred perspective all events and incidents in the group are now viewed as types and forms of communication about the group, both conscious and unconscious, verbal and behavioural. The group worker does not attempt to control members' behaviours but focuses on them as communications that can be thought about by the worker and members in order to make more meaningful and exchangeable interactions. This is a profound conceptual shift in thinking and in practice on the part of the group worker.

The group worker need no longer be afraid of the group nor does she need to micro-manage the group to keep it from flying out of control. The group worker is liberated to make the group their co-worker!

The group is seen as a natural partner or co-worker and as having an investment in taking responsibility for its own behaviour and success. Difficult and challenging behaviour is actively brought to the group's attention and the group is expected and encouraged to take responsibility to manage its own behaviour and experience. Concepts such as ownership and partnership take on a new and more authentic meaning as they are now embodied in active group interaction and participation. This view of the group as a natural co-worker reinforces for members the principle that groupwork is based on explicit agreements and contracts. I asserted earlier that the basic group contract was a psychological skin that contains natural conflicts within the group and promotes group collaboration (page 95). You can see how this emphasis on agreements and contracts underpins and stresses the primacy of group communal life and action.

Example

A psychoeducational group was in its second session of a 12 session course when a particular male member was observed to constantly talk about his problems and how he had tried various solutions without success. He talked over the facilitator and interrupted other members when they tried to come in and speak. After a time group members became silent and let him have the floor to himself. After the end of the session a female member approached the facilitator and said that she wouldn't return to the group as the talkative male member was monopolizing the time. The facilitator persuaded her to return and promised to sort out the situation.

In the third session the male member proceeded to monopolize the session again with constant talking. After some time of this the facilitator interrupted to address the man:

'John, you are doing a lot of work for the group.'

And then to the group:

'I wonder what the group is getting out of this? Could we think together about this?'

This had the immediate effect of stopping John continuing to speak and engaging the group in reflecting on what might be occurring and why. A brief discussion ensued which indicated that

- Some members were happy for John to talk as it saved them from having to talk
- They were shy and anxious at the beginning of this new experience
- Some members were afraid of being rejected or ridiculed if they talked
- Some members were afraid of saying anything to John in case it started a row

The facilitator was able to suggest to the group that the talkative John was in fact performing a necessary function for this new group and asked John what he thought about his talking. John said that he did not like silences and actually was usually uncomfortable in groups. It appeared that he was really trying to keep the group going and himself safe. The facilitator was now able to help the group members reflect on the anxious and uncomfortable feelings that get stirred up in a new and public situation and encourage them to talk together about this and what they might need to feel a little more relaxed in the group. This enabled the group to engage with each other and recommit to the task. No one dropped out of the group.

What this example demonstrates is a facilitator adopting a group-centred perspective and refusing to allow an individual to be the problem. The facilitator looks for an appropriate opportunity to make the group her co-worker and collaborate in thinking about the monopolizing talking as a communication that serves the group in some way and must be examined by the group. The group is seen as colluding with the behaviour which can then be reframed as a communication about the feelings stirred up when participating in a new group with strangers.

A less experienced facilitator unused to a group-centred perspective might have tried to control or contain the talkative member and missed completely the group dimension of the individual behaviour. The group would have continued with the unrecognized anxieties and membership would have dropped and participation reduced.

Example

A male member of a psychotherapy group persisted in coming late to the session. When challenged on this he claimed that as he came from a distance to attend the group he couldn't always predict traffic conditions. The group appeared to accept this and make allowance for him. The group therapist brought this recurring problem to supervision and was encouraged to take a group-centred approach. The next time the member arrived late the group therapist addressed him:

> 'Henry, you seem to be in two minds about being in the group. Part of you doesn't want to be here and arrives late and part of you does want to attend because you are here.'

And then to the group:

> 'The group seems to go along with this and even accept this. I wonder what the group is getting out of this?'

This intervention was successful in engaging the group in reflecting on what might be occurring and why. In the ensuing discussion it emerged that

- Group members quite admired Henry for defying the group therapist
- Henry was aware of the members' esteem for him and liked their attention
- They also had ambivalent feelings about being in the group

- They would also like to defy the therapist but were afraid of the consequences
- Unresolved feelings about earlier parental conflicts were being activated
- Henry was like the eldest child in a family and the other members were like watchful younger siblings

The group therapist was now able to help the group think about the way they related to Henry and how they used him to express some of their secret wishes. Together they were able to explore how the behaviour of lateness was actually a vehicle for communication about conflicts with parental authority and adolescent rebellion. The session was very satisfying for members who could now talk about their own ambivalent feelings more openly for the first time. Henry was able to reflect on his difficult adolescent experience with his father and see that he could make different choices as an adult and not simply repeat redundant behaviour.

Again, we see a group worker adopting a group-centred perspective and refusing to allow an individual to be the problem. The therapist looks for an appropriate opportunity to make the group her co-worker and collaborate in thinking about the timekeeping conflict as a communication that serves the group in some way and must be examined by the group. The group is helped to see that it is colluding with the behaviour and is getting something out of it. This group-centred intervention helped the group engage in a more mature discussion of important concerns and was successful in helping Henry make more adult choices and come to the group punctually.

And one more

A new female joined a longstanding psychotherapy group. Jan had addiction problems with alcohol and food and was very obese. From the beginning she demanded a lot of attention and disclosed a lot of personal material. She stirred up difficult feelings in the other members and particularly in a younger woman. Sue was slim and athletic and regularly worked out with her football team. The two women soon began to conflict with each other and Sue was particularly incensed when Jan called her a 'gym bunny'. Their deteriorating relationship began to affect other members. Some members started to absent themselves from sessions saying that the group was too aggressive and argumentative to bear. Others would keep silent and avoid being drawn into the conflict. The group therapist was unable to make any headway with the difficult conflict in the group and finally brought the situation to supervision. She was advised to remind the group that they had made an agreement to take responsibility to think about and manage their own behaviour and experience and that the conflict in the group was an important communication that needed to be understood.

The next time the conflict flared up the group therapist intervened and said to the group:

'This disagreement keeps occurring so I think we are not understanding something important here. You know that I think the nature and quality of the interpersonal relations between members is a central focus of group therapy, because these relationships frequently imitate important earlier relationships in members' family of origin, and feelings, attitudes, and fantasies about other members are an important means of identifying and exploring how previous experiences continue to distort the present, so let's see if we can think about what is really going on here.'

This intervention was helpful in stimulating discussion about how the group members felt and thought about what was happening in their group. It emerged that:

- The two female antagonists were unconsciously seeing in each other something that they could not see in themselves and were attacking this unwanted aspect of themselves
- Jan was helped by the group to recognize that she envied Sue's slim physique and her discipline around diet and exercise
- Sue was helped to recognize that she was terrified by Jan's obesity and lack of discipline around diet and disclosed that she had suffered from bulimia as a teenager
- The group members began to disclose their difficulties with managing alcohol, food, and smoking
- There was expanding awareness in the group as members came to recognize unwanted aspects of themselves and accept this without shame or reproach
- Most important, it emerged that through her attention seeking and aggressive behaviour Jan was actually unconsciously seeking help by provoking others to control her impulses. This wish for help was obviously not understood or read by the group and so she progressed to more aggressive behaviour that eventually did result in the behaviour being discussed in the group. The failure of the group to understand what was happening was a repetition of a failure of earlier maternal empathy

Once again, we can see how a difficult conflict in the group was only amenable to resolution when the group worker was encouraged to adopt a group-centred perspective. The therapist actively sought the group's help in addressing the problem. She reframed the conflict as a communication that had to be understood as a repetition of much earlier familial relationships and since this was distorting current relationships in the group it had to be thought about if the group was to be helpful and not damaging to its members. The group was enlisted as a co-worker and engaged in examining its own experience and behaviour.

Review

These examples emphasize the importance of thinking systemically about difficult behaviour in the group and indicate how you can intervene from this perspective.

- Do not be frightened by or avoid difficult behaviour in the group
- Do not allow an individual to be the problem

- Consider behaviour or an incident as a communication from the group about the group
- Understand that the group has some investment in the problem
- Remember that groupwork is based on explicit agreements and contracts
- Make the group your co-worker and ask them for help with the problem
- Expect and encourage the group to take responsibility to manage its own behaviour and experience
- Keep thinking systemically and look for opportunities to promote ownership and partnership

Chapter 17

Keeping your practice going

Putting together all the skills and attitudes that we have been talking about is not an easy business. It takes a great deal of concentration, persistence, and hard work. It means constantly reviewing your practice to see how and where you need to develop next. It means staying in touch with your purpose, refining your vision, and allowing your whole being to be involved in the undertaking. In order to start working with groups and keep your practice going, you must aim to develop a structure which will foster this sort of awareness and generate appropriate strategies for change and learning. Such a structure should rest upon four supporting principles:

- Recording
- Evaluation
- Consultation
- Peer support and training

Let us examine each of these principles and see what is involved.

Recording

Recording is essential and cannot be ignored and yet is an area that seems to present difficulties for both the novice and the more experienced group worker alike. There appears to be a number of reasons for this.

- Dislike of writing and office work – recording is 'tedious', 'passive', 'boring'
- 'Working' with the group is more exciting
- Recording is synonymous with 'spying', 'surveillance', and 'control'
- The purpose and function of recording is not always clearly thought out and accepted

Whatever the difficulties or objections the importance of recording cannot be stressed sufficiently. Recording serves the following purposes:

- It develops the powers of observation
- It is a means of examining individual and group behaviour and relating this to theoretical knowledge and advice
- It is a means of assessment and evaluation, documenting the growth and development in individuals, groups, and the worker, and providing evidence of action taken and material for future reflection and work
- Recording enables a worker to clarify his thoughts, express feelings, and can create deeper awareness and understanding of group situations
- Recording forms a basis for analyzing work method, focusing on skills, improving practice, and furthering member involvement and satisfaction
- It is an agency record which indicates the circumstances which precipitated contact, records the work done, over what length of time, and under what conditions, etc.

It is clear then that recording is a tool that can be used to help group members accomplish their goals and to help workers engage in this task. It is not a method of surveillance geared to generate yet more personal information for the authorities nor is it a tiresome chore to get through as quickly as possible. Recording is a way of staying in touch with your vision, developing skills, and learning how to co-operate with members to achieve the purposes for which the group was originally set up.

Guidelines for recording

Useful questions

A lot depends on the purpose of the recording, so ask yourself:

- Who is the recording for – agency, supervisor, colleagues, worker's use, member's use?
- What do these people need to know?
- What is the minimum material to be recorded – individual and group behaviour, performance, interaction; particular incidents; worker interaction, interventions?
- Who will have access to the recordings?

Purpose and objectives

Now make a clear statement about the purpose and objectives of your recording.

Consider who is to record

In some groups, especially when working with children, I find it valuable to involve the group in the recording process. It is a useful way of contextualizing sessions, summarizing work, and teaching skills of process analysis. You can use a rota for recording in the group diary so that each member takes a turn at describing events, or the recording can be made collectively at the end of each session.

Normally, however, this recording does not suit the analysis of worker interventions or group dynamics that you may wish to undertake so a more appropriate record is called for. This record is made by one worker as soon after the session as possible, according to a predetermined format. Where a number of workers co-lead in a group it is important that each worker write a brief personalized account of the session which can be used, or not, to help compile the official history of the session.

Consider the method of recording

In deciding the method that you wish to employ to record it is important to think about:

- The time available to record
- Your ability to recall after the event
- Your ability to summarize
- The availability, relevance, and expertise with technology – video recording, tape recording
- The use to which the recording is to be put

You may feel more comfortable writing up what happened in a session or may prefer to rely on the memory and accuracy of a tape recorder or video camera to capture the essence of the session. If introducing the latter be sure to check out members' fantasies and anxieties about how the material will be used and stored.

I personally prefer the traditional discipline of writing up the session and believe it to be the best method of recording and learning for the novice because in my experience:

- It develops a reflective, critical ability
- Writing stimulates and builds memory retention and recall
- It enables you to mentally rerun the group, clarifies thinking, and develops understanding of process and interaction
- It is a marvellous method of self-evaluation and training in the absence of a suitable supervisor
- Writing builds discipline, rigour, and concentration
- It helps formulate future objectives and strategies
- It provides opportunities for expression of feeling, resolution, and the emergence of meaning

Recording what goes on in groups

There are many ways of recording and analyzing what people do in groups. You can use sociograms, analyze interaction according to certain categories, observe the task- and group-oriented behaviours of members (see Chapter 3, page 70), and the like. The following framework can be used as a general guide to recording with your group:

- *Basic identifying information*: State name of group, date, time of session, those present, absent.
- *State session objectives*: Your desired outcomes and what you hope to accomplish in the session.
- *State the session programme and methodology you intend to use.*
- *Content analysis of session*: This is a straightforward narrative account of what occurred in the session. This gives a context for exploring process or particular incidents and interventions later on.
- *Process analysis of session*: This section allows for consideration and reflection of group dynamics. It is a qualitative analysis of what was happening. It can focus on:

  o   Process analysis of individual and group interaction in the session
  o   A particular event or the major incidents
  o   Themes such as communication, participation, relationships, power and influence, trust
  o   A set of actions or interventions undertaken by workers

The section on working with process on page 168, Chapter 9, will give you headings and advice on what to write and how to organize this portion of the record.

The following headings are also useful as a framework for recording:

- *Individual commentaries*: Include a brief description of each member's progress in that session. Consider their investment in the group, behaviour, performance, attitudes, and relationships. How are they working towards their personal goals and what help do they need?
- *Workers' intervention*: Consider the contribution and interventions of workers in the group. What was good, valuable, what was ill-timed, irrelevant, or off the mark? What skills do you need to develop or train up? How did you get on with co-workers? What was good about this? What was avoided? What needs to be reviewed?
- *Evaluative comment on session*: This is a general résumé of what took place, perhaps locating the session in some developmental context or stages theory. Indicate whether session objectives were achieved, what remains to be done, or needs to be renegotiated. How did programme work? What needs to be reviewed? What are your future objectives, plans?

By recording in this way you will have a full and comprehensive picture of what is happening in your group and can assess how your practice is hindering or facilitating this. In the absence of a supervisor or peer support, recording is an invaluable tool and may well be the only method available for training, so do begin now to pay more attention to the contribution that recording can make to keeping your practice going.

Evaluation

There are two aspects of evaluation which are of direct relevance to your ability to keep your practice going. The first concerns the way in which you evaluate change or progress within the group and this is group- or member-oriented. The second has to do with how you evaluate your own practice and performance and is worker-oriented. Let us look at this more closely.

Evaluating the group

The idea dies hard that evaluation is something that you only do at the end of the group. In Chapter 2 I suggested that evaluation has to be considered during the planning phase and before the group has been set up (see page 46).

Evaluation is a way of assessing:

> - Outcomes – the extent to which the group has achieved its goals in producing change/learning, etc.
> - Service delivery – the relevance, quality, acceptability of groupwork in a particular setting
> - Structure and process of the group – what actually happened in the group, how it was organized, how resources were used, and the like

Do not allow yourself to be put off by the thought of evaluating the group experience. It need not be complicated. The basic requirements for an evaluation study are:

> - The establishment of a baseline from which the programme starts
> - A record of the input of effort
> - An account of any movement from the baseline
> - Follow-up to see if change has been maintained

Within these principles you have a great deal of latitude in terms of how you go about assessing the group contribution. Even if not required to by your agency, it is worthwhile evaluating because it will provide you with thoughtful and rich insights into the nature and power of groups and will give you plenty of material to think about in terms of your own practice.

Here are some things to think about when considering how to evaluate the group.

What kind of information is needed?

The only rationale for collecting information is to answer specific questions which have been thought out well in advance. Inevitably a lot more information will be collected in the course of normal recording than will be used so it is worthwhile composing definite questions at the start or working to a framework through which information can be filtered. (See section on recording in this chapter.)

Ask yourself: what is it specifically that I want to know about the individual or group?

> - Behaviour
> - Skills
> - Attitudes

- Values
- Feelings
- Goals

Make a list of questions that you can work with.

Consider if particular questions, frameworks, or measurements are

- Appropriate
- Reliable
- Valid
- Easy to use and understand

It should be clear by now that the first step in the evaluation process is the early and explicit identification of the outcomes that the group is being set up to produce. These outcomes can refer to goal attainment, improved functioning, or effectiveness, and to certain specified changes in the targets of intervention. Outcomes should be defined operationally and should state as correctly as possible:

- Just how you could tell if a person had developed more self-awareness and insight

or

- What a person would do who had acquired new social skills

or

- How you would know if members had benefited from group support and caring

Consider who will be your sources of information

You can collect information from:

- Group members
- Worker observations
- Co-workers
- Significant others – parents, teachers, peers, colleagues, etc.

Consider how the information is to be obtained

There is a great diversity and range of methods for data collection. Amongst other methods, you can use:

- Direct observation of behaviour
- Surveys and questionnaires
- Personality tests and self-rating scales
- Formal or informal interviews
- Analysis of records, documents, and projects
- Sociometric devices

The important thing to remember here is that the instruments used must actually measure what you want them to, so do link the instruments specifically to your questions.

When will the information be obtained and recorded?

The purpose of evaluation will help you decide the timing and sequence of data collection. If you are measuring outcomes you will need a baseline at the start of the group which can be contrasted with information gathered at the end of the group. Evaluating the process of the group will require much more frequent and periodic assessment.

It is usually best to record information as close to the event as possible so anticipate that you will require a recording period after sessions and allow sufficient time.

Consider how you intend to use the information

You need to summarize the information collected and draw conclusions, create meaning, make statements, comparisons, and predictions and show if the work has value or not. Generally I use the information to:

- Abstract generalizations and relationships
- Generate working principles
- Adjust programme, goals, methodology
- Provide feedback and comparison for members, agency, significant others
- Provide learning, training, skill development
- Determine success, relevance, etc., of group

You can use collected information at the end of the group to make a thorough and final evaluation of the experience. It is also worth considering the building in of review periods every six to eight sessions in order to:

- See if plans are being carried out
- Determine if objectives are being met

- Reassess needs
- Realign to purpose
- Set fresh or more realistic objectives and plans

This can become a cyclical process which contributes to group functioning, and can if the reviews are recorded generate much valuable material for comparison and analysis later.

Involve members

Consider ways of encouraging the active participation of members where possible in the evaluative process. Any evaluation is time-consuming and depends on its respondents for its richness and relevance, so involving members is a good way of sharing the load and enriching the results. You may have to negotiate issues about confidentiality with group members and set boundaries on how the information being collected will be used and presented so as to preserve anonymity and the like. Make appropriate contracts and agreements which will reassure people and engage them in a process of ongoing assessment and realignment.

Encourage members to keep a personal journal where they can record, draw, or describe significant events, experiences, and insights in the group. These contemporaneous records can be augmented by the group diary records of project work, and periodic reviews to help determine whether change or improvement occurred during the life of the group. They also create a climate in which people experience evaluation as an integral part of group membership and see it contributing to group well-being and improved functioning.

Evaluating and teaching yourself

Once you begin to work with a group you can both evaluate yourself and get feedback from members and others on how you are doing. In this way you can begin to initiate a programme of self-training which will enable you to keep your practice fresh, innovative, and relevant.

The important thing to remember, however, is that you have to work at it – hard! Your practice will develop in an orderly and comprehensible manner only if you take responsibility for it and that means approaching your handling of groups in a thoughtful and organized way. Here are some guidelines which will help you evaluate and change your practice.

Keep a journal

Keep a personal journal in which you can jot down your thoughts, feelings, experiences, and insights in the group. Reread it constantly. Gradually you will find certain themes recurring. It may be something that you become aware you are avoiding or mishandling. It could be a situation which makes you anxious or uncomfortable.

Choose one problem area that you wish to work on

Without altering or changing in any way, begin to be more conscious of how this behaviour, attitude, or feeling manifests in the group. Gather information about this problem area. Try to identify stages, elements, or parts in the process. Can you recognize the imminence of the behaviour or feeling? What happens as the situation develops? What is it like for you afterwards? If it is appropriate, invite feedback from members or others on how they see you in a particular situation:

> I'm wondering if I come in too quickly sometimes to help you sort things out. What do you think about this?

Subsequent feedback will create a bigger, more detailed, and specific picture of what you are doing and may suggest options and possibilities.

You can also obtain feedback by asking members to fill in reaction forms or short questionnaires about specific topics at the end of sessions. Best of all is to cultivate an environment in which members feel it is permissible and even a friendly act to comment in a mature way about aspects of your practice.

Create a vision

Ask yourself why you want to develop your skill or ability in a particular area.

- Why do you need to change?
- What is the problem?
- Why is it a problem?
- Why is it a problem now?

Your answers to these questions serve two valuable functions:

- *They tell you what, specifically, you are dissatisfied with and why this is so.* Knowing what you want to develop or change begins to open up possibilities and can create a vision or sense of how you might behave differently. And as we have seen in Chapter 8, page 140, vision creates goals.
- *Goals are always important and never more so than when you are trying to maintain yourself in your practice.* Goals motivate because they promise rewards. Only the promise of behaving or intervening in a more effective way is going to get you to put in the necessary work to alter or modify an existing behaviour. So spend some time motivating yourself and determining why it is worthwhile to change.

Make your vision concrete

Rather than trying to change a number of things in your practice, work on one area at a time. To do this, sit down with pen and paper and write down a statement of the problem, your goal, or vision. Do a short brainstorming session and write down whatever ideas come to your mind as good possibilities. Do not think too hard about it. Just let the ideas come. Now take another sheet of paper and write at the top, 'My ideal model'. Write a paragraph or two describing an ideal image of yourself behaving or acting in a particular way.

I often find it useful at this stage to use some of the visualization techniques discussed in Chapter 10, page 187. A few minutes imagining or visualizing myself performing in a certain way gives the feel of the behaviour, affirms its value, and engages the will to change in the desired direction.

Now read over what you have written, then take a fresh sheet of paper. Based on what seems most meaningful from the ideal scene you have created above, make a list of three or four important goals in the problem area. You can then prioritize these goals in terms of what is most urgent, easiest, or worthy of attention. Choose one aspect and resolve to start with it.

Planning the change

The next thing to do is to acknowledge any feelings you may have about your specific goal which could hinder your progress. Feelings of fear, inadequacy, shame, and the like can create impotence and despair if not dealt with. An important way of handling such feelings is to reconnect to your original vision and draw strength from it. This affirms the value and rightness of your course.

It can also be useful to make a list of the things that will prevent you reaching your goal as it may well be that there are certain factors or a particular sequence of actions that must be considered before you start to initiate change.

Be sure to compile an equal list of things that will help you move forwards to your goal so that you can utilize and build on your positive abilities. It is worth reviewing the section on problem solving in Chapter 5, page 109 and in particular the discussion of 'force-field analysis' as there are some ideas which will help you plan a change programme.

From your programme determine your next realistic step and then initiate your change strategies one move at a time.

Evaluate progress

Because you have been specific at the goal-setting stage you can, after a predetermined period, assess how you have been getting on with altering or modifying your practice. If you find that you have not made as much progress as you thought, which will sometimes happen, do not get disheartened or assume that you have failed. Acknowledge to yourself that you still have not achieved your goal and consider whether it really is something that you want. You may have to repeat several of the above steps (choosing a problem area, creating a vision, and making it concrete) to determine whether you want to set the goal again or let it go.

It is important to acknowledge and work with unaccomplished goals in this way. Otherwise they will accumulate and leave you with a sense of inadequacy and failure which will eventually result in you avoiding evaluation and change in your practice. The key is always to choose only those goals that you genuinely want and will give you satisfaction.

When you find that you have achieved a goal, even it is small, be sure to acknowledge this and find a way of rewarding yourself. Rewards are what will motivate you and give you the strength and desire to continue developing your practice.

The process which I have outlined is an invaluable and essential part of your professional practice with groups and – particularly in the absence of supervision or training – will help you.

- See evaluation as an integral part of your work
- Obtain practice in goal setting and the management of change
- Get in touch with and clarify the important purposes and direction in your practice

---

Do try to develop the habit of constantly evaluating and monitoring your own practice. You will find that it pays very rich dividends.

Consultation

You must assume responsibility for your own professional growth and evolution. No one can develop your practice for you. You must do the work yourself. But at times it can be a painful and difficult experience and you will need support, guidance, and encouragement. So assuming responsibility for your professional growth involves setting up a support system which will contain you while you question and examine your practice. This is where the consultant comes in.

I use the word consultant instead of supervisor because I want to stress the importance of your personal choice and volition in keeping your practice going. The supervisor is one who is primarily obliged to hold you to account for your work, although he may help you unfold your practice. While being accountable for one's work is essential it is more your responsibility for developing and promoting your practice that I want to emphasize here. So the idea of a consultant as one who is sought out, as opposed to the supervisor who seeks out the practitioner, is more appropriate.

In order to keep your practice going and growing it is important that you engage with a more experienced worker who is prepared to help you look critically at what you do in groups. Ideally such a worker will have worked with groups and will be aware of the process and dynamics of collective behaviour. This worker will know from his own experience what is likely to happen at certain times in the group, may have some helpful ideas about current and apparently incomprehensible events, and will usually be able to guide you through the sandbars, shallows, and rapids of groupwork.

Often, however, it may not be possible to find someone in your agency experienced enough or willing to act as a consultant for you.

In these circumstances look around for a worker that you admire – someone who attracts you by virtue of his excellence or competence in his own field. A person like this can still help you a great deal even if he has not worked in groups. His experience and ability in his own sphere of activity will enable him to ask penetrating and stimulating questions which will give you a novel and fresh perspective on your practice.

Your practice consultant should be able to provide you with a safe, stimulating, and supportive environment in which you can:

- Consider an alternative, rational, and objective viewpoint on your practice
- Analyze the process and dynamics of group membership
- Consider and align with your purpose or vision
- Work from the known to the unknown, from the apparent to the hidden
- Learn to recognize inappropriate reactions and behaviours
- Explore your inner conflicts
- Experience your hidden feelings
- Experiment with new behaviour and attitudes
- Plan and execute strategies
- Find refreshment, strength, and nourishment

Using consultation

Before the session

Prepare yourself and your consultant by writing up the group session that you want to look at or forwarding any appropriate notes, tapes, or video recordings. It is useful to review your practice and identify any concerns or areas of work that you want to examine. Make an agenda for yourself. Sometimes in consultation you may find that there are issues or feelings that you avoid discussing or which emerge after your session. It is important to bring this unfinished business with you to the next session as your consultant cannot read your mind and this material can get in the way. It is up to you to keep the lines of communication open and clear.

During the session

Agree with the consultant an agenda of mutual concerns about your practice that can be discussed in the session. Clear any unfinished business. Be alert for any tendency on your part to impress, over-react, or try to change your consultant. If you are doing this with him you are probably doing this in your group or experiencing this with members and it is important to explore the motivations and feelings behind this behaviour. Some of the more common patterns that I have seen in my role as consultant are:

- Demand that the consultant give a prescription, magic formula, or answer endless questions
- Avoid, neglect, or ignore the consultant's suggestions
- Pretend to accept the consultant's suggestions when they seem incorrect or incomprehensible
- Fantasize that he can read your mind
- Blame him because he cannot understand you
- Keep the discussion at a safe or superficial level

Very often I have seen workers bring to the consultation and act out the behaviours and resistances that they themselves manifest or experience with members in the group. For this reason, it is wise to be alert to your feelings about the consultant since how you manage them between you will offer valuable insight and suggestions for handling similar feelings and behaviours in your group.

After the session

The consultant will stir up emotions, stimulate, and provide you with a wealth of material and advice. Plan to take some quiet time afterwards where you can sit and write in your journal. Make notes under headings such as:

- What I am doing well
- What I am weak in
- What I missed/avoided in the group
- What I am going to watch for/work with in the next group session
- Goals: short, medium, long-range
- How I felt about consultation/consultant
- Unfinished business
- What I appreciate about myself in consultation/last group session

The point is to give some time to planning how and what you are going to do about what came up in the consultation because if it is to be meaningful, you have to act on what you learned in these sessions. Genuine change in your practice comes about from the combination of insight plus new behaviour so do take time to consider specifically how you intend to use what is emerging in consultation.

In deciding to work with groups, resolve to build in a consultative dimension for your practice. But remember, consultation is an aid and support to your practice. It is not a substitute for hard work. It will enhance but not replace your responsibility for keeping your practice going.

Peer support and training

Another source of support, guidance, and encouragement for your practice is your colleagues and fellow workers. It is really important that you acquaint people in your work setting of your intention to run a group in order to secure their co-operation and ensure that you have the time and resource to work. As the group meets and starts to unfold, keep your colleagues informed of what is going on. Consider giving occasional verbal reports at a staff meeting, informal discussion of how you experience working with a group, short written reports, and the like. In this way you will involve other colleagues and interest them in your work. You will find then that in times of crisis or difficulty you have a sympathetic and knowledgeable support group to fall back on. Be careful, however, not to bore other people or flood the market with accounts of your work!

Outside your immediate work setting look for other group workers or people who are interested in working with groups. Get to know them, ask for advice with problems, and talk to them about their philosophy, technique, and style. Exchange views, books, tips, and begin to develop an informal network of support and resource. Try to set up a peer support group if possible. Even if there are only three or four members, such a group can be a valuable means of challenging yourself, puzzling out problems in your practice, and developing a sense of community. This sense or feeling of belonging to a groupwork community is very important. Very often novice group workers can feel isolated or separate from their colleagues by virtue of their interest in groups. In addition the characteristics and peculiarities of groupwork practice can also heighten the sense of separateness or difference. So contact and exchange with other group workers is a way of preserving and maintaining your practice particularly in adverse or hostile conditions. It is also worthwhile joining local or national groupwork associations which not only offer support, but also provide opportunities for further training.

These associations often offer short training courses which will help you develop your skills, reflect on your practice, and make new contacts. A word of advice: do not 'collect' two or three training courses in the hope of suddenly acquiring instant skills. Do one course and then aim to give yourself six months to a year to decide that in the next two groups you will experiment with and try out what you have been taught. In this way each training course that you do deepens and expands your practice in a mature and systematic manner.

Consider joining an experiential group which will give you the opportunity to feel what it is like to be a member amongst others in the group. This will provide rich insights and perceptions into interpersonal dynamics that will serve you well in your own practice. Join groups where you know good leaders are to be found. Study closely the style and technique of as many group leaders across as broad a spectrum as you can. Ask yourself continually:

- Why did he do/say that?
- What would I have said/done in that situation?
- What makes this leader good?
- What do I like about him?
- What do I not like about him?
- What can I borrow/adopt/modify from his style?

You do not have to give up your own individuality or become a clone of a certain group leader in order to adapt from his style. Give yourself permission to borrow parts of other people's way of working and then piece them together in your own unique style.

Look constantly for ways of being in contact with other people doing groupwork and learn from them. In this way you can minimize and cushion yourself from the inevitable hurts and challenges of working with a group of people, while at the same time ensuring that your practice is innovative, vital, and alive.

Survival procedures for creative group workers

Rule 1: Avoid crucifixions

This rule counsels against over-involvement or self-sacrifice in any cause which you do not wish to be your last. You are not a messiah nor are group members your disciples. So do not try to save, protect, rescue, or work it out for everyone all of the time. It is difficult to watch another person in pain or see them make what appears to be an avoidable error but often this is an essential part of their growth and you can best help by allowing it to happen. Avoid being seen as a saviour, guru, or charismatic leader because we crucify our messiahs, shoot our presidents, and forget our pop stars more quickly than you would find comfortable.

Rule 2: Don't push the river upstream

The essence of this rule is that you should learn to avoid working in any way which will energize resistance to the course or path that you believe is desirable. There seems to be a law of inverse effort which applies when you work in groups. People seem to be contrary. The more you do the less they do; the more helpful you try to be, the more they cling to their unhelpful beliefs. What is required is a light and sensitive touch because it is insistence, short-sightedness, and dogmatism on your part which will generate resistance among group members. So do not force encounters or tell people what to do. Learn to work from where the group is at. Go with the flow.

Rule 3: Wait quietly until the mud settles

Learn to wait and watch and listen. In this way your awareness is focused on the group and not just on your needs. Do not feel you should intervene immediately – stand back until you know what is happening in a situation. Keep quiet, remain attentive, and take things as they come. When you know what people want – or are repulsed by – then you can move and show them how they can get what they want by doing what you want them to do.

Rule 4: Learn to forgive yourself

In the course of working with groups it is inevitable that you will make mistakes and feel inadequate at times. Feelings of helplessness and confusion, shame, anger, and pain will frequently arise and threaten to overwhelm unless you can cultivate a sense of right proportion and be compassionate with yourself.

Be respectful of yourself as someone who is learning a difficult and demanding craft. Begin to see and use mistakes as a source of creativity and an opportunity to learn new skills and try out new behaviours. Learn to forgive yourself since if you cannot permit your own frailty and inadequacy you will really be unable to allow it in your group. Learn how to connect to the power of your own helplessness!

Rule 5: Cultivate goodwill

Keep in awareness why you thought the group was a good idea originally and use this vision to express goodwill towards group members. At various times members will attempt to please, shock, manipulate, and help you. There is no point in getting angry or hurt at this and rejecting them. This will only compound matters. Learn to accept members and help them explore these self-defeating behaviours and discover more positive and creative ways of being. Your job is to guide and facilitate the group, not join members in destructive relationships. So act with optimism and goodwill and teach by example.

Rule 6: Make up your own rules

No book or course can give you the complete prescription for working with a group. Every group is different, though there are similar patterns and themes. You will find yourself in situations which are not covered in this work and are new to you. Do not be afraid to improvise, break the normal rules, or go against the conventional wisdom. Use your imagination and intuition to guess at what is the best thing to do. If it doesn't work, fall back on rules 1, 3, and 4. If it does work incorporate it into your repertoire and forget about it! The important thing to remember is that you do the best you can and let it go at that. Rule 6 could have been rewritten as 'there are no rules'. It is your group so adapt, modify, create in your own fashion. If it works, use it! If it fails to work, use that too!

The last word

Writing this book has been for me analogous to working with a group. I entered the work full of vision, hope, and optimism. After a time the going became very tough and it was tempting to give up. But I persevered and as you see the work is complete. As always the difficulties arose from my attempts to make the work go where I wanted it to go. It is only to the degree that I have succeeded in letting go of my needs to impress, control, and expound that I have learned to co-operate with the process of the writing. Just like working with a group. May you learn the same lesson.

Name index

Subject index